Sport-Specific Testing and Training Methods in Youth

Sport-Specific Testing and Training Methods in Youth

Guest Editors

Alessandra Amato
Andrea Fusco
Cristina Cortis

MDPI

Basel • Beijing • Wuhan • Barcelona • Belgrade • Novi Sad • Cluj • Manchester

Guest Editors

Alessandra Amato
Department of Biomedical and Biotechnological Sciences
University of Catania
Catania
Italy

Andrea Fusco
Department of Medicine and Aging Sciences
University "G. D'Annunzio" of Chieti-Pescara
Chieti
Italy

Cristina Cortis
Department of Human Sciences, Society and Health
University of Cassino and Lazio Meridionale
Cassino
Italy

Editorial Office
MDPI AG
Grosspeteranlage 5
4052 Basel, Switzerland

This is a reprint of the Special Issue, published open access by the journal *Sports* (ISSN 2075-4663), freely accessible at: https://www.mdpi.com/journal/sports/special_issues/1N5CW332F5.

For citation purposes, cite each article independently as indicated on the article page online and as indicated below:

Lastname, A.A.; Lastname, B.B. Article Title. *Journal Name* **Year**, *Volume Number*, Page Range.

ISBN 978-3-7258-7653-2 (Hbk)
ISBN 978-3-7258-7654-9 (PDF)
https://doi.org/10.3390/books978-3-7258-7654-9

Contents

About the Editors

Alessandra Amato

Alessandra Amato is currently an assistant professor in sport science at the Department of Biomedical and Biotechnological Sciences, Section of Anatomy, Histology and Movement Science, School of Medicine, University of Catania (Italy). She obtained a Ph.D. in health promotion and cognitive sciences at the University of Palermo (Italy), receiving the title of Doctor Europaeus. She spent part of her doctoral studies at the University of Colorado Boulder (USA). She currently teaches Basketball Teaching Theory and Practice at Fujian Normal University (China).

Andrea Fusco

Andrea Fusco is currently an assistant professor in movement science at the Department of Medicine and Aging Sciences of the University "G. d'Annunzio" of Chieti-Pescara, Italy. He obtained a Ph.D. in the field of sport and health sciences at the University of Cassino and Lazio Meridionale, Italy, receiving the title of Doctor Europaeus. He was also a visiting researcher at the Human Performance Laboratory of the University of Wisconsin-La Crosse (USA) and the Biomechanics Laboratory in the Department of Sport Science and Kinesiology of the University of Salzburg, Austria. Dr. Fusco was recognized as a fellow of the European College of Sport Science in 2025.

Cristina Cortis

Cristina Cortis is currently a full professor in sports science at the Department of Human Sciences, Society, and Health of the University of Cassino and Lazio Meridionale, Italy. She obtained her Ph.D. in 2009 in sport and health sciences at the University of Rome "Foro Italico", Italy. She was a visiting researcher at the Human Performance Laboratory of the University of Wisconsin-La Crosse, USA, and at the University of Connecticut, USA. Prof. Dr. Cortis was recognized as a fellow of the American College of Sports Medicine in 2020 and a fellow of the European College of Sport Science in 2024.

sports

MDPI

Editorial

Sport-Specific Testing and Training Methods in Youth

Alessandra Amato [1], Andrea Fusco [2,*] and Cristina Cortis [3,4]

1 Department of Biomedical and Biotechnological Sciences, Section of Anatomy, Histology and Movement Science, School of Medicine, University of Catania, Via S. Sofia n°97, 95123 Catania, Italy; alessandra.amato@unict.it
2 Department of Medicine and Aging Sciences, University "G. d'Annunzio" of Chieti-Pescara, 66100 Chieti, Italy
3 Department of Human Sciences, Society and Health, University of Cassino and Lazio Meridionale, 03043 Cassino, Italy; c.cortis@unicas.it
4 European University of Technology EUt+, 03043 Cassino, Italy
* Correspondence: andrea.fusco@unich.it

1. Introduction

Research on the best athletic performance is undergoing a paradigm shift, characterized by a progressive decline in the age of specialization in numerous sports [1–4], while providing the opportunity for accelerated skill acquisition. This trend also presents a significant challenge for sports scientists, coaches, and physicians. The common belief among coaches, parents, and young athletes is that early and year-round specialization in a single sport can lead to elite performance and may also have a different influence on the development of a specific skill that affects everyday life, such as manual dexterity [5,6]. However, a growing number of studies contradict this theory, suggesting that such a limited approach may instead restrict children's exposure to diverse sporting experiences, impair the development of fundamental motor skills, and compromise the foundations for an active lifestyle [7–9]. In addition, recent studies have suggested that early specialization is associated with an increased risk of injury in various sports, for both boys and girls, as well as burnout and dropping out [10,11]. The key principle underlying this Special Issue is that young athletes represent a distinct population, not simply miniature adults. Their biological and psychological landscape is defined by ongoing processes of growth, maturation, and development, which profoundly influence their responses to training, susceptibility to injury, and long-term athletic outcomes [12–14]. The evidence consistently shows that the plastic neuromuscular system of a child or adolescent responds differently to aerobic and anaerobic stimuli than that of mature athletes. There are periods of accelerated adaptation, often conceptualized as "windows of opportunity" or sensitive periods, for components such as speed, strength, and skill acquisition [14,15]. Furthermore, the immature skeletal system, with the presence of growth cartilage, is more vulnerable to overload injuries, particularly under the repetitive high-load volumes typical of early specialization [16,17]. From a psychological perspective, the increasingly professionalized youth sports environment can contribute to burnout and anxiety, necessitating approaches that balance performance development with psychological well-being [18,19]. For these reasons, increasingly original research is investigating training and assessment strategies designed and adapted specifically for young athletes in different sports disciplines. For example, in a sport such as volleyball, recent studies have shown that differential training can improve technique and performance in the spike-jump, even in young athletes, highlighting the importance of interventions targeted at the specific technical and biomechanical needs of athletes with specific characteristics [20]. This Special Issue has brought together contemporary approaches to the management of young athletes, with a focus on the adaptation and specificity of methodologies, prioritizing the physiological and psychological demands of this population. Thirteen original articles have been published, generally classified into two key areas: training, which focuses on the application of specific interventions to improve athletic performance in young athletes, and testing, which explores the tools and methods used to assess physical abilities, monitor load, and validate new protocols in youth populations.

2. An Overview of the Published Articles

Results from training interventions demonstrate the impact of structured sport-specific training on young athletes, highlighting that specific programs can cause significant improvements in both physical and cognitive domains. Teteris et al. (Contribution 1) provide a neurophysiological perspective, showing that a 12-week reaction training program can enhance the choice reaction time in under-20 fencers. This is particularly relevant in sports where split-second decisions are a key skill and underscores the trainability of cognitive functions alongside physical skills during a crucial developmental period. On the other hand, Vasilescu and colleagues (Contribution 2) provide a reproducible evidence-based intervention tailored to the neuromotor development of children aged 10 to 12 years, designed specifically to improve lower limb strength in junior combat sports, recognizing that explosive strength is crucial for performing technical and decisive actions during combat. The intervention also addresses the essential need for training to be tailored to be effective. In basketball, three studies offer complementary insights. Amato et al. (Contribution 3) compared core and mobility training in youth players, finding that both 8-week interventions effectively improved the dynamic balance, overhead squat depth, and agility, pointing to the specific neuromuscular benefits of such training. However, Sansone et al. (Contribution 4) centered their research on another pivotal factor influencing basketball performance: the pre-competition warm-up. The study entailed a detailed comparative analysis of two distinct warm-up protocols administered to the same cohort of adolescent basketball athletes, demonstrating that warm-ups incorporating small-sided games more accurately replicate sport-specific match conditions. However, the findings also underscore the necessity of monitoring the external load parameters and ensuring sufficient physiological readiness within such protocols. This investigation thus yields practical evidence-based guidance for optimizing warm-up strategies in 16-year-old basketball players. On a longer timeline, Castro-Collado et al. (Contribution 5) demonstrated the holistic benefits of a structured school-based basketball program over 38 weeks. Their findings revealed not only improved physical fitness (a 45% increase in aerobic capacity) but also positive changes in body composition in prepubertal boys, advocating for such programs as a public health and athletic development tool. The importance of specificity is further emphasized by Herbert et al. (Contribution 6) in another team sport: handball. Their 11-week professional training program for elite adolescent players led to significant gains in sport-specific defense and offense times, with under 17 players also showing remarkable improvements in the VO_2 peak, ball velocity, and jump height. This study powerfully argues that targeted sport-specific training during adolescence is a key point for a professional career. Sagat similarly demonstrated how structuring specific sports training, such as sprint intervals with change of direction in soccer players, could significantly improve the explosive power, agility, speed, anaerobic capacity, and maximal oxygen uptake (VO_2max) in male under-17 soccer players (Contribution 7). Finally, Perazzetti et al. (Contribution 8) shifted the focus to the critical aspect of recovery and load management. Monitoring under-16 water polo players during a congested match schedule, they found that the internal load was correlated with

https://doi.org/10.3390/sports14030103

increased fatigue and decreased well-being, highlighting how recovery is a crucial part of training.

These papers focused on training offer a balanced approach between the importance of planning adequate training in terms of volume and also scheduling adequate recovery, which is crucial in this phase of growth for developing technical and physical skills. Reliable and valid testing is the foundation through which effective training is built. Other contributions of our Special Issue focused on advancements in testing and assessment, validated new protocols, compared testing environments, and explored the underlying physiological and biomechanical factors of performance. A key practical question was addressed by Carron et al. (Contribution 9), who found that run-based performance tests (sprints, agility, and fitness) in adolescent rugby league players yielded comparable results on both indoor and outdoor surfaces, offering valuable flexibility for practitioners working in varied environments. Despot and Plavec (Contribution 10) made a significant contribution by validating a new Ballroom Aerobic Test (BAT) for dance sport couples. The BAT showed strong agreement with gold-standard laboratory tests, providing a feasible and accurate field-based and sport-specific method to assess the aerobic capacity of dancers, a population often overlooked in sport science. The theme of specificity continues in the work of Crisafulli et al. (Contribution 11), who described the power–load relationship in elite canoeists and kayakers. Their data on bench press, ballistic bench press, and prone bench pull exercises provide coaches with preliminary benchmarks for designing strength and power training tailored to the unique "pull-dominant" demands of paddling sports. At a more fundamental physiological level, Massini et al. (Contribution 12) investigated the agreement between different high-intensity endurance indexes (Critical Speed, Respiratory Compensation Point, and 50%Δ) in young male runners. Their finding that these indices are broadly similar, though not entirely interchangeable at an individual level, refines our understanding of how to demarcate and target key training intensities in youth running. Two studies examine the long-term development of athletes. Marcelli et al. (Contribution 13) explored the relative age effect in a youth soccer academy, confirming that the birth month can influence motor performance and ball skills within annual age groups. This highlights the need for individualized training programs that account for biological maturity and not just chronological age. Meanwhile, Ouergui et al. (Contribution 14) demonstrated that interlimb asymmetry and bilateral deficit indexes measured in vertical jumps are significant predictors of sport-specific kicking performance in taekwondo athletes. This underscores the importance of balanced strength development and targeted neuromuscular training, even in sports dominated by unilateral actions.

The papers aimed to explore testing in this population, highlighting the importance of assessing by means of field-based and sport-specific methods before planning specific sports training and training load progression and the need to make the assessment more practical and applicable even outside laboratory settings, which may differ from real-world performance.

3. Conclusions

The findings of this Special Issue underline that the effective management of the young athlete requires a specific and dual-focused approach. It demands training that is not only structured and intense but also cognitively engaging, sport-specific, and carefully balanced with recovery. It equally depends on testing that is valid, reliable, practical, and sensitive to the specific demands of the sport and the individual characteristics of the developing athlete. The career path of a young athlete is a complex mix of growth, training, and competition. The research presented here provides coaches, athletic trainers, and sports scientists with insights and tools that are essential for approaching this path more effectively.

https://doi.org/10.3390/sports14030103

Given the success of this Special Issue, we have launched a second edition and hope to receive contributions focusing on other sports so that we can provide an increasingly comprehensive and specific overview of the metabolic and technical requirements of different disciplines, whether they are individual or team sports, indoor or outdoor, power or endurance performance. This will allow us to deepen our knowledge in these areas and to better achieve our goal: to promote an environment that improves performance, ensures well-being, and cultivates a lifelong passion for sport.

Conflicts of Interest: The authors declare no conflicts of interest.

List of Contributions:

1. Teteris, L.E.; Saulite, S.; Licis, R.; Greve, M.; Boobani, B. Application of the Vienna Test System to Measure Training-Induced Changes in Choice Reaction Time in U20 Fencers: A 12-Week Training Program Pilot Study. *Sports* **2025**, *13*, 400.
2. Vasilescu, F.; Leonte, N.; Porfireanu, C.M.; Tudor, V. Applied Research on the Impact of a Neuromotor Development Program on the Lower Limb Strength of Junior Athletes in Greco-Roman Wrestling. *Sports* **2025**, *13*, 428.
3. Amato, A.; Cortis, C.; Tropea, M.; Politi, M.; Fusco, A.; Musumeci, G. Comparison of the Core Training and Mobility Training Effects on Basketball Athletic Performance in Young Players: A Comparative Experimental Study. *Sports* **2025**, *13*, 398.
4. Sansone, P.; Vanacore, M.; Lorenzo-Calvo, J.; Bustamante-Sánchez, Á.; Vaquera, A.; Conte, D. Warming Up for Basketball: Comparing Traditional vs. Small-Sided Game Approaches in Youth Players. *Sports* **2025**, *13*, 452.
5. Castro-Collado, C.; Jurado-Castro, J.M.; Gil-Campos, M.; Pastor-Villaescusa, B.; Quintana-Navarro, G.M.; Llorente-Cantarero, F.J. Effects of After-School Basketball Program on Physical Fitness and Cardiometabolic Health in Prepubertal Boys. *Sports* **2025**, *13*, 291.
6. Herbert, W.; Vanja, R.; Matthias, H. Effectiveness of Specific Professional Training in Male Elite Adolescent Team Handball Players. *Sports* **2025**, *13*, 193.
7. Sagat, P. Pairwise Comparison of Effects of Linear vs. Change of Direction Short Bout Sprint Intervals on Physical Performance of Youth Male Soccer Players. *Sports* **2026**, *14*, 44.
8. Perazzetti, A.; Kaçurri, A.; Gjaka, M.; Pernigoni, M.; Lupo, C.; Tessitore, A. Impact of a Congested Match Schedule on Internal Load, Recovery, Well-Being, and Enjoyment in U16 Youth Water Polo Players. *Sports* **2025**, *13*, 286.
9. Carron, M.A.; Dalbo, V.J. Run-Based Tests Performed on an Indoor and Outdoor Surface Are Comparable in Adolescent Rugby League Players. *Sports* **2025**, *13*, 351.
10. Despot, T.; Plavec, D. The Criterion Validity of a Newly Developed Ballroom Aerobic Test (BAT) Protocol Against Objective Methods. *Sports* **2025**, *13*, 337.
11. Crisafulli, O.; Fortunati, M.; Gemelli, T.; Febbi, M.; Drid, P.; Ramat, S.; D'Antona, G. Power–Load Relationship of Bench Press, Ballistic Bench Press, and Prone Bench Pull in International Medal-Winning Canoeists and Kayakers. *Sports* **2025**, *13*, 191.
12. Massini, D.A.; Caritá, R.A.C.; Almeida, T.A.F.; Macedo, A.G.; Hernández-Beltrán, V.; Gamonales, J.M.; Espada, M.C.; Pessôa Filho, D.M. Physiological Correspondence Between Different Indexes of High-Intensity Endurance Exercise in Young Male Runners. *Sports* **2025**, *13*, 167.
13. Marcelli, L.; Silvestri, F.; Di Pinto, G.; Colombo, A.; Marzoli, F.; Gallotta, M.C.; Guidetti, L.; Perroni, F.; Curzi, D. Does Birth Month Matter? Effects of Birth Subgroupings on Motor Performance and Ball-Involving Tests in a Youth Soccer Academy. *Sports* **2025**, *13*, 382.
14. Ouergui, I.; Delleli, S.; Apollaro, G.; Messaoudi, H.; Kons, R.L.; Bridge, C.A.; Chtourou, H.; Franchini, E.; Faelli, E.; Ardigò, L.P. Relationships Between Sport-Specific Anaerobic Tests, Interlimb Asymmetry, and Bilateral Deficit as Measured from Vertical Jump Performances in Highly Trained Taekwondo Athletes. *Sports* **2025**, *13*, 103.

https://doi.org/10.3390/sports14030103

References

1. Güllich, A.; Barth, M. Effects of Early Talent Promotion on Junior and Senior Performance: A Systematic Review and Meta-Analysis. *Sports Med.* **2024**, *54*, 697–710. [CrossRef] [PubMed]
2. Johnston, K.; Wattie, N.; Schorer, J.; Baker, J. Talent Identification in Sport: A Systematic Review. *Sports Med.* **2018**, *48*, 97–109. [CrossRef] [PubMed]
3. Born, D.P.; Lorentzen, J.; Björklund, G.; Stöggl, T.; Romann, M. Variation vs. specialization: The dose-time-effect of technical and physiological variety in the development of elite swimmers. *BMC Res. Notes* **2024**, *17*, 48. [CrossRef] [PubMed]
4. Jayanthi, N.; Pinkham, C.; Dugas, L.; Patrick, B.; Labella, C. Sports specialization in young athletes: Evidence-based recommendations. *Sports Health* **2013**, *5*, 251–257. [CrossRef] [PubMed]
5. Amato, A.; Giustino, V.; Patti, A.; Proia, P.; Trivic, T.; Drid, P.; Obradovic, A.; Manojlovic, M.; Mondoni, M.; Paoli, A. Young basketball players have better manual dexterity performance than sportsmen and non-sportsmen of the same age: A cross-sectional study. *Sci. Rep.* **2023**, *13*, 20953. [CrossRef] [PubMed]
6. Pasulka, J.; Jayanthi, N.; McCann, A.; Dugas, L.R.; LaBella, C. Specialization patterns across various youth sports and relationship to injury risk. *Physician Sportsmed.* **2017**, *45*, 344–352. [CrossRef] [PubMed]
7. Myer, G.D.; Jayanthi, N.; DiFiori, J.P.; Faigenbaum, A.D.; Kiefer, A.W.; Logerstedt, D.; Micheli, L.J. Sports Specialization, Part II: Alternative Solutions to Early Sport Specialization in Youth Athletes. *Sports Health* **2016**, *8*, 65–73. [CrossRef] [PubMed]
8. Jayanthi, N.; Schley, S.; Cumming, S.P.; Myer, G.D.; Saffel, H.; Hartwig, T.; Gabbett, T.J. Developmental Training Model for the Sport Specialized Youth Athlete: A Dynamic Strategy for Individualizing Load-Response During Maturation. *Sports Health* **2022**, *14*, 142–153. [CrossRef] [PubMed]
9. Post, E.G.; Trigsted, S.M.; Schaefer, D.A.; Cadmus-Bertram, L.A.; Watson, A.M.; McGuine, T.A.; Brooks, M.A.; Bell, D.R. Knowledge, Attitudes, and Beliefs of Youth Sports Coaches Regarding Sport Volume Recommendations and Sport Specialization. *J. Strength Cond. Res.* **2020**, *34*, 2911–2919. [CrossRef] [PubMed]
10. d'Hemecourt, P.; Sugimoto, D.; Stracciolini, A.; Whitney, K. Youth Sport Specialization: Current Concepts and Clinical Guides. *HSS J.® Musculoskelet. J. Hosp. Spec. Surg.* **2024**, *20*, 416–423. [CrossRef]
11. McLellan, M.; Allahabadi, S.; Pandya, N.K. Youth Sports Specialization and Its Effect on Professional, Elite, and Olympic Athlete Performance, Career Longevity, and Injury Rates: A Systematic Review. *Orthop. J. Sports Med.* **2022**, *10*, 23259671221129594. [CrossRef] [PubMed]
12. Brenner, J.S. Sports Specialization and Intensive Training in Young Athletes. *Pediatrics* **2016**, *138*, e20162148. [CrossRef] [PubMed]
13. Tingelstad, L.M.; Raastad, T.; Till, K.; Luteberget, L.S. The development of physical characteristics in adolescent team sport athletes: A systematic review. *PLoS ONE* **2023**, *18*, e0296181. [CrossRef] [PubMed]
14. Lloyd, R.S.; Cronin, J.B.; Faigenbaum, A.D.; Haff, G.G.; Howard, R.; Kraemer, W.J.; Micheli, L.J.; Myer, G.D.; Oliver, J.L. National Strength and Conditioning Association Position Statement on Long-Term Athletic Development. *J. Strength Cond. Res.* **2016**, *30*, 1491–1509. [CrossRef] [PubMed]
15. Balyi, I.; Hamilton, A. Long-term athlete development: Trainability in childhood and adolescence. *Olymp. Coach.* **2004**, *16*, 4–9.
16. Bergeron, M.F.; Mountjoy, M.; Armstrong, N.; Chia, M.; Côté, J.; Emery, C.A.; Faigenbaum, A.; Hall, G.; Kriemler, S.; Léglise, M.; et al. International Olympic Committee consensus statement on youth athletic development. *Br. J. Sports Med.* **2015**, *49*, 843–851. [CrossRef] [PubMed]
17. Chen, D.L.; Meyers, R.N.; Provance, A.J.; Zynda, A.J.; Wagner, K.J., 3rd; Siegel, S.R.; Howell, D.R.; Miller, S.M. Early Sport Specialization and Past Injury in Competitive Youth Rock Climbers. *Wilderness Environ. Med.* **2022**, *33*, 179–186. [CrossRef] [PubMed]
18. Brenner, J.S.; Watson, A. Overuse Injuries, Overtraining, and Burnout in Young Athletes. *Pediatrics* **2024**, *153*, e2023065129. [CrossRef] [PubMed]
19. Bianco, A.; Ravalli, S.; Maugeri, G.; D'Agata, V.; Vecchio, M.; D'Amico, A.G.; Pavone, V.; Lucenti, L.; Amato, A.; Gentile, A.; et al. The "Journal of Functional Morphology and Kinesiology" Journal Club Series: Highlights on Recent Papers in Overtraining and Exercise Addiction. *J. Funct. Morphol. Kinesiol.* **2019**, *4*, 68. [CrossRef] [PubMed]
20. Fuchs, P.X.; Fusco, A.; Bell, J.W.; von Duvillard, S.P.; Cortis, C.; Wagner, H. Effect of Differential Training on Female Volleyball Spike-Jump Technique and Performance. *Int. J. Sports Physiol. Perform.* **2020**, *15*, 1019–1025. [CrossRef] [PubMed]

https://doi.org/10.3390/sports14030103

sports

MDPI

Article

Application of the Vienna Test System to Measure Training-Induced Changes in Choice Reaction Time in U20 Fencers: A 12-Week Training Program Pilot Study

Lukass Edmunds Teteris [1], Sergejs Saulite [1], Renars Licis [1], Mara Greve [2] and Behnam Boobani [1,*]

[1] RSU Latvian Academy of Sport Education, Riga Stradins University, LV-1006 Riga, Latvia; lukass16@inbox.lv (L.E.T.); sergejs.saulite@rsu.lv (S.S.); renars.licis@rsu.lv (R.L.)
[2] Statistics Unit, Riga Stradins University, LV-1007 Riga, Latvia; mara.greve@rsu.lv
* Correspondence: behnam.boobani@rsu.lv

Abstract: This pilot study examined the effects of a 12-week reaction training program on physical and cognitive performance (choice reaction) in U20 Latvian fencers. Five qualified right-handed male fencers (aged 14.8–18.6 years) completed the Vienna Test System choice reaction task at baseline and after 12 weeks while cycling through five heart rate zones (1–5). Reaction speed (RS), motor speed (MS), choice reaction time (CR), and heart rate (HR) were recorded. Paired-sample *t*-tests indicated no significant group-level changes: RS (t = 1.46, $p = 0.21$, d = 0.65, 95% CI [−36.92, 118.92]), MS (t = 2.37, $p = 0.07$, d = 1.06, 95% CI [−3.14, 40.34]), CR (t = 1.70, $p = 0.16$, d = 0.76, 95% CI [−37.30, 156.26]), and HR (t = −2.69, $p = 0.054$, d = −1.20, 95% CI [−12.53, 0.17]). Individual responses revealed that three athletes improved CR in low- to moderate-intensity zones (−12.66% to −27.18%), whereas heart rate increased modestly (1.35% to 9.60%). Given the critical age for developing choice reaction, these findings should be considered as preliminary and exploratory, offering initial insights into how training might influence cognitive performance in young fencers and demonstrating that responses can differ across heart rate zones and among individuals.

Keywords: young athletes; fencing; training methods; choice reaction time; performance

1. Introduction

Fencing, which involves attacking and defending using a sword, is included in the Olympic Games [1]. It is a combat sport that demands open-skill strategies, complex body movements, and tactical play. Athletic performance in fencing reflects how effectively an athlete can execute actions. Like other sports, success relies on multiple physical and mental factors, including reaction time, agility, flexibility, coordination, and decision-making skills [2,3]. Fencing specifically requires athletes to respond quickly to tactile, visual, and auditory stimuli, which are the primary types of stimuli in fencing [4,5]. The blade, considered the second fastest object in sports competition, demands extremely rapid reactions. Typically, scoring actions last about 5 s in foil and 15 s in épée [6]. Therefore, responding effectively is an essential skill and performance [7,8].

Reaction time (RT) is a fundamental skill influencing success in fencing [9]. Reacting to a moving object involves several steps: perceiving the stimulus, estimating its speed, adopting an appropriate posture, and making a decision. In situations where multiple responses are possible, athletes rely on choice reaction time, which requires selecting the correct action under time pressure. This advantage is linked to shorter motor response times, which contribute to superior physical performance and, ultimately, better competitive results [9]. Furthermore, RT acts as an indicator of the efficiency of the cognitive system in processing information [10]. Cognitive processes are usually evaluated through behavioral measures like reaction time.

Cognitive skills and decision-making are essential for athletic performance in competitive sports, especially in combat sports like fencing [11,12]. In fencing, athletes need to constantly anticipate their opponent's moves by interpreting cues or patterns in their behavior [13,14]. Research indicates that physical exertion and exercise can impact both cognitive performance and reaction time, but individual responses differ [15–18]. Studies using computer-based tasks indicate no significant differences between groups, or that elite or well-trained fencers typically have faster reaction and choice reaction times than less experienced athletes [18,19].

Some studies indicate that reaction time (RT) in fencers can be improved through training [20–22]. Conversely, other research contends that genetic factors mainly influence RT and are less affected by training [23]. To anticipate attacks, respond, and stay accurate, fencers must extract relevant information from an opponent's constantly changing posture, distance, movements, or even the current match status [13]. Therefore, fencing demands quick and accurate decision-making under ongoing competitive pressure, along with an evolving perception of physical effort 18]. Since athletes are always under time limitations, both decision-making and sensorimotor reaction times need to be minimized to increase performance [8]. Improving the fencing training system involves identifying and justifying new methods for organizing training, based on modern scientific evidence. The Vienna test system (VTS) [24] is a psychological assessment device that includes tests of many different constructs, such as reaction time and attention, used by applied practitioners to conduct psychological testing in fencing [19,24,25]. Physical preparation is a key part of fencing performance, including explosive starts, sustained readiness for the right moment to attack, and the ability to make quick decisions [26]. Reactions are a crucial part of performance and are closely related to cognitive performance in fencers [27]. Several studies highlight the importance of improving reaction time and response speed to both auditory and visual stimuli, dual-task conditions, the role of speed in a fencer's hand movements, and various training interventions [2,19,26,28–32]. This pilot study aimed to assess the effects of a 12-week reaction training program on physical and cognitive performance (choice reaction) in U20 Latvian fencers. We hypothesized that the targeted training program would improve choice reaction performance.

2. Materials and Methods

2.1. Participants

Five qualified young right-handed male foil fencers from the Latvian national U20 team, all ranked among the top athletes nationally, participated in the study (Table 1). The inclusion criteria included (a) age ranging from 14 to 20 years, which is a critical period for developing choice reaction [28], and (b) training at least 4 times per week. Exclusion criteria were (a) use of drugs, medications, or any conditions (neuromuscular diseases), or musculoskeletal injuries that could affect test outcomes, and (b) previous experience with the VTS. A qualified athlete in this study is defined as a fencer who is in the top 10 of the Latvian rankings, has participated in national and international competitions, and has an EFC (European Fencing Confederation, https://www.eurofencing.info/rankings/individual-rankings, URL accessed on 23 October 2025) or FIE (International Fencing Federation, https://fie.org/athletes, URL accessed on 23 October 2025) ranking. Participants ranged in age from 14.8 to 18.6 years (m = 17.04, SD = 1.43), with an average height of 179.2 cm (SD = 6.87) and body weight of 66.02 kg (SD = 10.33). The study followed the ethical regulations of the Declaration of Helsinki. Information about the purpose of the study was given to the participants, and they voluntarily consented to take part. For underage athletes, written informed consent was additionally obtained from parents or legal guardians. The research protocol was approved by the Ethical Committee of Riga Stradins University, Latvian Academy of Sport Education (protocol no. 8/3/51813, and approval date 30 July 2023). Participants could withdraw at any time without consequence.

Table 1. Individual characteristics and ranking of fencers.

Subject	Age (Years)	Height (cm)	Body Mass (kg)	HR Rest (bpm)	EFC Rank *	FIE Rank *
S1	17.9	186	60	62	-	47
S2	17.1	178	62	79	328	-
S3	18.6	186	82.1	85	-	477
S4	16.8	170	56	76	48	549
S5	14.8	176	70	76	469	-

* cm: centimeter; kg: kilogram; bpm: beat per minute. * Ranking for the years 2023–2034; EFC: European Fencing Confederation; FIE: International Fencing Federation.

2.2. Procedures

The experimental protocol included a baseline assessment (pre-test) and a follow-up assessment after 12 weeks (post-test). None of the participants had previous experience with the cognitive tasks of the Vienna choice reaction test. Therefore, before the intervention, all athletes completed two familiarization sessions, during which they practiced the choice reaction (CR) test while cycling for 30 min on a stationary bike [33]. This ensured that participants were familiar with the test procedures. One week later, the baseline assessment was conducted. At both pre- and post-test, participants performed the CR test five times while cycling on a cycle ergometer (Wattbike Pro/Trainer, Wattbike Ltd., Nottingham, UK) across five heart rate zones (Z1–Z5), monitored using a Polar heart rate system (Polar Team Pro, Polar Electro Oy, Kempele, Finland). The zones were defined according to a previous study [34] and Tanaka's age-based prediction equations for maximal heart rate [35]: zone 1 (50–59% HRmax), zone 2 (60–69% HRmax), zone 3 (70–79% HRmax), zone 4 (80–89% HRmax), and zone 5 (90–100% HRmax).

Upon arriving at the laboratory, participants sat and rested for 10 min. They first did a 10 min warm-up on the cycle ergometer. The protocol was performed in stages, with each stage corresponding to one heart rate zone. Each stage and the CR test lasts between 3 and 5 min. A total of five CR tests were performed. At the end of each stage, participants increased their pedaling intensity to reach the next target zone. During testing, the CR response panel was mounted on the ergometer. Workload progression was not standardized by resistance settings but was instead guided by heart rate response and self-selected pedaling intensity. The entire test took approximately 25–30 min.

Participants were advised to refrain from alcohol, caffeine, and vigorous physical activity for at least 24 h prior to testing. Participants were asked verbally to confirm they followed the pre-test instructions and reported full compliance. If they were noncompliant, testing would be rescheduled.

The Vienna Test System (VTS) is a popular computerized tool used for objectively assessing various psychological constructs. It is commonly employed in sports science to examine how different factors influence cognitive performance [24]. During the CR test, stimuli include yellow and red circles, auditory tones, and combinations of these. The key stimulus combination requires participants to respond when both a yellow and a red circle appear simultaneously. Two output variables from the CR test were recorded.

Reaction speed (RS) is the time elapsed from when the relevant stimulus appears to when the participant's finger lifts from the rest position button. It indicates how quickly an individual perceives a stimulus and initiates a response. Motor speed (MS) represents the second component of CR and is defined as the interval from when the finger lifts off the rest button to when the designated response is pressed. MS provides an index of processing and motor execution speed. The CR test lasts between 3 and 5 min. All procedures were non-invasive and supervised by the researcher and fencing coach.

2.3. Intervention

The modified reaction training program [21,36] was conducted twice weekly for 12 weeks (July–September 2024), with each session lasting 30 min and including 10 exercises (Appendix A, Tables A1–A3). This program was performed alongside participants' regular fencing and general training. The training protocol involved both general and fencing drills and was adapted from different sports to improve reaction time and cognitive performance [Table 2]. Each general and regular fencing session, without emphasizing reaction exercises, began with a standardized warm-up and continued with stretching, jogging, footwork, and tactical and technical training. Special training consisted of 10 reaction exercises using various equipment, including balls of different sizes and weights, tennis balls, jump ropes, and agility ladders. Exercises included catching balls, performing single-leg hops, cone-color reaction tasks, fencing drills, and combined movement and cognitive challenges such as jumping while catching a glove and shuttle runs. Sessions ended with cool-down exercises. The first author and a fencing coach oversaw all training sessions. Every fencer participated in each session.

Table 2. The weekly training schedule.

Day	Monday	Tuesday	Wednesday	Thursday	Friday
Trainings	General training (60 min)	General (30 min) + special training (30 min)	Rest	General (30 min) + special training (30 min)	General training (60 min)

2.4. Statistical Analysis

Data were analyzed using Microsoft Excel 2016 and Jeffreys's Amazing Statistics Program (JASP) version 0.18.3. Due to the limited sample size and based on earlier research [14,37], descriptive statistics, including the minimum (Min), maximum (Max), mean (m), standard deviation (SD), effect sizes (Cohen's d), confidence intervals (CIs), and percentage change (%Change), were calculated. Data normality was assessed using the Shapiro–Wilk test. A paired *t*-test (t) was used for data analysis. The significance level was $p < 0.05$. Percentage change (%Change) was calculated using the following formula:

$$\%Change = [(mpost - mpre)/mpre] * \times 100. \quad (1)$$

3. Results

The results are divided into two parts: (1) overall pre–post changes in reaction speed (RS), motor speed (MS), choice reaction (CR), and heart rate (HR), and (2) individual zone-based profiles showing within-athlete changes over the 12-week training period. For RS, MS, and CR, lower values and reduction (milliseconds, ms) indicate faster responses, while HR values are given as average beats per minute (bpm).

3.1. Overall Pre–Post Results of RS, MS, CR, and HR

Reaction Speed (RS). Descriptive statistics for RS across participants are presented in Table 3. Overall post-test results showed a decrease in RS for S1, S3, and S5, indicating faster responses. The most improvement was seen in S1, with RS decreasing from m = 560.4, SD = 63.85 ms at pre-test to m = 415.4, SD = 27.55 ms at post-test, a −25.87% change. S3 and S5 showed moderate improvements of −12.45% and −8.67%, respectively. Conversely, S2 exhibited an increase in RS (3.49%), indicating slower responses, while S4 remained unchanged.

Table 3. Overall RS results (n = 5).

Variable	Sub	Test Phase	m ± SD	95% CI Lower, Upper	Min	Max	%Change
RS (ms)	S1	Pre	560.4 ± 63.85	481.11, 639.69	467	625	−25.87
		Post	415.4 ± 27.55	381.18, 449.61	371	444	
	S2	Pre	440.6 ± 40.78	389.96, 491.23	397	504	3.49
		Post	456 ± 36.47	410.70, 501.29	428	518	
	S3	Pre	345.2 ± 24.89	314.29, 376.11	317	380	−12.45
		Post	302.2 ± 14.09	284.69, 319.70	288	325	
	S4	Pre	308.4 ± 34.81	265.17, 351.62	255	343	0
		Post	308.4 ± 33.97	266.21, 350.58	272	346	
	S5	Pre	373.6 ± 4.03	368.58, 378.61	367	378	−8.67
		Post	341.2 ± 30.77	302.98, 379.41	308	388	

RS: reaction speed; ms: milliseconds; Sub subject; m mean, SD: standard deviation; CI: confidence interval; Min: minimum, Max: maximum.

The motor speed (MS). Table 4 shows the results of MS, which demonstrated consistent improvements in four athletes. S1 indicated the greatest change, decreasing from m = 127.4, SD = 21.36 ms to m = 85.40, SD = 17.53 ms, reflecting a −32.96% and a large reduction. Notable decreases were also observed in S5 (−26.64%), S3 (−17.14%), and S2 (−15.36%). S4 showed an increase (4.85%).

Table 4. Overall MS results (n = 5).

Variable	Sub	Test Phase	m ± SD	95% CI Lower, Upper	Min	Max	%Change
MS (ms)	S1	Pre	127.4 ± 21.36	100.87, 153.92	96	155	−32.96
		Post	85.40 ± 17.53	63.63, 107.16	66	103	
	S2	Pre	82 ± 5.29	75.43, 88.57	75	89	−15.36
		Post	69.4 ± 5.03	63.15, 75.64	62	75	
	S3	Pre	84 ± 8.45	73.50, 94.49	74	97	−17.14
		Post	69.6 ± 3.05	65.81, 73.38	65	72	
	S4	Pre	90.6 ± 4.03	85.58, 95.61	85	95	4.85
		Post	95 ± 10.52	82.53, 108.67	85	112	
	S5	Pre	106.6 ± 9.42	94.89, 118.30	96	120	−26.64
		Post	78.2 ± 4.32	72.83, 83.56	73	84	

MS: motor speed; ms: milliseconds; Sub: subject; m mean, SD: standard deviation; CI: confidence interval; Min: minimum, Max: maximum.

Choice reaction (CR) and heart rate (HR). CR followed a similar trend (Table 5), with S1 decreasing substantially (m = 687.8, SD = 76.02 ms to m = 500.8, SD = 38.80 ms), resulting in a −27.18% reduction in post-test. The HR was increased from m = 124.9, SD = 26.4 to m = 141.4, SD = 28.5 bpm (8.85%). CR improvements were also evident in S3 (−13.37%), with improvements in HR (9.6%) and S5 (−12.66%), as well as HR (2.39%) in the post-test. Conversely, CR in S2 (0.53%), with a HR (1.35%), and S4 (1.25%), HR (1.5%) showed negligible increases.

Table 5. Overall CR and HR results in pre- and post-tests (n = 5).

Variable	Sub	Test Phase	m ± SD	95% CI Lower, Upper	Min	Max	%Change
CR (ms)	S1	Pre	687.8 ± 76.02	593.39, 782.20	563	760	−27.18
		Post	500.8 ± 38.8	452.61, 548.98	437	539	
	S2	Pre	522.6 ± 45.88	465.62, 579.57	472	593	0.53
		Post	525.4 ± 39.51	476.33, 574.46	497	591	
	S3	Pre	429.2 ± 31.09	390.59, 467.80	398	477	−13.37
		Post	371.8 ± 13.55	354.97, 388.62	360	393	
	S4	Pre	399 ± 31.49	359.89, 438.10	350	432	1.25
		Post	404 ± 25.65	327.14, 435.85	371	435	
	S5	Pre	480.2 ± 7.69	470.64, 489.75	470	487	−12.66
		Post	419.4 ± 28.97	383.42, 455.37	383	461	
HR (bpm)	S1	Pre	124.93 ± 26.4	92.14, 157.72	90	154	8.85
		Post	141.43 ± 28.53	105.99, 176.86	106	171	
	S2	Pre	133.2 ± 21.12	106.97, 159.42	113	163	1.35
		Post	135 ± 23.72	105.53, 164.46	106	168	
	S3	Pre	125 ± 13.15	108.66, 141.33	116	148	9.6
		Post	137 ± 19.72	112.51, 161.48	118	162	
	S4	Pre	138.8 ± 23.47	109.64, 167.95	113	169	1.5
		Post	(141 ± 26.58)	107.99, 174	108	175	
	S5	Pre	142.2 ± 23.13	113.47, 170.92	113	173	2.39
		Post	145.6 ± 24.77	114.83, 176.36	112	175	

CR: choice reaction; ms: milliseconds; HR: heart rate; bpm: beats per minute; Sub: subject; m mean, SD: standard deviation; CI: confidence interval; Min: minimum, Max: maximum.

Group level. Paired-sample t-tests (Table 6) examined pre- and post-test differences in RS, MS, CR, and HR. Shapiro–Wilk tests indicated normal distributions for all variables ($p > 0.05$). No significant changes were observed for RS, t(4) = 1.46, p = 0.218, d = 0.65, or CR, t(4) = 1.70, p = 0.163, d = 0.76. However, effect sizes indicate moderate changes in cognitive-motor performance. MS showed a trend toward improvement, t(4) = 2.37, p = 0.076, d = 1.06, and HR approached significance, t(4) = −2.69, p = 0.054, d = −1.20.

Table 6. t-test results for RS, MS, CR, and HR.

Sub	Test Phase	m ± SD	95% CI Lower, Upper	t	p	d
RS (ms)	Pre	405.64± 99.13	−36.92, 118.92	1.46	0.218	0.65
	Post	364.64 ± 68.07				

Table 6. *Cont.*

Sub	Test Phase	m ± SD	95% CI Lower, Upper	t	*p*	d
MS (ms)	Pre	98.12 ± 19	−3.14, 40.34	2.37	0.076	1.06
	Post	79.52 ± 10.91				
CR (ms)	Pre	503.76 ± 113.26	−37.30, 156.26	1.70	0.163	0.76
	Post	444.28 ± 65.7				
HR (bpm)	Pre	133.82 ± 6.86	−12.53, 0.17	−2.69	0.054	−1.20
	Post	140 ± 4.13				

Sub: subject; RS: reaction speed; MS: motor speed; CR: choice reaction; HR: heart rate; ms: milliseconds; bpm: beats per minute; m: mean; SD: standard deviation; CI: confidence interval; t: *t*-test; *p*: *p*-value < 0.05; d: Cohen's effect size.

3.2. Individual Zone-Based Profiles of Athletes

The results of individual zones are shown in Figure 1. Subject 1 showed consistent and substantial cognitive performance improvements across all zones (Figure 1a). RS decreased by −17% to −34% across Z1–Z5, with the largest in Z2 (−34%). MS is dramatically affected, especially in Z4 (−47.6%) and Z1 (−38.7%). Correspondingly, CR decreased between −21.9% and −32.4%. However, HR responses increased by 10–18% across all zones. S2's profile (Figure 1b) was more mixed. RS was reduced in Z1 (−13%) and Z3 (−4.7%), but increased in Z2 (24.8%) and Z4 (10%). MS consistently improved (−7% to −30%), with the greatest change in Z1. Results for CR show a reduction in Z1 (−15.7%) and Z3 (−6.9%) but an increase in Z2 (19.4%) and Z4 (7%). HR responses were stable to slightly elevated (−6% to 5.6%).

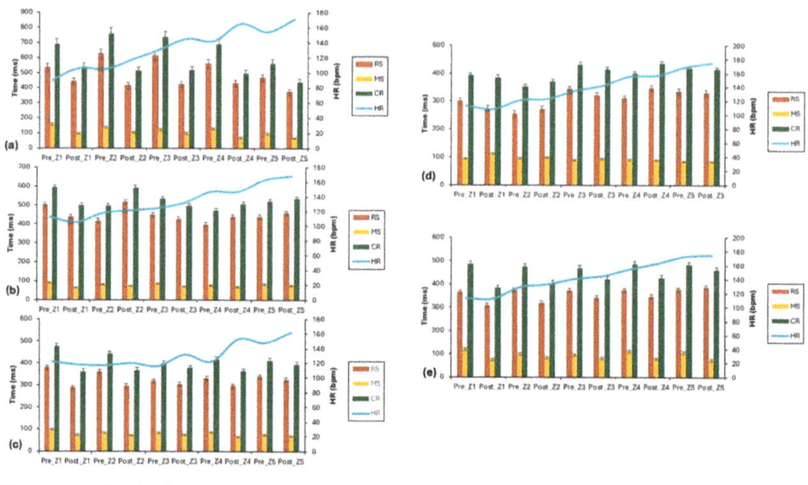

Figure 1. Individual zone profiles per athlete (*n* = 5); subfigures (**a–e**) correspond to subjects 1–5, respectively.

S3 showed a strong and generalized reduction across most zones (Figure 1c). RS decreased by −24% in Z1, −17.8% in Z2, and around −4% in Z3–Z5. MS shows a reduction in all zones (−8% to −25%), with the best in Z1. CR decreased by −24.5% in Z1, −17% in Z2, and moderately in Z3–Z5. HR patterns, however, indicated modest decreases in Z1 (−3.3%) but increases up to 25% in Z4. The results for S4 show the most variable profile (Figure 1d). RS decreased in Z1 (−8.7%) and Z3 (−6.4%), but increased in Z2 (6.7%) and Z4 (11.6%). MS increased in Z1 (19.1%) and Z2 (4.2%), and stability was maintained in Z5. CR showed small changes (−2% to 8.8%). HR increased modestly across most zones (0.6% to 5.2%). The results of RS for S5 show a reduction in Z1–Z4 (−7% to −16%), but Z5 increased by 2.6%. MS decreased across all zones (−16% to −37.5%), with the largest reduction in Z1. CR also decreased across the zones (−4.7% to −21.3%). HR changes were minimal (−0.9% to 5.2%).

4. Discussion

This study examined the effects of a 12-week reaction training program on physical and cognitive performance in U20 fencers. The main findings indicate that at the group level, paired-samples *t*-tests for reaction speed (RS), motor speed (MS), choice reaction (CR), and heart rate (HR) did not reach statistical significance. Nevertheless, individual-level analyses revealed that choice reaction performance improved post-intervention in athletes S1, S3, and S5, while it decreased for athletes S2 and S4, particularly when tested at different heart rate zones, highlighting individual variability. Heart rate changes were modest across participants, indicating that improvements in choice reaction performance were not strongly associated with cardiovascular responses. These findings should be interpreted as preliminary and exploratory, providing initial insights into how training may influence cognitive performance in young fencers and illustrating that responses can vary across heart rate zones and among individuals.

The cognitive performance is influenced by variables such as training intensity, duration, and the task, interacting to create complex effects on performance outcomes [38]. McMorris [39] proposed that exercise influences cognition by activating the hypothalamic and sympathetic–adrenal systems, thereby increasing catecholamine release. These biochemical changes affect neural processes involved in attention and information processing, though the exact relationship between exercise intensity and cognitive performance remains complex and not fully understood. Specifically, post-intervention CR decreased across fencers (m = 500.8, SD = 38.8 to m = 419.4, SD = 28.97 ms) compared to baseline (m = 687.8, SD = 76.02 to m = 480.2, SD = 7.69 ms), corresponding to percentage changes ranging from 0.53% to −27.18%. These findings indicate that although individual results varied, the group results, including the lack of a significant effect ($p > 0.05$) due to sample size, all participants completed the 12-week reaction training without dropouts, indicating that this training protocol is feasible to implement and support in future, larger-scale studies. Concurrently, changes in heart rate responses varied among participants (Table 4), highlighting individual differences in physiological adaptation to the intervention.

Furthermore, individual optimal heart rate zones for achieving faster choice reaction times were observed in zones 1–2 (HR range: 106–118 bpm), with noticeable variation among participants (Figure 1). This result is consistent with earlier studies [40–44], which have shown that low to moderate intensity exercise improves response speed to choice reaction and visual stimuli. Specifically, the relationship between reaction time and exercise intensity seems to follow an exponential pattern: reaction time decreases as exercise intensity increases to the aerobic threshold (around 120 bpm), then plateaus between 130–155 bpm, and gradually rises again beyond the anaerobic threshold, continuing up to maximal effort. Stimuli further influence the impact of higher intensities (above 160 bpm).

In contrast to our findings, some studies have shown that low-intensity exercise does not significantly influence cognitive task performance, while higher intensities may improve reaction speed [15–18]. This partially aligns with previous research suggesting a U-shaped relationship of training intensity and cognitive performance, where moderate exercise has a beneficial effect but high-intensity training may impair performance [45]. However, the inverted-U model has faced criticism, and newer studies highlight that the impact of training on cognitive performance is related to the task [35]. Furthermore, athletes and non-athletes respond differently to exercise. Several studies comparing experienced athletes with novices indicate that athletes tend to benefit more from exercise, likely because of their greater familiarity with high physiological stress and the substantial physical, emotional, and cognitive demands involved [46–49].

In this study, we also investigated the effect of a 12-week training program on heart rate (HR). The increase was modest, ranging from 1.35% to 9.60% across participants, with the largest increase observed in S3 (9.60%) and the smallest in S2 (1.35%). Exercise is known to trigger both immediate and long-term adaptations in HR [50]; however, the relatively low training load of the current program may explain the limited HR changes in some athletes. Although sessions were held twice weekly for 30 min over 12 weeks, the ten exercises included were not enough to produce significant cardiovascular adaptation. Endurance training causes significant changes in cardio-autonomic regulation [51], which were not achieved in the current intervention. Importantly, improvements in CR performance observed in S1, S3, and S5 occurred despite modestly elevated HRs. This aligns with dual-task paradigms [33,44], where athletes must maintain cognitive performance while performing physical tasks, reflecting adaptations relevant to the training and fencing competition. Previous research has also shown that fatigue caused by high-intensity exercise generally leads to increased and longer reaction times [41].

Task complexity is another key factor affecting how exercise influences cognitive performance. Cognitive load results from the interaction between exercise, brain catecholamines, which increase arousal by activating the reticular formation, and the cognitive task. In this study, athletes S2 and S4 showed increased CR, aligning with previous findings [38]. A likely reason is that the combination of pedaling for 30 min and performing the test created a higher cognitive and physical load, leading to longer reaction times. Conversely, other fencers (S1, S3, and S5) completed these complex tasks with shorter CRs. The longer CRs seen in S2 and S4 may be related to the wait-and-see strategy [52], where additional cognitive processes like decision-making and information integration extend reaction time. Therefore, the amount and type of information needed to generate a response depend on the task and help explain individual differences in CR performance [53]. Moreover, caution is advised when comparing results from different studies, especially when the CR or experimental setup varies [54]. In this study, we used the CR test on a bicycle, a new laboratory measure for this group, since fencers usually do not use the VTS in their regular training. The familiarization was limited to 2 sessions, which may explain differences in cognitive performance. This could make measurements reflect the effect of being new to an unfamiliar dual task, where cycling demands much cognitive capacity and could interfere with other tasks (VTS), rather than measuring true cognitive impact.

Attention, which depends on executive functions like inhibitory control and working memory, also affects choice reaction time and overall performance [55,56]. In fencing, cues can appear anywhere in the visual field, requiring athletes to use peripheral vision and quickly move their gaze through rapid eye movements. Previous research shows that elite fencers are generally better at focusing on these cues [14]. In this study, two athletes (S2 and S4) showed longer choice reaction times, possibly indicating reduced or distracted attention, which can hinder information processing and fencing performance. Importantly, the critical age for developing CR is between approximately 15 and 20 years old [28]. In this study, the fencers were in a crucial age period when differences in reaction time and related variables are most likely to be detected. However, it is important to recognize that multiple factors, including age, ambient temperature, type of stimulus, nerve conduction quality, and receptor sensitivity, influence individual differences in outcomes. While the findings partly support the hypothesis that 12 weeks of training could improve choice reaction, there are several limitations. First, the small sample size of five males was determined by participant availability and by the inclusion and exclusion criteria of the study during data collection, rather than by predefined sample size calculations. Especially considering the critical age for developing choice reaction [28] and the fact that athletes (under 20 years old) and competing at the national or international level. Although they represent a rare and highly selective group, this complicates the recruitment of larger cohorts. Additionally, this study's limitations include the lack of a control group and the absence of randomization. Future studies should increase the number of participants (including left-handed fencers) and add other specific weapons (such as épée and saber), which would be beneficial. Future research with larger sample sizes and longer data collection periods could provide more solid insights into the effects observed in this study. Second, the results obtained in a controlled laboratory setting may not directly apply to field environments [57] or actual competitions, as the procedures used here do not consider key factors in fencing, such as dynamic interaction with an opponent [58]. While this study focused on cognitive performance, which is crucial for executing fencing skills, a full understanding of how physical load influences cognitive expertise requires examining the underlying neurophysiological mechanisms. The present study included only male foil fencers aged 14–18. Future studies should expand the sample to include female athletes, athletes of different ages, and various levels of expertise. Because of differences in segment length and muscle mass, sex-related variations in execution speed could also be worth exploring. Since competitive fencing has been linked to cognitive fatigue, examining how it affects execution speed and accuracy could be valuable. Additionally, since the 12-week training program was tested with a small group, adding a control group would help provide clearer conclusions about its effect on cognitive performance, especially choice reaction. Results cannot establish causality. Observed changes may reflect learning or familiarization.

5. Conclusions

The present pilot study examined the effects of a 12-week reaction training program on physical and cognitive performance (choice reaction) in U20 Latvian fencers. While the group results showed no significant changes in the variables, some individual changes suggested that a 12-week training program may improve choice reaction time. Also, the current program's low training load may explain the limited HR changes in some athletes. Given the critical age for developing choice reaction, a small sample size may limit the study, and these findings should be interpreted as preliminary and exploratory, providing initial insights into how training may influence cognitive performance in young fencers and illustrating that responses can vary across heart rate zones and among individuals. However, it is important to recognize that multiple factors, including age and stimulus type, influence individual differences in outcomes. These points emphasize the need for future research with highly controlled designs, including clear definitions of participant expertise, specific exercise protocols, and well-defined cognitive tasks.

Author Contributions: Conceptualization, L.E.T., S.S., R.L., M.G. and B.B.; methodology, L.E.T., M.G. and B.B.; formal analysis and data curation, L.E.T., M.G. and B.B.; investigation, L.E.T. and B.B.; writing—review and editing, L.E.T., S.S., R.L., M.G. and B.B.; visualization, L.E.T. and B.B.; supervision, S.S., R.L. and B.B. All authors have read and agreed to the published version of the manuscript.

Funding: This research was funded within the framework of the European Union Recovery and Resilience Mechanism Plan and the state budget-funded project "RSU internal and RSU with LASE external consolidation" (No. 5.2.1.1.i.0/2/24/I/CFLA/005), implemented under a Doctoral Grant.

Institutional Review Board Statement: The study was conducted in accordance with the Declaration of Helsinki and approved by the Ethical Committee of Riga Stradins University, Latvian Academy of Sport Education (protocol code no. 8/3/51813, and approval date 30 July 2023).

Informed Consent Statement: Informed consent was obtained from parents or legal guardians.

Data Availability Statement: Data are available upon request to the correspondence author. An anonymized dataset/code will be open access (for reproducibility).

Acknowledgments: We are thankful to the athletes for participating in this study.

Conflicts of Interest: The authors declare no conflicts of interest. The funders had no role in the design of the study; in the collection, analyses, or interpretation of data; in the writing of the manuscript; or in the decision to publish the results.

Abbreviations

The following abbreviations are used in this manuscript:

RT	Reaction time
VTS	Vienna test system
CR	Choice reaction
RS	Reaction speed
MS	Motor speed
m	mean
SD	Standard deviation
%Change	Percentage change
ms	milliseconds
Sub	subject
Min	minimum
Max	maximum
HR	Heart rate
bpm	beats per minute
Z	Zone

Appendix A

Table A1. The 12-week training program description (2× a week), month 1.

No.	Instructions	Dosage
1	Launch a tennis ball, let it bounce, and catch it with one hand while extending your arm (from the guard position)	2 × 1 min + rest 30 s
2	Throw a reaction ball and grab it with one hand after it hits the ground.	2 × 1 min + rest 30 s
3	In the same exercise, catch the ball during the drill, then immediately perform a forward lunge.	2 × 1 min + rest 30 s
4	Agility leather exercises: step forward, then move your right foot outside the square boundary.	2 × 1 min + rest 30 s
5	Agility leather exercises: step ahead, then shift your left foot beyond the edge of the box.	2 × 1 min + rest 30 s
6	Begin in a defensive stance, take two strides forward, and one step back.	2 × 1 min + rest 30 s
7	Start from the guard position, walk to the first marker, then retreat to the next, repeat this relay-style movement.	2 × 1 min + rest 30 s
8	Practice fencing footwork from a ready stance, changing direction whenever the coach claps.	2 × 1 min + rest 30 s
9	Moving into the fighting stance, the individual responds to cones of various colors.	2 × 1 min + rest 30 s
10	Jogging in place in a fencing stance and striking the fencing target on a coach's command.	2 × 1 min + rest 30 s

Table A2. The 12-week training program description (2× a week), month 2.

No.	Instructions	Dosage
1	Throw the tennis ball up, catch it smoothly, and stretch your arm forward quickly.	2 × 1 min + rest 30 s
2	Put two colored objects in front. When the coach says a color, touch the one that matches.	2 × 1 min + rest 30 s
3	Two athletes stand apart 2 m and step forward to tap the object in front of them.	2 × 1 min + rest 30 s
4	Each athlete has two colored items. When the coach gives the signal, they race to grab the right one (reaction play).	2 × 1 min + rest 30 s
5	Agility leather exercises: Jump into each box using only the right foot.	2 × 1 min + rest 30 s
6	Agility leather exercises: jump onto each box using only the left leg.	2 × 1 min + rest 30 s
7	From the guard position, when told, take two fast steps forward and wait for the next signal.	2 × 1 min + rest 30 s
8	Move around freely. When signaled, lunge forward, go back to ready stance, take two quick steps back, and repeat	2 × 1 min + rest 30 s
9	Running in place in the fencing stance and catching the fencing glove with a lunge.	2 × 1 min + rest 30 s
10	Jumping rope and catching the fencing gloves.	2 × 1 min + rest 30 s

Table A3. The 12-week training program description (2× a week), month 3.

No.	Instructions	Dosage
1	Place two colored posts in front. When the coach says a color, the athlete quickly taps that one using their strong hand.	2 × 1 min + rest 30 s
2	Two athletes stand facing each other with a post between them. When the coach gives the signal, they race to grab it—whoever gets it first wins.	2 × 1 min + rest 30 s
3	Exercise no. 2 is repeated, and the coach shouts different commands: hand on knee, hand on head, etc. When he shouts and puts his hand on the pole, the athletes must quickly grab the pole.	2 × 1 min + rest 30 s
4	While jumping rope, reach out and catch the fencing glove during the movement.	2 × 1 min + rest 30 s
5	Step forward and backward like in fencing. When signaled, sprint in place with high knees from the guard position.	2 × 1 min + rest 30 s
6	Do jumping jacks, then catch the fencing glove when prompted.	2 × 1 min + rest 30 s
7	Run back and forth between two points, and catch tennis balls during the drill (Shuttle running).	2 × 1 min + rest 30 s
8	Move freely. When the coach signals, take two fast steps back, then lunge forward with power.	2 × 1 min + rest 30 s
9	Jump from a distant spot toward a closer one using agility leather.	2 × 1 min + rest 30 s
10	Make two forward jumps with both feet, then jump backward once.	2 × 1 min + rest 30 s

References

1. Chen, T.L.W.; Wong, D.W.C.; Wang, Y.; Ren, S.; Yan, F.; Zhang, M. Biomechanics of fencing sport: A scoping review. *PLoS ONE* **2017**, *12*, e0171578. [CrossRef]
2. Torun, V.; Ince, G.; Durgun, B. The effects of basic fencing studies and velocity training on reaction time in the 9–12-year-old beginners of fencing. *Sport Sci.* **2012**, *5*, 59–66.
3. Witkowski, M.; Bojkowski, Ł.; Karpowicz, K.; Konieczny, M.; Bronikowski, M.; Tomczak, M. Effectiveness and Durability of Transfer Training in Fencing. *Int. J. Environ. Res. Public Health* **2020**, *17*, 849. [CrossRef] [PubMed]
4. Borysiuk, Z.; Markowska, N.; Konieczny, M.; Kręcisz, K.; Błaszczyszyn, M.; Nikolaidis, P.T.; Knechtle, B.; Pakosz, P. Flèche versus Lunge as the Optimal Footwork Technique in Fencing. *Int. J. Environ. Res. Public Health* **2019**, *16*, 2315. [CrossRef]
5. Gutiérrez-Cruz, C.; Rojas, F.J.; Gutiérrez-Davila, M. Effect of defence response time during lunge in foil fencing. *J. Sports Sci.* **2015**, *34*, 651–657. [CrossRef]
6. Sorel, A.; Plantard, P.; Bideau, N.; Pontonnier, C. Studying fencing lunge accuracy and response time in uncertain conditions with an innovative simulator. *PLoS ONE* **2019**, *14*, e0218959. [CrossRef]

7. Chtara, H.; Negra, Y.; Chaabene, H.; Chtara, M.; Cronin, J.; Chaouachi, A. Validity and Reliability of a New Test of Change of Direction in Fencing Athletes. *Int. J. Environ. Res. Public Health* **2020**, *17*, 4545. [CrossRef]
8. Milic, M.; Nedeljkovic, A.; Cuk, I.; Mudric, M.; García-Ramos, A. Comparison of reaction time between beginners and experienced fencers during quasi-realistic fencing situations. *Eur. J. Sport Sci.* **2020**, *20*, 896–905. [CrossRef]
9. Balkó, S.; Zbigniev, B.; Simonek, J. The influence of different performance levels of fencers on simple and choice reaction time. *Rev. Bras. Cineantropometria Desempenho Hum.* **2016**, *18*, 391–400. [CrossRef]
10. Jensen, A.R. *Clocking the Mind: Mental Chronometry and Individual Differences*, 1st ed.; Elsevier Science & Technology: Chantilly, VA, USA, 2006. [CrossRef]
11. Van Maarseveen, M.J.J.; Savelsbergh, G.J.P.; Oudejans, R.R.D. In Situ Examination of Decision-Making Skills and Gaze Behaviour of Basketball Players. *Hum. Mov. Sci.* **2018**, *57*, 205–216. [CrossRef]
12. Chang, C.L.; Lin, F.T.; Li, K.W.; Jou, Y.T.; Huang, C.D. A study of optimal handle shape and muscle strength distribution on the lower arm when holding a foil. *Percept. Mot. Skills* **2009**, *108*, 524–530. [CrossRef]
13. De Quel, Ó.M.; Bennett, S.J. Perceptual-Cognitive Expertise in Combat Sports: A Narrative Review and a Model of Perception-Action/Habilidades Perceptivo-Cognitivas En Deportes de Combate: Una Revisión Narrativa y Un Modelo de Percepción-Acción. *RICYDE Rev. Int. Cienc. Deporte* **2019**, *15*, 323–338. [CrossRef]
14. Bagot, P.; Fournier, J.F.; Kerivel, T.; Bossard, C.; Kermarrec, G.; Martinent, G.; Bernier, M. Visual Search Strategies of Elite Fencers: An Exploratory Study in Ecological Competitive Situation. *J. Funct. Morphol. Kinesiol.* **2023**, *8*, 106. [CrossRef]
15. Llorens, F.; Sanabria, D.; Huertas, F. The influence of acute intense exercise on exogenous spatial attention depends on physical fitness level. *Exp. Psychol.* **2015**, *62*, 9–21. [CrossRef]
16. Cereatti, L.; Casella, R.; Manganelli, M.; Pesce, C. Visual attention in adolescents: Facilitating effects of sport expertise and acute physical exercise. *Psychol. Sport Exerc.* **2009**, *10*, 136–145. [CrossRef]
17. Delignières, D.; Brisswalter, J.; Legros, P. Influence of physical exercise on choice reaction time in sports experts: The mediating role of resource allocation. *J. Hum. Mov. Stud.* **1994**, *27*, 173–188.
18. Mouelhi Guizani, S.; Bouzaouach, I.; Tenenbaum, G.; Ben Kheder, A.; Feki, Y.; Bouaziz, M. Simple and choice reaction times under varying levels of physical load in high-skilled fencers. *J. Sports Med. Phys. Fitness* **2006**, *46*, 344–351. [PubMed]
19. Johne, M.; Poliszczuk, T.; Poliszczuk, D.; Dąbrowska-Perzyna, A. Asymmetry of Complex Reaction Time in Female Épée Fencers of Different Sports Classes. *Pol. J. Sport Tour.* **2013**, *20*, 25–29. [CrossRef]
20. Di Martino, G.; Giommoni, S.; Esposito, F.; Alessandro, D.; della Valle, C.; Iuliano, E.; Fiorilli, G.; Calcagno, G.; di Cagno, A. Enhancing Focus and Short Reaction Time in Épée Fencing: The Power of the Science Vision Training Academy System. *J. Funct. Morphol. Kinesiol.* **2024**, *9*, 213. [CrossRef]
21. Magyar, P.; Faur, M.; Nita, V.; Dintica, G.; Oravitan, M. Developing the speed of fencers at the level of the lower and upper limbs through a combined program of non-specific and fencing-specific exercises. *Ann. Appl. Sport Sci.* **2023**, *11*, 1–12. [CrossRef]
22. Johne, M. The impact of fencing training symmetrisation on simple reaction time. *Biomed. Hum. Kinet.* **2021**, *13*, 231–236. [CrossRef]
23. Roca, A.; Williams, A.M. Expertise and the Interaction Between Different Perceptual-Cognitive Skills: Implications for Testing and Training. *Front. Psychol.* **2016**, *7*, 792. [CrossRef]
24. Schuhfried, G. *Vienna Test System: Psychological Assessment*; Schuhfried: Moedling, Austria, 2013.
25. Patócs, Á.; Melia, L.; Kovács, S.; Fózer-Selmeci, B.; Révész, L.; Tóth, L. Reactive Stress Tolerance and Personality Characteristics of Hungarian Elite Fencers. *Cogn. Brain Behav.* **2016**, *20*, 171–184.
26. Nesen, O.; Klimenchenko, V. Indicators of speed and strength abilities of young fencers 12–13 years old. *Pedagog. Health* **2022**, *1*, 23–28. [CrossRef]
27. Aydın, Ö.; Doğan, E.; Sevilmiş, E.; Sağlam, Ç.K. Examining the effects of attention and concentration levels on reaction time in fencing. *Phys. Educ. Stud.* **2024**, *28*, 90–96. [CrossRef]
28. Balkó, S.; Rous, M.; Balkó, I.; Hnízdil, J.; Borysiuk, Z. Influence of a 9-week training intervention on the reaction time of fencers aged 15 to 18 years. *Phys. Act. Rev.* **2017**, *5*, 146–154. [CrossRef]
29. Witkowski, M.; Tomczak, E.; Bojkowski, Ł.; Borysiuk, Z.; Tomczak, M. Do Expert Fencers Engage the Same Visual Perception Strategies as Beginners? *J. Hum. Kinet.* **2021**, *78*, 49–58. [CrossRef]
30. Gutiérrez-Davila, M.; Rojas, F.J.; Gutiérrez-Cruz, C.; Navarro, E. Effect of dual-attention task on attack and defensive actions in fencing. *Eur. J. Sport Sci.* **2017**, *17*, 1004–1012. [CrossRef]
31. Petronijević, S.; Petrović, A.; Ćopić, N.; Jovanović, S.; Gajić, I. The influence of maturation on the speed of the individual hand movements in fencing. *Homo Sport.* **2019**, *21*, 1–5.
32. Johne, M. The influence of three-year symmetrical training on the precision and frequency of the fencers' movement. *Cent. Eur. J. Sport Sci. Med.* **2023**, *1*, 5–12. [CrossRef]
33. Torbeyns, T.; de Geus, B.; Bailey, S.; De Pauw, K.; Decroix, L.; Van Cutsem, J.; Meeusen, R. Cycling on a Bike Desk Positively Influences Cognitive Performance. *PLoS ONE* **2016**, *11*, e0165510. [CrossRef]

34. Oates, L.W.; Campbell, I.G.; Iglesias, X.; Price, M.J.; Muniz-Pumares, D.; Bottoms, L.M. The physiological demands of elite épée fencers during competition. *Int. J. Perform. Anal. Sport* **2019**, *19*, 76–89. [CrossRef]
35. Tanaka, H.; Monahan, K.D.; Seals, D.R. Age-Predicted Maximal Heart Rate Revisited. *J. Am. Coll. Cardiol.* **2001**, *37*, 153–156. [CrossRef]
36. Turna, B. The Effect of Agility Training on Reaction Time in Fencers. *J. Educ. Learn.* **2020**, *9*, 127–135. [CrossRef]
37. Sellés-Pérez, S.; Arévalo-Chico, H.; Fernández-Sáez, J.; Cejuela, R. Training Characteristics, Performance, and Body Composition of Three U23 Elite Female Triathletes throughout a Season. *Sports* **2024**, *12*, 53. [CrossRef] [PubMed]
38. McMorris, T.; Turner, A.; Hale, B.J.; Sproule, J. Beyond the catecholamines hypothesis for an acute exercise-cognition interaction: A neurochemical perspective. In *Exercise-Cognition Interaction: Neuroscience Perspectives*; McMorris, T., Ed.; Academic Press: New York, NY, USA, 2016; pp. 65–104. [CrossRef]
39. McMorris, T. Exercise and Cognitive Functions: A Neuroendocrinological Explanation. In *Exercise and Cognitive Function*; McMorris, T., Tomporowski, P.D., Audiffren, M., Eds.; John Wiley & Sons: Hoboken, NJ, USA, 2009; pp. 41–68.
40. Zemková, E.; Miklovič, P.; Hamar, D. There is a relationship between intensity of exercise and reaction time on laterally concordant and discordant stimuli. *Acta Kinesiol.* **2009**, *3*, 59–63.
41. Zemková, E. Effects of acute and chronic exercise on agility skills. *Vidyabh. Int. Interdiscip. Res. J.* **2021**, *12*, 500–504.
42. Levitt, S.; Gutin, B. Multiple Choice Reaction Time and Movement Time During Physical Exertion. *Res. Q. Am. Assoc. Health Phys. Educ. Recreat.* **1971**, *42*, 405–410. [CrossRef]
43. Mekari, S.; Fraser, S.; Bosquet, L.; Bonnéry, C.; Labelle, V.; Pouliot, P.; Lesage, F.; Bherer, L. The relationship between exercise intensity, cerebral oxygenation, and cognitive performance in young adults. *Eur. J. Appl. Physiol.* **2015**, *115*, 2189–2197. [CrossRef]
44. Horváth, D.; Négyesi, J.; Győri, T.; Szűcs, B.; Tóth, P.J.; Matics, Z.; Ökrös, C.; Sáfár, S.; Szabó, N.; Takács, B.; et al. Application of a reactive agility training program using light-based stimuli to enhance the physical and cognitive performance of car racing drivers: A randomized controlled trial. *Sports Med. Open* **2022**, *8*, 113. [CrossRef]
45. Davey, C. Physical exertion and mental performance. *Ergonomics* **1973**, *16*, 595–599. [CrossRef]
46. Pesce, C.; Cereatti, L.; Forte, R.; Crova, C.; Casella, R. Acute and chronic exercise effects on attentional control in older road cyclists. *Gerontology* **2011**, *57*, 121–128. [CrossRef] [PubMed]
47. Boobani, B.; Grants, J.; Glaskova-Kuzmina, T.; Zidens, J.; Litwiniuk, A. Effect of green exercise on stress level, mental toughness, and performance of taekwondo athletes. *Arch. Budo J. Innov. Agonol.* **2024**, *20*, 29–40.
48. Boobani, B.; Grants, J.; Litwiniuk, A.; Boge, I.; Glaskova-Kuzmina, T. Effect of Walking in Nature on Stress Levels and Performance of Taekwondo Athletes in the Competition Period. *J. Kinesiol. Exerc. Sci.* **2024**, *34*, 17–27. [CrossRef]
49. Boobani, B.; Kalnina, Z.; Glaskova-Kuzmina, T.; Erina, L.; Liepina, I. Utilizing Facial Emotion Analysis with FaceReader to Evaluate the Effects of Outdoor Activities on Preschoolers' Basic Emotions: A Pilot Study in e-Health. *Int. J. Online Biomed. Eng.* **2025**, *21*, 61–75. [CrossRef]
50. Van de Vegte, Y.J.; Tegegne, B.S.; Verweij, N.; Snieder, H.; van der Harst, P. Genetics and the heart rate response to exercise. *Cell Mol. Life Sci.* **2019**, *76*, 2391–2409. [CrossRef] [PubMed]
51. Yamamoto, K.; Miyachi, M.; Saitoh, T.; Yoshioka, A.; Onodera, S. Effects of endurance training on resting and post-exercise cardiac autonomic control. *Med. Sci. Sports Exerc.* **2001**, *33*, 1496–1502. [CrossRef] [PubMed]
52. Navia, J.A.; Avilés, C.; López, S.; Ruiz, L.M. A current approach to anticipation in sport. *Stud. Psicol.* **2018**, *38*, 1–19. [CrossRef]
53. Hagemann, N.; Schorer, J.; Canal-Bruland, R.; Lotz, S.; Strauss, B. Visual perception in fencing: Do the eye movements of fencers represent their information pickup? *Atten. Percept. Psychophys.* **2010**, *72*, 2204–2214. [CrossRef]
54. Badau, D.; Baydil, B.; Badau, A. Differences among Three Measures of Reaction Time Based on Hand Laterality in Individual Sports. *Sports* **2018**, *6*, 45. [CrossRef]
55. Varesco, G.; Sarcher, A.; Doron, J.; Jubeau, M. Striking a balance: Exploring attention, attack accuracy and speed in fencing performance. *Eur. J. Sport Sci.* **2024**, *24*, 1278–1286. [CrossRef] [PubMed]
56. Posner, M.I.; Dehaene, S. Attentional Networks. *Trends Neurosci.* **1994**, *17*, 75–79. [CrossRef] [PubMed]
57. Sirotic, A.C.; Coutts, A.J. The reliability of physiological and performance measures during simulated team-sport running on a non-motorised treadmill. *J. Sci. Med. Sport* **2008**, *11*, 500–509. [CrossRef] [PubMed]
58. Voss, M.W.; Kramer, A.F.; Basak, C.; Prakash, R.S.; Roberts, B. Are Expert Athletes 'Expert' in the Cognitive Laboratory? A Meta-Analytic Review of Cognition and Sport Expertise. *Appl. Cogn. Psychol.* **2010**, *24*, 812–826. [CrossRef]

sports

MDPI

Article

Applied Research on the Impact of a Neuromotor Development Program on the Lower Limb Strength of Junior Athletes in Greco-Roman Wrestling

Florentin Vasilescu [1], Nicoleta Leonte [2,*], Cristiana Maria Porfireanu [3] and Virgil Tudor [4]

[1] Sportive Club No. 5, 010241 Bucharest, Romania; iuliu81@yahoo.co.uk
[2] Department of Physical Education and Sport—Physical Therapy, National University of Science and Technology Politehnica Bucharest, 060042 Bucharest, Romania
[3] Department of Physical Education and Sport, Academy of Economic Studies Bucharest, 010374 Bucharest, Romania; criss.porfi@gmail.com
[4] Faculty of Physical Education and Sport, National University of Physical Education and Sport, 060057 Bucharest, Romania; virgiltudor@yahoo.com
* Correspondence: nicoleta.leonte@upb.ro

Abstract: This study investigates the effects of a structured motor intervention program on the development of lower limb strength in junior athletes practicing Greco-Roman wrestling. Recognizing the crucial role of explosive strength in performing technical and decisive actions during combat, the research introduces a progressive, applied training protocol tailored to the neuromotor development of children aged 10 to 12 years (control group: M = 11.14, SD = 1.10; experimental group: M = 11.07, SD = 0.83). Conducted over 17 months, the study involved two groups of 14 registered wrestlers each from School Sports Club No. 5 in Bucharest. The experimental group participated in a complementary motor training program emphasizing plyometric drills, bodyweight strength exercises, and wrestling-specific movements, while the control group continued with the standard training routine. The intervention's impact was evaluated using the OptoJump Next system, a biomechanical analysis tool measuring key indicators of explosive strength—jump height, ground contact time, flight time, and reactive strength index (RSI)—through the single-leg counter-movement jump (CMJ) test. Comparative analysis of pre- and post-intervention results showed significant improvements in neuromotor performance among athletes in the experimental group, confirming the effectiveness of the proposed methodology. This research thus provides a reproducible, evidence-based intervention model with direct applicability in optimizing the training of young Greco-Roman wrestlers.

Keywords: explosive strength; juniors; Greco-Roman wrestling; intervention program; OptoJump

1. Introduction

In Olympic wrestling—particularly in the Greco-Roman style—motor qualities such as explosive strength, reaction speed, and postural stability are fundamental to both technical and tactical performance. These attributes rely heavily on lower-body efficiency, which underpins balance, attack initiation, counteractions, and rapid phase transitions during combat [1,2].

The period of middle childhood and preadolescence (ages 10–12) represents an optimal window for neuromotor development interventions due to the heightened plasticity of the central nervous system and the increased adaptability of the musculoskeletal system to training stimuli [3,4]. At this stage, the foundation for reactive and explosive strength can be effectively developed through functional, age-appropriate methods that avoid excessive loading.

Recent studies have shown that well-structured and supervised plyometric training programs can significantly enhance young athletes' neuromotor performance, directly influencing sport-specific abilities [5,6]. In Greco-Roman wrestling, lower-limb explosive strength is essential for executing rapid lifts, disengagements, blocks, and pivots from unstable positions. Therefore, developing this capacity during formative years has a lasting impact on athletic performance and helps prevent neuromuscular imbalances or injuries [7].

The assessment of these motor qualities has evolved from subjective evaluation toward the use of advanced technologies that provide precise, reproducible data. Among the most widely used tools in performance laboratories is the OptoJump Next system, which enables objective analysis of reaction speed, coordination, motor control, and neuromuscular balance. Based on optical sensors, the system allows biomechanical assessment of vertical jumps and other reactive movements. Measured parameters such as jump height, flight time, ground contact time, and the reactive strength index (RSI) serve as key indicators for evaluating lower-limb explosive power [2,8].

Contemporary literature further emphasizes the importance of tailoring motor interventions for junior athletes according to their individual profiles, developmental levels, and wrestling style. Experimental studies support the integration of plyometrics, bodyweight strength exercises, and sport-specific drills within a safe, progressive, and well-structured framework [1,9].

In wrestling, technical efficiency depends on the integration of multiple physical qualities. Explosive strength enables rapid attack initiation (projections, throws, leg entries), facilitates breaking grips and counterattacks, supports sudden changes in direction, and provides the energy "burst" needed at decisive moments. Lower-limb strength, as a combination of force and speed, generates the main impulse for lifts, projections, and pushes; ensures stability in defensive and ground positions; and maintains pressure in clinches or edge-of-mat situations. Balance allows athletes to resist pushes and pulls without losing position, recover quickly after directional changes, and maintain control during throws. Coordination ensures smooth transitions between techniques (e.g., attack to counterattack), accuracy in pivots and releases, and efficient movement that minimizes unnecessary energy expenditure.

This study aligns with current scientific approaches by proposing an applied neuromotor development program aimed at enhancing lower-limb explosive strength in junior Greco-Roman wrestlers [10,11]. The 17-month intervention was objectively evaluated through repeated OptoJump testing, providing a solid quantitative basis for assessing the effectiveness of the applied methodology.

The research seeks to strengthen the scientific foundation of training for junior athletes by offering coaches a validated, reproducible model with practical applicability. It also presents an integrated perspective on how explosive strength can be safely and effectively developed and monitored without compromising the health or natural growth of young wrestlers.

The study is guided by two central research questions:

What is the effect of a specific intervention program on the development of lower-limb explosive strength in junior Greco-Roman wrestlers, as measured by the OptoJump system?

Which training methods (exercises and techniques) are most effective for optimizing lower-limb explosive strength in young wrestlers, considering their age and the demands of the Greco-Roman style?

To address these questions, the study is based on the hypothesis that implementing a structured neuromotor development program—centered on plyometric exercises, functional strength training, and wrestling-specific applications—will produce significant improvements in the lower-limb explosive strength of junior athletes compared to those following a standard training regimen. The effectiveness of this program is expected to be demonstrated through objective data obtained from the OptoJump testing system, revealing statistically significant gains in the experimental group relative to the control group.

2. Materials and Methods

2.1. Participants

Research Conditions

The participants included in this experimental research were organized into two distinct groups of junior athletes: an experimental group (EG) and a control group (CG), each composed of 14 subjects (n = 14). These athletes, aged between 10 and 12 years, were registered and actively training in the Greco-Roman wrestling section of School Sports Club No. 5 in Bucharest (Table 1).

Table 1. Subjects of the Research Groups (Control and Experimental)—Anthropometric Parameters in the Initial Phase of the Study.

Variables	Mean		Standard Deviation	
	CG *	EG *	CG *	EG *
Age (ani)	11.14	11.07	1.10	0.83
Body mass (kg)	53.79	54.64	13.71	18.85
Height (cm)	154.57	156.86	13.19	13.92
BMI	22.4	20.8	3.58	5.1
Variable	**t-statistic**	**df**	***p*-value**	
Age	0.19	24.18	0.851	
Body mass	−0.14	23.75	0.893	
Height	−0.45	25.92	0.659	
BMI	0.96	23.31	0.347	

CG *—Cotrol group. EG *—Experimetal group. All p-values > 0.05, meaning no statistically significant differences exist between the control and experimental groups at baseline for age, body mass, height, or BMI. The groups can be considered comparable before the intervention.

The choice of this size took into account:

A. Available population and selection criteria

The study took place within the School Sports Club no. 5 Bucharest, the Greco-Roman wrestling section, where the number of athletes aged 10–12 years and comparable level of training was limited. The inclusion of 28 subjects allowed coverage of the entire eligible population, while maintaining the practical relevance of the research.

B. Randomisation to remove bias

After identifying the eligible athletes, they were randomly assigned (randomised) to the two groups using a draw procedure.

Randomization was designed to reduce the influence of subjective factors (e.g., coach preferences, past performance) and increase the internal validity of the study.

In this way, the initial differences between the groups have been minimised and any observed effects can be attributed with greater confidence to the experimental programme.

To be eligible, athletes had to meet all of the following conditions:

- Age between 10 and 12 years at the start of the study.

- Active membership in the Greco-Roman wrestling section of School Sports Club No. 5 Bucharest, with regular attendance at training sessions.
- Minimum training experience (e.g., at least 6 months–1 year) to ensure a basic level of technical and motor skills.
- Good health status, confirmed by a sports medical certificate, with no conditions that would prevent participation in high-intensity physical effort.
- Informed consent from parents/legal guardians for participation in the study.

Exclusion Criteria Athletes were excluded if they met any of the following conditions:

- Acute or chronic musculoskeletal injuries, or other medical conditions limiting physical activity (e.g., cardiac, respiratory problems).
- Frequent absences from training sessions, which could affect the implementation of the experimental program.
- Concurrent participation in other special training programs or competitions that might influence the studied variables.
- Lack of informed consent from parents/legal guardians.
- Failure to meet age criteria or club membership requirements.

The two groups were carefully balanced in terms of initial morphological, functional, and motor characteristics to ensure optimal homogeneity. This homogeneity was essential for objectively conducting the experimental intervention and created favorable conditions for comparing the effects of the specific intervention program applied to the experimental group with those of the standard training program followed by the control group. Additionally, age, height, weight, and body mass index (BMI) indicators of the children in both research groups were analyzed. All subjects were declared medically fit for specific physical effort, according to their sports medical records. Their participation in the study was conducted in strict compliance with current ethical standards regarding research involving minors. The experimental protocol was approved by the Ethics Committee of School Sports Club No. 5 Bucharest (499/11 June 2025), and informed consent was obtained in writing from the athletes' parents or legal guardians before the commencement of any research procedures.

2.2. Study Design

The research was carried out at School Sports Club No. 5 in Bucharest, within a controlled environment specifically adapted to the training requirements of junior Greco-Roman wrestlers. The experimental procedures were conducted under real training conditions, while maintaining the methodological rigor characteristic of a systematically planned intervention study.

The independent variable—the specific intervention program—was applied to the experimental group over a period of approximately 17 months, from March 2023 to September 2024 (see Table 2). During this time, athletes in the experimental group participated in a structured training program designed to complement the classical training method, with a particular focus on developing lower-limb explosive strength. In contrast, the control group continued to follow the club's standard training regimen, without any additional exercises or interventions related to the research objectives.

Throughout the study, all working conditions were carefully controlled. The sports infrastructure (wrestling mats, strength training equipment), training schedule, and coaching staff remained constant for both groups to minimize the potential influence of external variables. Both the initial and final assessments were conducted under identical conditions—within the same training facility and using the same technological equipment (OptoJump Next system)—to ensure the validity, reliability, and comparability of the collected data.

Table 2. Research Stages.

Period	Activity
March 2023	Initial Testing
April 2023–August 2024	Implementation of the Intervention Program
September 2024	Final Testing

2.3. Research Content

The present research followed an applied experimental design aimed at evaluating the influence of a specific neuromotor development program on lower-limb strength in two groups of junior athletes practicing Greco-Roman wrestling. The intervention program was structured to enhance explosive strength and motor control through the integration of plyometric exercises and wrestling-specific techniques.

The research process was organized into four main stages:

1. Documentation and Research Design Stage

During this initial stage, recent specialized literature was analyzed to establish the theoretical foundation of the study. The research hypothesis and objectives were formulated, the intervention methods were defined, and the biomechanical indicators relevant for evaluating lower-limb strength were selected.

2. Initial Evaluation Stage (Pretesting)

The pretesting phase took place at the beginning of the experimental period (March 2023) at the training facility of School Sports Club No. 5 in Bucharest. All participating athletes were evaluated using the OptoJump Next system, performing the countermovement jump (CMJ) to establish baseline measurements for jump height, ground contact time, and reactive strength index (RSI).

Previous studies have reported a coefficient of variation (CV%) from 1 to 5% and an intra-class correlation coefficient (ICC) greater than 0.90 for test–retest assessments using this system, confirming its high accuracy and reliability in evaluating neuromotor performance.

3. Applied Intervention Stage

The intervention phase was conducted over approximately 17 months (March 2023–September 2024) and involved the implementation of a progressive neuromotor development program applied exclusively to the experimental group.

The decision to extend the program to 17 months was based on two primary considerations:

Gradual and safe adaptation: Adequate time was needed for the athletes to progressively develop fundamental motor capacities—strength, speed, endurance, and mobility—while minimizing overload and injury risk.

Structured periodization: The 17-month duration allowed for division into macrocycles (annual) and mesocycles (monthly or bimonthly), ensuring a logical progression through the main phases of preparation: general, specific, competitive, and transition training.

The program incorporated plyometric exercises, wrestling-specific movements aimed at lower-limb strength development, and functional activities aligned with the technical demands of the Greco-Roman style. The control group, in parallel, continued their standard club training program without additional interventions related to the research objectives.

All training sessions were conducted at the facilities and laboratories of School Sports Club No. 5 in Bucharest under continuous supervision and methodological control.

4. Final Evaluation Stage (Post-testing)

The post-testing phase was carried out at the end of the intervention period (September 2024) under identical conditions to the pretest. The same equipment, testing protocols, and evaluation procedures were applied to ensure consistency and data comparability.

The collected results were statistically analyzed to determine the effectiveness of the intervention and to identify performance differences between the experimental and control groups.

Through this structured approach, the research seeks to provide scientific validation for a specific intervention program aimed at developing lower-limb strength in junior Greco-Roman wrestlers. By utilizing objective, technology-assisted evaluation methods, the study contributes to strengthening the methodological foundation of physical training for this age category and offers practical insights for optimizing athletic development in Greco-Roman wrestling.

2.3.1. Training Methods Used in the Research

Experimental Group—Intervention Focused on Lower Limb Strength Development and Standing Wrestling Techniques

The program designed for the experimental group targeted specific neuromotor development, directly enhancing lower limb explosiveness, reactivity, and stability through a functional integration of strength components into wrestling techniques performed in a standing position. Accordingly, the program included advanced plyometric exercises, functional partner training, tactical and technical applications, and specialized thematic sequences for Greco-Roman wrestling.

Specific Plyometric Exercises were aimed at increasing reactive capacity and explosive strength, including:

- Jumps on a mat from a guard position
- Drop jumps with immediate takeoff and repositioning for engagement
- Lateral jumps over a partner, followed by rapid penetration into attack position
- Squat jumps combined with partner lifting exercises

Functional Strength Training Included

- Squats with a partner on the back, for posterior chain development and stability
- Pulls and pushes from a clinch position
- Repeated mannequin lifts using a belt grip
- Circuit exercises incorporating "sumo walks," lunges with grip, and balance drills simulating wrestling movements

Technical-Tactical Elements Specific to Greco-Roman Wrestling

- Takedowns via belt grip, lifting, and swinging, emphasizing force impulse synchronization
- Rotations from torso grasp, placing opponents in disadvantageous positions
- Low-guard penetrations, adjusting center of gravity and efficient lower limb positioning
- Thematic applications where athletes executed techniques immediately after securing a grip

Reactive and Stability Components Were Developed Through

- Tandem exercises (pushes, resistance, holding)
- Repetitions of low-guard throws using mannequins
- Medicine ball drills (e.g., vertical and lateral throws from strength positions)
- Video feedback and biomechanical corrections regarding lower limb positioning and technique execution

This set of methods aimed to optimize physical qualities and wrestling-specific motor skills simultaneously, ensuring a real transfer between neuromotor development and competitive performance in Greco-Roman wrestling (see Table 3).

Table 3. The weekly training program.

Day/Focus	Warm-Up (10–15 Min)	Plyometrics	Functional Strength	Technical–Tactical	Reactive & Stability	Session Duration
Day 1—Explosiveness	Dynamic mobility, wrestling drills	• Jumps from guard 3 × 10 • Drop jumps 3 × 8 • Lateral jumps + penetration 3 × 6/side • Squat jumps + partner lift 3 × 8	Squats w/partner 3 × 10 Mannequin lifts 3 × 6	Belt-grip takedowns 4 × 5 Torso rotations 3 × 6	-	~75–80 min
Day 2—Strength & Stability	Dynamic warm-up, balance drills	• Jumps from guard 2 × 10	Squats w/partner 3 × 10 Clinch pulls/pushes 3 × 20 s Circuit: sumo walks, lunges w/grip, balance (3 rounds, 30 s each, 30 s rest)	Low-guard penetrations 3 × 8	Tandem pushes/pulls 3 × 20 s Low-guard mannequin throws 3 × 6 Med ball throws (vertical 3 × 8, lateral 3 × 8/side)	~80–90 min
Day 3—Integration & Simulation	Wrestling-specific mobility, dynamic partner drills	• Drop jumps 3 × 8 • Lateral jumps + penetration 3 × 6/side	Circuit: sumo walks, lunges, balance (3 rounds, 30 s/30 s)	Thematic sequences: grip → immediate technique 4 × 30 s Belt-grip takedowns 3 × 5	Tandem drills 3 × 20 s Med ball throws 3 × 8 each	~80–90 min

Control Group—Standard Training Program for the Greco-Roman Style

The control group was trained using a traditional program commonly applied in beginner or intermediate-level athlete preparation, without biomechanical analysis or technology-assisted interventions. The training focused on learning and reinforcing fundamental techniques of the Greco-Roman style using conventional general and specific training methods.

General Physical Component Included

- Linear runs and obstacle runs, push-ups, sit-ups, pull-ups
- Basic squats, stationary or dynamic jumps, mobility drills

Technical Exercises Focused On:

- Learning and repeating takedown techniques such as basic belt grip and balanced throws
- Controlled projections with a partner, without explosive or reactive elements
- Mannequin drills to reinforce fundamental techniques in takedowns and lifts

Tactical Applications Were Conducted Through

- Thematic training fights (engagements without ground transition, responses to slow attacks)
- Attack/counterattack simulations from fixed guard positions or in restricted spaces
- Paired drills in repeated series, without progressive difficulty increments

Motor Skill Games Targeted:

- Balance maintenance, controlled opposition, gripping and postural stability exercises
- Wrestling-themed games adapted to the athletes' age

This program ensured a standard training framework without additional optimization elements, making it ideal for comparing the effectiveness of the intervention applied to the experimental group.

2.3.2. Research Variables

In the experimental research conducted at School Sports Club No. 5 in Bucharest, two groups of young junior athletes followed differentiated training programs designed to examine the impact of neuromotor development on lower-limb strength parameters. The methodological design involved the application of an independent variable to the experimental group, while the control group continued with the standard training program, in order to highlight potential functional and motor adaptations.

The independent variable was represented by the neuromotor intervention program applied to the experimental group. This program integrated plyometric exercises, functional strength development methods, and standing wrestling techniques specific to the Greco-Roman style. It was designed to stimulate the development of explosive strength and lower-limb reactive capacity, and was carefully adapted to the athletes' age and training level.

The dependent variable consisted of the level of lower-limb strength development, objectively measured using the OptoJump Next system through countermovement jump (CMJ) testing. The analyzed indicators included jump height, flight time, ground contact time, and the Reactive Strength Index (RSI), which reflects neuromuscular efficiency and the ability to generate force rapidly.

By analyzing these variables, the research aims to provide an objective foundation for evaluating the effectiveness of a targeted strength development program within a specific wrestling context. Ultimately, the study seeks to contribute to the scientific substantiation of methodological decisions in the training of young performance athletes.

2.3.3. Statistical Analysis

The data were analyzed using the Statistical Package for the Social Sciences (SPSS, version 29.0.2.0; IBM, Armonk, NY, USA). The data collected from various measurements and tests were subjected to statistical processing using the following procedures and indicators.

For group comparisons, Analysis of Variance (ANOVA) and dependent-samples *t*-tests were applied where appropriate. For ANOVA, F-values, *p*-values, and effect sizes (η^2) were reported, while for dependent-samples *t*-tests, t-values and *p*-values were presented. In addition, Pearson correlation coefficients (r) were calculated to examine relationships between key variables.

The normality of data distributions was verified using the Shapiro–Wilk test, and the homogeneity of variances was assessed. All assumptions required for the applied statistical tests were satisfied.

The sample size was determined a priori using power analysis (G*Power, version 3.1.9.8). Assuming a medium effect size (f = 0.25), an alpha level of 0.05, and a statistical power of 0.80, the required sample size was calculated as N = 28 participants. Accordingly, the study included 28 junior athletes (14 in the experimental group and 14 in the control group), meeting the minimum sample size requirement [12,13].

3. Results

During testing with the OptoJump analysis system, vertical jumps (5JS2D) were performed, with five repetitions for each leg (right and left). These measurements provided conclusive data for our research (Figure 1).

Five vertical jumps were performed for each lower limb, with the OptoJump computerized program objectively measuring the following indicators:

- T Cont—ground contact time with the force plate, measured in fractions of a second
- T Flight—flight time (time spent in the air), measured in fractions of a second
- Height—jump height (calculated in cm)

- RSI—Reactive Strength Index—"The reactive strength index (RSI) is an effective marker of reactive force due to the rapid shortening caused by prior activation in the DJ—Drop Jump, also known as the stretch-shortening cycle" [10].
- Pace—jump cadence
- Power—strength (watts/kg)

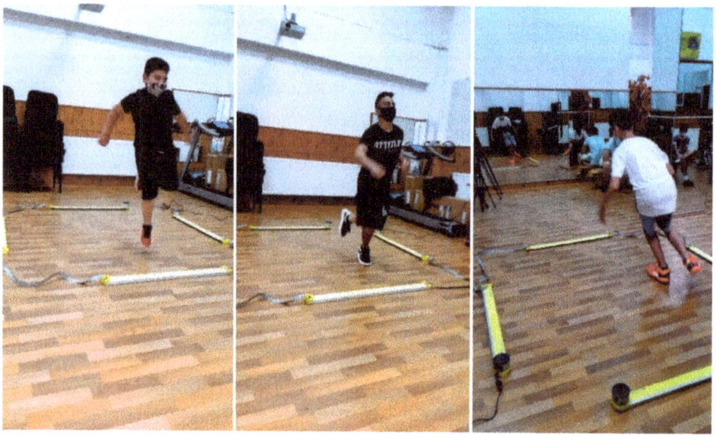

Figure 1. Images of OptoJump Next Testing.

We considered vertical jump performance to be the most relevant indicator for Greco-Roman wrestling, given the specificity of techniques in this discipline. For this reason, we conducted all comparative analyses between the subjects of the two research groups based on this parameter.

3.1. Descriptive Statistics

Control Group vs. Experimental Group

The program produced major improvements in height and power variables (the core performance parameters), with a large effect size and a clear Group × Time interaction; the Experimental group progressed significantly more than the Control group.

For Tcont, TFlight, and RSI variables, moderate effects were observed (the Experimental group shows a better tendency, but not as strong).

Pace variable remained stable → it was not affected by the intervention (see Table 4).

Table 4. Statistical indicators—Control Group and the Experimental Group in the Initial and Final Testing.

Variable	Group	IT *** (Mean ± SD)	FT *** (Mean ± SD)	ANOVA (Time, Group)	η^2	Interpretation
TCont.	CG *	0.53 ± 0.19	0.63 ± 0.36	F(1,26) = 4.8, p = 0.038 (T) ns (G)	0.16	GC increases, EG decreases at FT
	EG *	0.49 ± 0.20	0.42 ± 0.15			
TFlight	CG	0.16 ± 0.07	0.22 ± 0.10	F(1,26) = 6.4, p = 0.018 (T) ns (G)	0.12	Both groups increase, more in EG
	EG	0.14 ± 0.05	0.28 ± 0.09			
Height	CG	4.2 ± 2.5	11.7 ± 8.0	F(1,26) = 45.2, p < 0.001 (T) F(1,26) = 5.8, p = 0.024 (G)	0.36	Large effect, clear progress in EG
	EG	2.8 ± 1.5	12.6 ± 5.4			
Power	CG	6.1 ± 5.3	14.2 ± 12.0	F(1,26) = 39.1, p < 0.001 (T) F(1,26) = 6.2, p = 0.020 (G)	0.34	Strong increase, EG improves more

Table 4. *Cont.*

Variable	Group	IT *** (Mean ± SD)	FT *** (Mean ± SD)	ANOVA (Time, Group)	η^2	Interpretation
	EG	4.9 ± 2.1	13.9 ± 5.0			
Pace	CG	1.65 ± 0.30	1.60 ± 0.30	ns ** (T, G)	<0.05	Stable variable, no changes
	EG	1.74 ± 0.28	1.55 ± 0.19			
RSI	CG	0.12 ± 0.08	0.31 ± 0.28	F(1,26) = 5.9, p = 0.022 (T) ns (G)	0.14	Small increase, more accentuated in EG
	EG	0.07 ± 0.03	0.34 ± 0.17			

CG, EG *—control group, experimental group. ns **—not significant. FT, IT ***—Final test, Initial Test.

Inferential Statistics

T-Test—Control Group versus Experimental Group (Final Testing)

In order to find out whether there is a statistically significant difference between the initial and the final *t*-test, we apply the Paired Two Sample for Means (*t*-Test).

- Ground Contact Time (GCT):

The t-statistic obtained for this test was t(26) = 2.71, exceeding the two-tailed critical t-value (1.67) at a 95% confidence level. The result was statistically significant (p = 0.01 < 0.05). The mean value of GCT in the control group (0.55 s) was higher than that of the experimental group (0.37 s), indicating that the experimental training program effectively reduced ground contact duration. The differences between individual results and group means were statistically significant, confirming the robustness of this finding.

- Flight Time (FT):

For Flight Time, the test produced t(26) = 3.69, also exceeding the critical t-value (1.67) with a high level of significance (p < 0.001, 95% confidence). The mean value in the control group (0.21 s) was lower than that in the experimental group (0.29 s). This statistically significant difference supports the research hypothesis, indicating improved explosive performance among athletes in the experimental group.

- Group Consistency:

The control group displayed a higher standard deviation (SD = 0.12), reflecting greater variability in performance, whereas the experimental group showed a lower SD (0.01) and a very small coefficient of variation (CV = 0.01), demonstrating high internal consistency and stability of results.

Overall, the inferential statistical tests confirm that $t_{stat} > t_{(Crit)}$ and $p < 0.05$ for the analyzed parameters, allowing the results to be generalized to the broader population of junior Greco-Roman wrestlers. In other words, if the tests were repeated under similar conditions, comparable outcomes would be expected (see Table 5).

Table 5. Statistical indicators –Ground Contact Time and Flight Time (CG vs. EG).

Indicators		Mean	SD	CV	t Stat	P (T ≤ t) One-Tail	t Critical One-Tail	P (T ≤ t) Two-Tail	t Critical Two-Tail
Ground Contact Time	CG *	0.55	0.34	0.12	2.71	0.00	1.67	0.01	2.01
	EG **	0.37	0.09	0.01					
Flight Time	CG	0.21	0.09	0.01	−3.69	0.00	1.67	0.00	2.01
	EG	0.29	0.07	0.01					

CG *—control group; EG **—experimental group.

Based on the values of standard deviation (SD = 8.30; 11.56) and coefficient of variation (CV = 68.95; 133.7), the results of the control group showed substantial dispersion, indicating considerable variability in individual performances for both jump height and power. In contrast, the experimental group demonstrated higher and more consistent performance levels, reflecting improved homogeneity and training adaptation.

- Jump Height:

The test yielded t(26) = 2.10, which exceeds the two-tailed critical t-value (1.67) at the 95% confidence level. The result was statistically significant ($p = 0.01 < 0.05$). The mean jump height of the control group (7.61 cm) was lower than that of the experimental group (11.60 cm). This significant difference confirms the research hypothesis, indicating that the neuromotor intervention program effectively enhanced vertical jump performance.

- Power per kg of Body Weight:

For this indicator, the test produced t(26) = 1.21, which is below the two-tailed critical t-value (1.67). The result was not statistically significant ($p = 0.15 > 0.05$) at the 95% confidence level. Although the experimental group showed a higher mean power output (13.50 W/kg) compared to the control group (10.52 W/kg), the difference cannot be generalized to the entire population since $t_{stat} < t_{(Crit)}$ and $p > 0.05$.

Nevertheless, even statistically non-significant differences in explosive power can have practical importance in Greco-Roman wrestling, where subtle variations in force application often influence the outcome of competitive matches. These findings are summarized in Table 6.

Table 6. Statistical indicators—Height and Power (CG vs. EG).

Indicators		Mean	SD	CV	t Stat	P (T ≤ t) One-Tail	t Critical One-Tail	P (T ≤ t) Two-Tail	t Critical Two-Tail
Height	CG	7.61	8.30	68.95	−2.10	0.02	1.67	0.04	2.01
	EG	11.60	1.50	2.24					
Power	CG	10.52	11.56	133.70	−1.21	0.11	1.67	0.23	2.01
	EG	13.50	1.76	3.09					

- Jump Frequency (Cadence):

The test produced t(26) = 0.10, which is below the two-tailed critical t-value (1.67) at the 95% confidence level. The result was not statistically significant ($p = 0.15 > 0.05$). The mean jump frequency for the control group (1.56 jumps/s) was nearly identical to that of the experimental group (1.57 jumps/s), indicating no meaningful difference between the groups.

- Reactive Strength Index (RSI):

For the RSI, the test yielded t(26) = 0.56, which is also below the two-tailed critical t-value (1.68), with $p = 0.15 > 0.05$. The mean RSI in the control group (0.27) was slightly lower than that in the experimental group (0.32); however, this difference was not statistically significant.

Since $t_{stat} < t_{(Crit)}$ and $p > 0.05$ for both indicators, the inferential statistical tests do not allow these results to be generalized to the broader population. In other words, if the tests were repeated under similar conditions, comparable results might not be consistently observed.

- Two-Sample *t*-Test Summary:

When comparing the control and experimental groups, the two-sample *t*-test assuming equal variances revealed statistically significant differences for Ground Contact Time, Flight Time, and Jump Height. In contrast, no significant differences were found for Power, Jump Frequency (Cadence), or the Reactive Strength Index.

These findings indicate that the neuromotor intervention program applied to the experimental group had a stronger and statistically validated effect on explosive movement parameters (contact time, flight time, and jump height). Although notable numerical differences were observed for power, cadence, and RSI, they did not reach statistical significance. This suggests that while the training program improved several key aspects of explosive performance, further research is warranted to optimize its effects on power output and reactive strength (Table 7).

Table 7. Statistical indicators –Cadence and Reactive Strength Index—RSI (CG vs. EG).

Indicators		Mean	SD	CV	t Stat	P (T ≤ t) One-Tail	t Critical One-Tail	P (T ≤ t) Two-Tail	t Critical Two-Tail
Cadence	CG	1.56	0.37	0.14	−0.10	0.46	1.67	0.92	2.01
	EG	1.57	0.18	0.03					
Reactive Strength Index (RSI)	CG	0.27	0.50	0.24	−0.56	0.29	1.68	0.58	2.01
	EG	0.32	0.16	0.03					

3.2. Statistical Association

Correlation Coefficient—Control Group

A strong positive correlation was observed among the following indicators: Flight Time, Jump Height, Power per kg of body weight, and Reactive Strength Index (RSI) (Table 8). All these parameters represent distinct expressions of lower-limb force production.

Table 8. Correlation between Variables—Control Group.

Control	Test	T Cont.	T Flight	Height	Power	Pace	RSI
Test	1.00						
T Cont.	0.04	1.00					
T Flight	0.37	−0.03	1.00				
Height	0.33	−0.08	0.90	1.00			
Power	0.29	−0.16	0.81	0.92	1.00		
Pace	−0.08	−0.67	−0.42	−0.31	−0.20	1.00	
RSI	0.26	−0.19	0.72	0.88	0.99	−0.13	1.00

- Flight Time and Jump Height:

A very strong positive correlation was found between Flight Time and Jump Height (r = 0.90). In addition, Flight Time showed strong correlations with Power per kg of body weight (r = 0.81) and with the Reactive Strength Index (r = 0.72). Practically, this indicates that athletes who exhibit longer flight times also tend to achieve greater jump heights and higher levels of power output and reactive strength.

- Jump Height and Power/Reactive Strength Index:

Jump Height demonstrated a very strong positive correlation with both Power per kg of body weight (r = 0.92) and the Reactive Strength Index (r = 0.88). These findings suggest that athletes capable of achieving greater jump heights also display higher power output and greater reactive strength, emphasizing the interdependence of these performance indicators.

- Power per kg Body Weight and Reactive Strength Index:

An almost perfect positive correlation was identified between Power per kg of body weight and RSI (r = 0.99), indicating that increases in relative power are almost directly proportional to increases in reactive strength. This reinforces the notion that both variables capture closely related aspects of explosive neuromuscular performance.

- Jump Frequency and Ground Contact Time:

In contrast, a moderate negative correlation was found between Jump Frequency and Ground Contact Time (r = −0.67), suggesting that higher jump frequencies are associated with shorter ground contact times—a desirable feature in explosive athletic movements.

- Jump Frequency and Flight Time/Jump Height:

A small negative correlation was observed between Jump Frequency and both Flight Time (r = −0.42) and Jump Height (r = −0.42). This relationship is expected, as increases in Flight Time and Jump Height (indicating greater power generation) are typically accompanied by a reduction in jump cadence. Conversely, higher jump frequencies are associated with shorter flight times and lower jump heights, reflecting a trade-off between frequency and power expression (Table 8).

Correlation Coefficient—Experimental Group

In Table 9 a strong positive correlation is observed between:

- Flight Time and Height (r = 0.98), Flight Time and Power (r = 0.98), and Flight Time and Reactive Strength Index (r = 0.96): This indicates that high values of Flight Time are associated with high values of Height, Power, and the Reactive Strength Index.
- Height and Power (r = 0.98) and Height and Reactive Strength Index (r = 0.97): In other words, high jump heights are associated with high power output and high values of the reactive strength index (with a correlation of r = 0.99 reported in one instance).
- Power and Reactive Strength Index (r = 0.99): Very high power values are, therefore, almost perfectly associated with very high Reactive Strength Index values.

Table 9. Correlation between Variables—Experimental Group.

Experiment	Test	T Cont.	T Flight	Height	Power	Pace	RSI
Test	1.00						
T Cont.	−0.37	1.00					
T Flight	0.81	−0.32	1.00				
Height	0.78	−0.30	0.98	1.00			
Power	0.78	−0.37	0.98	0.98	1.00		
Pace	−0.35	−0.37	−0.63	−0.58	−0.57	1.00	
RSI	0.76	−0.40	0.96	0.97	0.99	−0.50	1.00

A moderate positive correlation is observed between:

- Jump Cadence and Reactive Strength Index (r = 0.50): This means that higher jump cadence values tend to be associated with moderate increases in the Reactive Strength Index.

On the other hand, there is a small negative correlation—without statistical significance—between:

- Ground Contact Time and Flight Time (r = −0.32)
- Ground Contact Time and Height (r = −0.30)
- Ground Contact Time and Power (r = −0.37)
- Ground Contact Time and Jump Cadence (r = −0.37)
- Ground Contact Time and Reactive Strength Index (r = −0.40)

These negative correlations indicate that longer Ground Contact Times are associated with lower values of Flight Time, Height, Power, Jump Cadence, and the Reactive Strength Index. In practical terms, when the expression of force (in the form of power) is lower, Ground Contact Time tends to be higher.

4. Discussion

This study contributes to the specialized literature on optimizing the physical and technical-tactical training of junior Greco-Roman wrestlers by introducing an intervention program focused on developing lower-body strength and executing techniques in a standing position. A distinctive feature of this research is the use of the OptoJump system for precise quantification of neuromotor performance, providing an objective evaluation framework [14–16].

According to recent studies, the performance of Greco-Roman wrestlers is closely linked to explosive strength and reaction ability, particularly in executing offensive maneuvers initiated from a standing position. These components are essential in an acyclic sport characterized by rapid alternation between maximum-intensity efforts and phases of control or energy conservation [17–20]. The findings of our research, which showed a significant increase in jump height and the Reactive Strength Index (RSI) in the experimental group, suggest that these characteristics may play a relevant role in athletic performance, although their direct contribution to competitive success requires further investigation.

The specific effort required in Greco-Roman wrestling places continuous demands on the neuromuscular system under conditions of constant contact with the opponent, where reaction speed and motor coordination are decisive factors [21,22]. Therefore, the selection of training methods such as plyometric jumps, dummy lifts, and clinch-position exercises facilitated a direct transfer between physical development and the application of sport-specific techniques.

Mocanu et al. (2023) [23] emphasize that junior competitive performance is determined not only by general physical preparation but also by its integration into tactical contexts similar to competition scenarios.

Furthermore, the homogeneity of performance within this group, observed in statistical analysis, aligns observations on the positive effects of sport-specific adapted programs in standardizing performance [24].

An additional explanation of the observed progress lies in the differentiated methodological approach. While the control group followed a conventional training regimen focused on general exercises and fundamental techniques, the experimental group benefited from functional stimuli tailored to competition demands. This methodological distinction also explains the more modest progress recorded by the control group, a finding supported by Nagovitsyn et al.'s (2019) [25] research on the necessity of adapting training programs to the neuromotor profile of young wrestlers.

Moreover, recent studies indicate that utilizing technological measurement systems such as OptoJump not only ensure objectivity but also enhance athletes' motivation and engagement in the learning process [26–29]. Although no direct questionnaire-based evaluation was conducted, this observation is indirectly supported by the behavior of the athletes in the experimental group, who consistently demonstrated active engagement and a more rapid adaptation to the technical and physical demands of training. This indirect evidence should, however, be interpreted with caution, as subjective measures of perception and motivation were not systematically collected.

Plyometric exercises combined with wrestling techniques, along with the inclusion of tactical sequences under opposition conditions, have facilitated a genuine transfer between the development of neuromotor qualities and their applicability in actual combat. The effectiveness of this training approach is supported by recent literature, which advocates for aligning physical preparation with the biomechanical and tactical demands of combat sports [30–33]. Additionally, integrated training methods that incorporate complex motor tasks within decision-making contexts have been shown to contribute to the development of advanced neuromotor control and the execution efficiency of techniques under competitive conditions [34–37].

In this context, it is essential to highlight that neuromotor development is not merely a consequence of increased exercise volume but, more importantly, of the quality of these stimuli and how they are integrated into the technical-tactical content specific to Greco-Roman wrestling [38–41].

Limits. While the findings provide valuable insights into the effectiveness of a structured motor intervention program for junior Greco-Roman wrestlers, several limitations should be acknowledged. First, the sample size was relatively small (n = 28), which may limit the generalizability of the results to larger or more diverse populations. Second, the participants were recruited from a single sports club, meaning that contextual factors such as coaching style, training culture, and facilities may have influenced the outcomes. Third, although the intervention spanned 17 months, longer-term follow-up was not conducted, so it remains unclear whether the observed improvements are maintained over time. Finally, the study focused primarily on explosive strength parameters (e.g., CMJ performance, RSI, flight and contact times), while other relevant dimensions of athletic performance, such as technical execution under fatigue or injury risk, were not assessed.

5. Conclusions

The study conducted on the impact of a structured neuromotor development program has highlighted significant advancements in lower-limb power among junior Greco-Roman wrestlers. Over a 17-month period, the experimental group, which engaged in a specialized training regimen that included plyometric exercises, body-weight strength applications, and wrestling-specific drills, showed marked improvements in key explosive power metrics. These results underscore the effectiveness of the proposed intervention model, providing coaches and trainers with a reproducible approach to optimize the training of young wrestlers. Future research should continue to explore the long-term benefits of such targeted training programs across various age groups and competitive levels in wrestling. The originality of this research lies in its integrative approach, which combines neuromotor development with sport-specific applications in Greco-Roman wrestling for young junior athletes. Furthermore, the research employs objective biomechanical monitoring tools, such as the OptoJump system and video feedback, to quantify performance changes and refine technical execution. By contrasting this with a control group following conventional methods, the study highlights the efficacy of the intervention and provides a practical, replicable methodological framework for coaches to support the athletic development of young wrestlers. This represents both the scientific innovation and applied expertise of the research.

Author Contributions: Conceptualization, F.V. and N.L.; methodology, F.V. and V.T.; software, C.M.P.; validation, N.L., F.V. and V.T.; formal analysis, C.M.P.; investigation, F.V.; resources, F.V.; data curation, N.L.; writing—original draft preparation, F.V.; writing—review and editing, N.L. and V.T.; visualization, C.M.P.; supervision, N.L.; project administration, F.V.; funding acquisition, All authors have read and agreed to the published version of the manuscript.

Funding: The APC was funded by PubArt.

Institutional Review Board Statement: The study was conducted in accordance with the Declaration of Helsinki, and approved by the Ethics Committee of School Sports Club no 5 (protocol code 499/11.06.2025) for studies involving humans.

Informed Consent Statement: Informed consent was obtained from all participants and the parents or legal guardians of minors involved in the study.

Data Availability Statement: Supporting raw data for the conclusions drawn in this article are available from the authors on demand.

Acknowledgments: Acknowledgements to the wrestling section of CSS5 Bucharest for participating in this research and to the parents for granting permission to include the results in this study.

Conflicts of Interest: Author Florentin Vasilescu collaborated with the Research and Innovation Center in Sport, Politehnica University of Bucharest. He participated in the design and implementation of the study, as well as in data collection and analysis. The role of the Center was to provide research infrastructure and institutional support. The remaining authors declare that the research was conducted in the absence of any commercial or financial relationships that could be construed as a potential conflict of interest.

Abbreviations

The following abbreviations are used in this manuscript:

CG	Control group
EG	Experimental group
** ns	not significant
*** FT, IT	Final test, Initial Test

References

1. Abbes, Z.; Chamari, K.; Mujika, I.; Tabben, M. Neuromuscular fitness and performance in young athletes: A scoping review. *Biol. Sport.* **2021**, *38*, 391–403.
2. Zemková, E.; Kováčiková, Z. Sport-specific training induced adaptations in postural control and their relationship with athletic performance. *Front. Hum. Neurosci.* **2023**, *16*, 1007804. [CrossRef]
3. Forte, R.; De Vito, G. Comparison of neuromotor and progressive resistance exercise training to improve mobility and fitness in community-dwelling older women. *J. Sci. Sport Exerc.* **2019**, *1*, 124–131. [CrossRef]
4. Pojskic, H.; Pagaduan, J.; Uzicanin, E.; Separovic, V.; Spasic, M.; Foretic, N.; Sekulic, D. Reliability, Validity and Usefulness of a New Response Time Test for Agility-Based Sports: A Simple vs. Complex Motor Task. J. Sports Sci. Med. **2019**, *18*, 623–635. [PubMed] [PubMed Central]
5. Ramirez-Campillo, R.; García-Hermoso, A.; Moran, J.; Chaabene, H.; Negra, Y.; Scanlan, A.T. The effects of plyometric jump training on physical fitness attributes in basketball players: A meta-analysis. *J. Sport Health Sci.* **2022**, *11*, 656–670. [CrossRef] [PubMed] [PubMed Central]
6. Sañudo, B.; de Hoyo, M.; Carrasco, L. The effectiveness of a neuromuscular training program on physical performance in youth athletes: A systematic review. *J. Strength. Cond. Res.* **2019**, *33*, 1367–1373. [CrossRef]
7. Pojskic, H.; Pagaduan, J.; Babajic, F.; Asceric, M. Effects of training on reaction time and agility in young male athletes. *J. Hum. Kinet.* **2022**, *82*, 179–188. [CrossRef]
8. Reigal, R.E.; Barrero, S.; Martín, I.; Morales-Sánchez, V.; Juárez-Ruiz de Mier, R.; Hernández-Mendo, A. Relationships between reaction time, selective attention, physical activity, and physical fitness in children. *Front. Psychol.* **2019**, *10*, 2278. [CrossRef]
9. Beck, D., Hossner, E.J.; Zahno, S. Mechanisms for handling uncertainty in sensorimotor control in sports: A scoping review. *Int. Rev. Sport Exerc. Psychol.* **2025**, *18*, 723–757. [CrossRef]
10. Ramirez-Campillo, R.; Sanchez-Sanchez, J.; Romero-Moraleda, B.; Yanci, J., García-Hermoso, A.; Manuel Clemente, F. Effects of plyometric jump training in female soccer players' vertical jump height: A systematic review with meta-analysis. *J. Sports Sci.* **2020**, *38*, 1475–1487. [CrossRef] [PubMed]
11. Rapotan, A.; Mihăilescu, L.; Mihai, I. The impact of OptoJump training on the power of lower limbs in female triple jumpers. *J. Phys. Educ. Sport* **2023**, *23*, 555–563. [CrossRef]
12. Montoro-Bombú, R.; de la Paz Arencibia, L.; Buzzichelli, C.; Miranda-Oliveira, P.; Fernandes, O.; Santos, A.; Rama, L. The validity of the Push Band 2.0 on the Reactive Strength Index assessment in Drop Jump. *Sensors* **2022**, *22*, 4724. [CrossRef]

13. Gravetter, F.J.; Wallnau, L.B. *Statistics for the Behavioral Sciences*, 10th ed.; Cengage Learning: Boston, MA, USA, 2017.
14. Grădinaru, L.; Mergheș, P.; Oravițan, M. The contribution of plyometric exercises assisted by sensory technology on vertical jump parameters in U15 female volleyball players. *Pedagog. Phys. Cult. Sports* **2024**, *28*, 156–167. [CrossRef]
15. Kittel, A.; Lindsay, R.; Le Noury, P.; Wilkins, L. The use of extended reality technologies in sport perceptual-cognitive skill research: A systematic scoping review. *Sports Med.-Open* **2024**, *10*, 128. [CrossRef] [PubMed]
16. Gierczuk, D.; Cieśliński, I.; Bujak, Z.; Sadowski, J. Relationship between selected strength and power variables and sports level in Greco-Roman wrestlers aged 14–18 years. *Int. J. Environ. Res. Public Health* **2021**, *18*, 4813. [CrossRef]
17. Zugaj, N.; Karnincic, H.; Baic, M. Differences in motor, functional, and sport-specific skills in gifted wrestlers with different acceleration of biological development. *Sport. Mont.* **2023**, *21*, 117–121. [CrossRef]
18. Tashnazarov, R.; Karimov, M.; Nasimov, M. The role of neuromuscular preparedness in tactical wrestling performance. *World J. Wrestl. Res.* **2022**, *1*, 33–39.
19. Akhmetov, R.; Khusainov, R.; Nurgaliev, A. Neuromuscular coordination and reaction speed in young wrestlers. *J. Phys. Educ. Sport* **2021**, *21*, 1485–1491. [CrossRef]
20. Petrov, M.; Dimitrov, T. Neuromotor training interventions in youth wrestling: Effects on explosive power. *Eur. J. Wrestl. Sci.* **2023**, *5*, 22–31.
21. Balsalobre-Fernández, C.; Romero-Franco, N.; Jiménez-Reyes, P. Performance assessment and monitoring using new technologies: A theoretical framework. *Sports* **2021**, *9*, 66. [CrossRef]
22. Longakit, J.; Aque, F.J.; Toring-Aque, L.; Lobo, J.; Ayubi, N.; Mamon, R.; Coming, L.; Padilla, D.K.; Mondido, C.A.; Sinag, J.M.; et al. The effect of a 4-week plyometric training exercise on specific physical fitness components in U21 novice volleyball players. *Pedagog. Phys. Cult. Sports* **2025**, *29*, 86–95. [CrossRef]
23. Mocanu, G.D.; Murariu, G.; Potop, V. Differences in explosive strength values for students of the faculty of physical education and sports (male) according to body mass index levels. *Pedagog. Phys. Cult. Sports* **2023**, *27*, 71–83. [CrossRef]
24. Bujalance-Moreno, P.; Fortes, V.; Gallardo, L. Effects of combined plyometric and specific wrestling training on performance in youth Greco-Roman wrestlers. *Int. J. Sports Sci. Coach.* **2020**, *15*, 686–694. [CrossRef]
25. Nagovitsyn, R.S.; Koryagina, I.A.; Kharisova, G.R. Adaptive models of training in combat sports for junior athletes. *J. Phys. Educ. Sport* **2019**, *19*, 1534–1540.
26. Suárez-Arrones, L.; Sáez de Villarreal, E.; Requena, B. Integrative strength and tactical training in combat sports: A pathway to improve transferability. *Strength Cond. J.* **2022**, *44*, 44–51. [CrossRef]
27. Chaabene, H.; Negra, Y.; Capranica, L.; Bouguezzi, R.; Hachana, Y.; Granacher, U. Specific physical training in young combat athletes: A systematic review and meta-analysis. *Front. Physiol.* **2020**, *11*, 1099. [CrossRef]
28. Slimani, M.; Miarka, B.; Briki, W.; Cheour, F. Comparison of Mental Toughness and Power Test Performances in High-Level Kickboxers by Competitive Success. *Asian J. Sports Med.* **2016**, *7*, e30840. [CrossRef] [PubMed] [PubMed Central]
29. Beato, M.; Drust, B. The importance of high-intensity training and neuromuscular specificity in youth combat athletes: A practical framework. *J. Funct. Morphol. Kinesiol.* **2021**, *6*, 36. [CrossRef]
30. Silva, A.F.; Ramirez-Campillo, R.; Sarmento, H.; Afonso, J.; Clemente, F.M. Effects of training programs on decision-making in youth team sports players: A systematic review and meta-analysis. *Front. Psychol.* **2021**, *12*, 663867. [CrossRef] [PubMed]
31. Tibana, R.A.; Sousa NMFd Prestes, J.; Feito, Y.; Ernesto, C.; Voltarelli, F.A. Monitoring Training Load, Well-Being, Heart Rate Variability, and Competitive Performance of a Functional-Fitness Female Athlete: A Case Study. *Sports* **2019**, *7*, 35. [CrossRef] [PubMed]
32. Aloui, G.; Dhahbi, W.; Ceylan, H.İ.; Stefanica, V.; Alneama, A.; Mami, M.; Hayes, L.; Muntean, R.I.; Hermassi, S. A Combined Balance and Plyometric Training Approach: Effects on Physical Performance Parameters in Youth Male Handball Players: A Randomized Controlled Trial. *Rev. Psicol. Deporte (J. Sport Psychol.)* **2025**, *34*, 1–12.
33. Latyshev, M.; Sergeev, N.; Kudinov, A. Individualization of physical training in youth wrestling based on motor characteristics. *Teor. Prakt. Fiz. Kult.* **2020**, *12*, 23–25.
34. Ramos-Campo, D.J.; Ávila-Gandía, V.; Martínez-Rodríguez, A. Specific physical conditioning in combat sports: A practical update for trainers. *Strength Cond. J.* **2022**, *44*, 52–60. [CrossRef]
35. Dreve, A.A.; Stoica, M.; Gheara, C.; Stoian, O.; Saftel, A. Physical Effort Monitoring with the Catapult Gps System in the Context of an Aerobic Endurance Testing of Rugby Players. *Elearning Softw. Educ.* **2021**, *3*, 328–337.
36. Aquino, R.; Carling, C.; Palucci Vieira, L.H.; Gonçalves, L.G.C.; Puggina, E.F. Tactical behavior and its relationship with physical and technical performance in youth combat sports. *Int. J. Perform. Anal. Sport* **2023**, *23*, 215–227.
37. Tarrit, B.; Garnier, Y.M.; Birat, A.; Ruas, C.V.; Estevam, E.; Rance, M.; Morel, C.; Nottin, S.; Mattiello-Sverzut, A.C.; Nosaka, K.; et al. Can neuromuscular differences manifest by early adolescence in males between predominantly endurance and strength sports? *Eur. J. Appl. Physiol.* **2024**, *124*, 2651–2663. [CrossRef]

38. Ojeda-Aravena, A.; Herrera-Valenzuela, T.; Valdés-Badilla, P.; Báez-San Martín, E.; Thapa, R.K.; Ramirez-Campillo, R. A systematic review with meta-analysis on the effects of plyometric-jump training on the physical fitness of combat sport athletes. *Sports* **2023**, *11*, 33. [CrossRef] [PubMed]
39. Abdullayev, I.X. Improvement of the special physical training model of greco-roman junior wrestlers. *Ment. Enlight. Sci.-Methodol. J.* **2023**, *4*, 9–20.
40. Petrov, A.; Zimkin, D. Standardization of physical performance in junior combat athletes: Methodological considerations. *Phys. Educ. Theory Pract.* **2020**, *26*, 87–91.
41. Mihaiu, C.; Stefanica, V.; Joksimović, M.; Ceylan, H.İ.; Pirvu, D. Impact of Specific Plyometric Training on Physiological and Performance Outcomes in U16 Performance Athletes Soccer Players. *Rev. Rom. Pentru Educ. Multidimens.* **2024**, *16*, 206–223. [CrossRef]

sports

MDPI

Article

Comparison of the Core Training and Mobility Training Effects on Basketball Athletic Performance in Young Players: A Comparative Experimental Study

Alessandra Amato [1], Cristina Cortis [2,3], Matteo Tropea [1], Marco Politi [1], Andrea Fusco [4,*] and Giuseppe Musumeci [1,5]

1 Department of Biomedical and Biotechnological Sciences, Section of Anatomy, Histology and Movement Science, School of Medicine, University of Catania, Via S. Sofia n°97, 95123 Catania, Italy; alessandra.amato@unict.it (A.A.); matteotp@gmail.com (M.T.); m.politi98@gmail.com (M.P.); g.musumeci@unict.it (G.M.)
2 Department of Human Sciences, Society and Health, University of Cassino and Lazio Meridionale, 03043 Cassino, Italy; c.cortis@unicas.it
3 European University of Technology EUt+, 03043 Cassino, Italy
4 Department of Medicine and Aging Sciences, University "G. d'Annunzio" of Chieti-Pescara, 66100 Chieti, Italy
5 Research Center on Motor Activities (CRAM), University of Catania, Via S. Sofia n°97, 95123 Catania, Italy
* Correspondence: andrea.fusco@unich.it

Abstract: This study compared the effects of core (CTG) or mobility training (MTG) on basketball-specific skills in youth players, focusing on dynamic balance. Both training modalities have a recognized role in enhancing performance, but few studies have examined their impact on this population. Thirty-one young (age 14.71 ± 2.27 years) males were assigned to an 8-week CTG or MTG. Overhead Squat, Y-Balance Test, Agility T-Test, Sit-and-Reach, Functional Hop Tests, and the Balance Error Scoring System were assessed before (pre) and after (post) the intervention for both dominant (D) and non-dominant (ND) limbs. Both groups improved the postero-lateral direction of the Y-Balance Test for the D (CTG, MD [95% CIs] = −8.108 [−15.620, −0.595], p = 0.035; MTG, MD [95% CIs] = −15.234 [−23.512, −6.956], p = 0.024) and ND (CTG, MD [95% CIs] = −9.110 [−16.150, −2.070], p = 0.013; MTG MD [95% CIs] = −13.899 [−21.657, −6.141], p = 0.001) limb and the medial reach for D (CTG, MD [95% CIs] = −17.279 [−26.364, −8.194], p = 0.001; MTG, MD [95% CIs] = −22.050 [−32.061, −12.039], p = 0.03) and ND (CTG, MD [95% CIs] = −9.309 [−17.093, −1.526], p = 0.021; MTG, MD [95% CIs] = −13.614 [−22.190, −5.037], p = 0.003), the Overhead Squat Test (CTG, MD [95% CIs] = −3.059 [−3.797, −2.321], p = 0.001; MTG, MD [95% CIs] = −3.643 [−4.456, −2.830], p = 0.001), and Agility T-Test (CTG, MD [95% CIs] = 0.572 [0.072, 1.073], p = 0.026; MTG, MD [95% CIs] = 0.696 [0.145, 1.248], p = 0.024) skills. Only CTG showed a significant improvement (MD [95% CIs] = −8.294 [−16.162, −0.426], p = 0.04) in single-leg hop performance for the ND limb. No significant improvements were observed in static balance or flexibility. No time × group effect was found. Both interventions improved key basketball-specific motor abilities and could be added to the basketball training session without adverse effect.

Keywords: team sport; performance; youth sport; neuromuscular control; balance; range of motion

https://doi.org/10.3390/sports13110398

1. Introduction

Basketball is a high-intensity, intermittent team sport characterized by frequent accelerations and decelerations, rapid changes in direction, and vertical jumps that impose specific physical demands on athletes, requiring speed, power, and endurance to perform effectively [1]. Advancements in training strategies and modifications to the game's rules have contributed to an increasingly fast-paced and physically demanding sport. Consequently, optimal physical conditioning, including good mobility, balance, agility, and, in general, the development of good neuromotor function [2], has become a key factor for basketball players, not only for maximizing performance but also for maintaining physical integrity and reducing injury risk. In response, physical conditioning programs have evolved to incorporate not only traditional sport-specific skills and general strength and endurance training, but also functional components designed to enhance these key motor abilities required for the game. Among these, core and mobility training have garnered increased attention in recent literature for their potential to both improve athletic performance and mitigate injury risk [3–9].

The core, which comprises the lumbopelvic–hip complex, functions as a central conduit for force transmission between the upper and lower extremities. In basketball, many movements originate in the lower limbs and culminate in upper-body execution (e.g., shooting, passing, rebounding). Sasaki et al. [10] examined the effect of core training in drop landings and single-leg squats in basketball players, reporting partial improvements in both. Hessam et al. [4] demonstrated that a 12-week core training program led to significant improvements in agility and dynamic balance in adolescent basketball players, directly linking core stability to these performances.

Mobility training, frequently mischaracterized as solely preventative, is increasingly recognized as a critical component of performance optimization. Mobility is not only related to joint range of motion but also gives information about neuromuscular control throughout that range under dynamic conditions [11]. Cook and colleagues demonstrated that exercises such as the deep squat are a predictive tool for evaluating the functional mobility of the hips, ankles, and shoulders, while also assessing motor control and core stability [12]. Limited joint mobility, particularly in the hips, shoulders, and ankles, has been associated with dysfunctional movement patterns, elevated injury risk, and decreased power output [13]. Enhancing mobility facilitates access to biomechanically advantageous positions, improves movement efficiency, and supports the execution of sport-specific skills such as the defensive stance or triple-threat position [14]. Mobility training, particularly focusing on the hips, has been shown to directly enhance functional range of motion and transfer to improvements in agility and sprint times in high school basketball players [15]. On the other hand, there are currently no studies linking hip mobility training with improved dynamic balance in young basketball players.

Therefore, the available evidence suggests that core training seems primarily to enhance the stability and efficiency of the kinetic chain, which is essential for powerful, coordinated movements such as jumping, cutting, and absorbing contact. In contrast, mobility training focuses on optimizing the range of motion and neuromuscular control around joints, which is a prerequisite for achieving optimal biomechanical positions and preventing movement restrictions that can lead to inefficiency or injury. However, a direct comparison of the effects of these two training methods on the same motor skill, assessed with standardized tests, is lacking. Addressing this gap is essential to determine whether each method has a specific efficacy, as they appear to target different yet complementary aspects of basketball performance. Such a comparison would allow for the optimal integration of each methodology, in terms of timing and objectives, alongside traditional sport-specific skill training. In basketball players, deficits in balance are a common risk factor for lower limb injuries [16]. For these reasons, the primary aim of our study will be to analyze the effect of the two training modalities on dynamic balance as assessed by a standardized test. Our secondary objective will be to compare any differences and simultaneous effects of the two modalities on the basketball-specific skills, agility, mobility, and flexibility.

By integrating these protocols into standard youth basketball practice, this study seeks to elucidate the most efficient training strategy for optimizing key physical qualities. The rationale for this comparison is not to determine a superior training modality per se, but to investigate whether core and mobility training elicit distinct, sport-specific adaptations. It is hypothesized that core training will preferentially enhance agility and dynamic balance by improving trunk stabilization and force transfer during rapid directional changes. In contrast, mobility training is expected to yield greater improvements in functional movement patterns by addressing joint kinematics and neuromuscular control, which are critical for achieving the deep stances and full ranges of motion required in basketball. The intervention protocols and the test battery proposed in this study have been specifically designed to reflect this rationale.

2. Materials and Methods

2.1. Participants

We recruited 36 basketball players belonging to the youth categories of the "Sporting Club Adrano A.S.D" basketball team (Catania, Italy). All the participants followed the same weekly basketball training routine, training three days per week for 90 min per session, for a total weekly basketball training volume of 270 min.

Individuals were eligible if they were without lesions or trauma to bones, ligaments, tendons, or muscles of the lower extremities in the previous 6 months, had no prior diagnosis of orthopedic disorders, and with at least 1 year of basketball experience. Participants were excluded if they did not meet the inclusion criteria, if they had stopped practicing basketball, or if they were regularly engaged in other sports disciplines. The study was conducted following the Declaration of Helsinki and was approved by the Scientific Committee of the 'Research Center on Motor Activities' at the University of Catania (Catania, Italy), protocol CRAM-57-2024, date of approval 17 July 2024. Before participation, all athletes read an informed consent form for the anonymous use of their data, which was then signed by their legal guardians and the adolescents themselves to participate in the study. They also completed a self-reported questionnaire, which served to confirm their eligibility and to gather personal information, lifestyle details, and information about their training habits. The "Waterloo Footedness Questionnaire" [17] was administered to identify the dominant (D) and non-dominant (ND) leg.

2.2. Study Design

Athletes were randomly distributed to two homogeneous groups: the core training group (CTG) (n = 18) or the Mobility Training Group (MTG) (n = 18). CTG conducted exercises that included concentric, eccentric, and isometric contractions targeting both deep and superficial core muscles. For the MTG, the protocol included static and dynamic stretching and targeted mobility exercises for key joints involved in basketball. We used block randomization [18], which provided a better guarantee that both groups would be of nearly equal size and have a similar age distribution. We defined the blocks according to three categories: U13, U15, and U19. Before participant enrollment, the primary investigator (A.A.) determined the sequence of random assignment to the two intervention groups (mobility training or core training) for the three blocks by using the Excel formula "=RANDOM ()". This allowed us to maintain the allocation concealment. Then, a research assistant (M.T.) randomly drew the names of the participants from a pool and assigned them sequentially to the pre-established group sequence. This ensured that the researchers involved in enrolling participants could not know the upcoming group assignment, thus preventing selection bias.

All participants completed a test battery that identified tests suitable for analyzing the specific skills for basketball performance. The outcome assessors, M.P., together with a research assistant, conducted the physical performance tests and were blinded to the group assignment of the participants. M.P. and the research assistant were not involved in the training interventions. Participants were also instructed not to disclose their training group affiliation to the assessors.

The battery test (adapted from Read et al. [19] and Bird et al. [20]) was performed before (T0) and after (T1) 8 weeks of training and included seven tests, covering the mobility, agility, and static and dynamic balance skills. The tests included the Overhead Squat Test (OST), the Back Scratch Test, Sit-and-Reach Test (SRT), Agility T-Test, Y-Balance Test (YBT), Functional Hop Test, and Balance Error Scoring System (BESS).

2.3. Mobility, Balance, and Agility Assessment

2.3.1. Overhead Squat Test

OST is a validated test included in the "Functional Movement Screen" that gives important information about the specific mobility of the basketball player and any motor dysfunction of the hips, knees, and ankles [19,21,22]. The specific scoring protocol used in this study is adapted from the original description by Cook et al. [12], and subsequent validation work by Minick et al. [23]. Participants had to perform eight consecutive squats with hands at the level of the iliac crests and two squats with arms extended above the head with feet not exceeding shoulder width. The operator was instructed to observe the behavior of the ankle joint, knee joint, and pelvis. A poor ability to maintain pelvic anteversion during movement, visibly impaired degrees of bending of the ankle and knee joints, and lateral movements of the latter (stance in valgus or varus). If none of these issues were present, each joint received a score of one. This phase of the test, performed with the hands placed on the hips, provided a maximum of 3 points available (one point for each of the three areas assessed: ankles, knees, and pelvis).

After one minute, the test was repeated with the arms extended above the head to assess the mobility of the shoulder joint and ankle dorsiflexion under closed kinetic chain conditions. In case the athlete's ear was visible during the squat, this meant poor mobility of this joint, so a score of zero was assigned; otherwise, a score of one was assigned. Ankle dorsiflexion was evaluated by observing whether the tibia remained parallel to the torso in the sagittal plane. If not, the score was zero; otherwise, the score was one. This second phase evaluated both left and right shoulders and ankles, for a maximum of 4 points. Finally, the scores from all 7 criteria (3 from the first phase and 4 from the second) were summed to obtain the total OST score. A higher score reflected better movement quality and control during the squat.

2.3.2. Back Scratch Test

The Back Scratch Test was developed and validated to evaluate upper-body flexibility [24]. We measured the total shoulder range of motion by recording the distance (negative value) or overlap (positive value) in cm between the middle fingers as they reached behind the back. The participants performed the test twice with each arm, alternating sides, with no recovery time between right and left limbs; the final score in cm was considered the best attempt from both arms. The operator measured laterally to the hand that was above, between the two extremities of the middle fingers, when there was an overlap between hands [25].

2.3.3. Sit-and-Reach Test

The SRT is a reliable and validated method for assessing the flexibility of the back muscle chain [26]. The assessment is carried out using a standardized box (Baseline 12-1085, Fabrication Enterprises, New York, NY, USA). Participants sat on the floor with their legs fully extended and the soles of their feet placed flat against the front of the box. From this starting position, participants were instructed to inhale, then exhale while bending forward at the waist with arms and fingers extended, reaching as far as possible along the centimeter scale positioned on top of the box. Three repetitions were performed, and the average of the three attempts was considered for data analysis. There was no recovery time between sets, as only the time needed to slowly return to the starting position was allowed. The effectiveness of doing three repetitions to obtain a reliable result in SRT has been previously demonstrated [27].

2.3.4. Agility T-Test

The most commonly used test to assess agility is the Agility T-Test. According to the protocol, originally described by Semenick [28] and validated for reliability and validity by Pauole et al. [29], participants were required to sprint forward from a starting line, touch the first cone 10 m in front of the starting line with the right hand, shuffle left 5 m and touch the second cone with the left hand, shuffle right 10 m and touch the third cone with the right hand, shuffle back 5 m to the first cone, then backpedal 10 m as fast as possible to the start line [30]. First, the test administrator explained and performed the test slowly. Then, the participants performed a familiarization repetition of the test, followed directly by a single test at maximum intensity, during which the time (in seconds) was recorded.

2.3.5. Balance Error Scoring System

The BESS is designed to assess an individual's ability to maintain static balance. The protocol and error scoring criteria used were based on the original development by Riemann et al. [31] and the subsequent widespread application and review by Bell et al. [32]. Participants had to maintain six conditions: double-leg stance, single-leg stance (on the ND leg), and tandem stance (ND foot behind the D one), for 20 s with eyes closed on both a firm and foam surface. A 20 s rest was provided between conditions. One error point was recorded for: opening the eyes; removing hands from the hips, stepping, stumbling, or falling; lifting the forefoot or heel; moving the hip into more than 30° of abduction; or remaining out of the test position for more than 5 s. The final BESS scores were the sum of errors for all conditions.

2.3.6. Y-Balance Test

The YBT is a valuable musculoskeletal screening tool to assess dynamic balance and the identification of lower limb and trunk movement dysfunction in basketball players [33]. Plisky et al. demonstrated that diminished performance on the YBT is associated with an increased risk of non-contact lower extremity injuries [34]. Its validity in basketball is further supported by its close approximation of the split-stance posture, a common and functional biomechanical position frequently adopted during gameplay.

We followed the methodology of Fullam et al. [35] and the original, foundational protocol described by Plisky et al. (2006) [36]. We constructed a "Y" with tape on the floor, one oriented anteriorly and the other two in the posteromedial and posterolateral directions, both at a 135-degree angle to the first. The three arms of the "Y" were then calibrated with the tape measure to simplify the collection of results. The athlete stood in the center of this "Y," with his toe resting at the point of convergence of the three pieces of tape, barefoot and with his hands on his hips. The goal was to move a reach block as far as possible with the non-supporting foot along the anterior directions (ANT), posteromedial directions (PM), and posterolateral directions (PL), without crushing it or putting pressure on the floor, without performing a push on the reach block to make it go farther, and return with the non-supporting foot to the supporting foot without touching the floor. The distance traveled by the reach block was then measured with a meter from the point of convergence of the arms of the "Y" to the nearest edge of the reach block in each direction and for both D and ND limbs. Therefore, the six derived measures (D ANT, D PL, D PM, ND ANT, ND PL, and ND M) in cm were considered separately for data analysis. To reduce confounding by anthropometry, normalized reach distances were calculated for each measure using the following formula: $Reach\ distance \div Limb\ length \times 100$. The YBT protocol and normalization procedure have demonstrated excellent inter-rater and test–retest reliability [34]. Participants completed a single familiarization trial before the test for both the D and ND limbs.

2.3.7. Functional Hop Tests

The Functional Hop Tests are a validated battery test [37] that offers valuable insight into lower limb strength, explosive power, and dynamic stability [38,39]. The specific procedures were implemented as per the original reliability studies by Ross et al. [37] and the normative data collection in basketball players by Myers et al. [39]. The test was conducted in 4 stages:

1. Single-Leg Hop for Distance: The athlete begins on the testing leg with his toe at the starting line and performs a forward hop, landing on the same leg. The distance is measured from the starting line to where the heel lands. The athletes were instructed to stabilize the landing with good control and minimal movement for at least three seconds.
2. Triple Hop for Distance: Starting on the testing leg with the toe at the start line, the athlete performs three powerful forward hops using the same leg. The total distance was measured from the start to the heel's landing point after the third hop. Athletes were instructed to maintain balance and hold the final landing position steadily for a minimum of three seconds.
3. Crossover Triple Hop for Distance: The athlete stands on the same side of a centerline tape as the leg being tested (e.g., right side for the right leg), with the toe at the start line. Each participant performs three continuous hops forward, crossing over the tape in a zig-zag pattern with each hop. The total distance was measured to the heel's landing after the third hop. The athlete was instructed to hold the final position with control and limited sway for at least three seconds.
4. Six-Meter Timed Hop on One Leg: The athlete started on the testing leg with the toe on the start line. On the command "3, 2, 1, go," he was instructed to hop as quickly as possible over a six-meter distance using only that leg. The timer was stopped when the athlete crossed the six-meter finish line.

Participants performed one submaximal trial for each stage to familiarize themselves with the task. Then, they performed three maximal trials for both D and ND limbs for each of the four stages. The best hop distance of the three trials for the first, second, and third stages was used for statistical analysis [39,40]. Participants had 30 s of rest between the trials of the same stage and one minute of rest between stages [41].

2.3.8. Training Programs

The exercise interventions are described in accordance with the Consensus on Exercise Reporting Template (CERT) guidelines [42] to enhance the clarity, reproducibility, and completeness of the intervention reporting. Participants performed the training session under the supervision of an Italian basketball federation coach (M.T.), who also collected information on adherence to exercise by calling the roll of all players involved in the study at each session. Additionally, during the session, M.T. was required to record any adverse events reported by participants, including the onset of pain or fatigue before, during, or after the protocol. Both groups trained three times per week for 8 weeks before their ordinary basketball training session for a total of 24 sessions.

2.3.9. Core Training Protocol

The protocol was adapted from Sasaki et al. [10] and consisted of three exercises: plank, side plank, and Nordic hamstrings exercise (NHEs). Planks and side planks were performed for two sets of 30 s, while the NHE was performed once for progressively 3 to 15 repetitions according to the protocol [10]. The recovery time between sets and between exercises was 30 s to maintain the basketball game's physiological demands of a 1:1 work-rest ratio of [43].

The plank was performed by resting the forearms and toes on the ground, keeping the pelvis tilted backward to increase the work of the abdominal muscles. The exercise consisted of two sets of thirty seconds each (Figure 1a). From week 5 to week 8, the difficulty level of the exercise increased, and the participant had to lift a limb and hold the position throughout the series (30 s). In the first series, one limb was kept lifted, and in the next series, the contralateral limb was kept lifted (Figure 1b). The side plank was performed by lying on the side on the ground, keeping the head, shoulders, torso, pelvis, and lower limbs aligned. The forearm was placed on the side on which the athlete rested, and the leg of the same side on the ground; then, a ninety-degree bend at knee level was performed. In addition, the hip closest to the ground was lifted to keep the obliques and transverse muscles in tension. The lower limb farthest from the ground was kept raised off the ground, in line with the rest of the body (Figure 1c). After the first 4 weeks, to increase the level of difficulty, the exercise was performed by stretching the lower limb resting on the ground (Figure 1d). The exercise consisted of two sets of thirty seconds per side. Plank exercises were included to target the anterior core stabilizers, critical for maintaining spinal alignment and facilitating force transfer during athletic movements [44]. To perform the NHE, athletes started from a kneeling position, with the support of a partner sitting on the athlete's legs, and they had to let themselves fall forward, slowing down the fall as much as possible and keeping the torso and pelvis vertical (Figure 1e). The NHE was included as a key component of the core training program, being an effective hamstring strengthener and putting high demand on lumbopelvic stabilizers. Electromyographic studies confirmed that the NHE elicits moderate-to-high activation of the erector spinae and internal oblique muscles, which are essential for maintaining a neutral spine and stable pelvis against the gravitational and inertial forces during the eccentric lowering phase [44–46], critical for the transfer of forces across the kinetic chain. We assumed that the NHE would enhance core stability under dynamic, high-load conditions, with a direct transfer to the functional outcomes assessed in this study. Specifically, improved lumbopelvic control is a known determinant of performance in dynamic balance tasks like the YBT [47] and contributes to more efficient force transfer during the deceleration and re-acceleration phases of agility and hopping tasks [48,49]. Therefore, the NHE was selected to improve the integrated stability and function of the posterior chain, which is fundamental to basketball performance. The repetitions ranged from three to five for the first level, five to ten for the second level, and ten to fifteen for the third level (reached progressively over the 8 weeks). The exercise was performed in a single set.

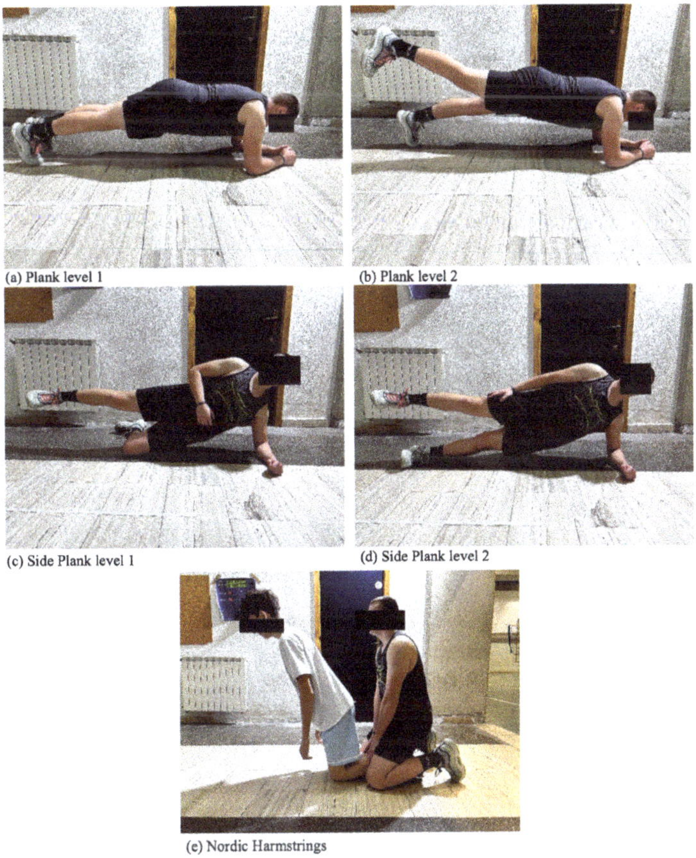

Figure 1. Core training exercises. The figure shows pictures of the Participant performing each exercise of the core training protocol: (**a**) Plank level 1; (**b**) plank level 2; (**c**) side plank level 1; (**d**) side plank level 2; (**e**) Nordic hamstring.

2.3.10. Mobility Training

The protocol, including a 30 s rest between each exercise, was adapted from Antoranz et al. [15].

The first exercise was the 1 min 90–90 hip rotation, focusing on stretching the hip flexors and increasing external hip rotation. The athletes were sitting on the floor with their legs in a 90–90 position. They gently rotated their hips outward, thus bringing their knees toward the ground (Figure 2a). The exercise lasted one minute for one repetition.

The second exercise was the half-kneeling ankle mobility. Athletes started from the lunge position with the knee on the ground, and they brought the front knee forward to induce a dorsal flexion of the tibio-tarsal joint. Athletes had to maintain the position for 30 s per leg for one repetition (Figure 2b). No recovery was allowed between left and right limb repetition. This drill targets ankle dorsiflexion, which is a known limiting factor in Overhead Squat performance and dynamic balance [50].

The third exercise was the half-kneeling hamstring stretch. From the starting position of the previous exercise, athletes extended the leg of the front knee forward to generate a stretch of the hamstrings, maintaining a 90 degree angle between the trunk and the extended leg. When they reached the maximum stretch phase, they kept it for 2 s, and then they returned to the starting position. The exercise lasted 30 s for each leg and was repeated once (Figure 2c).

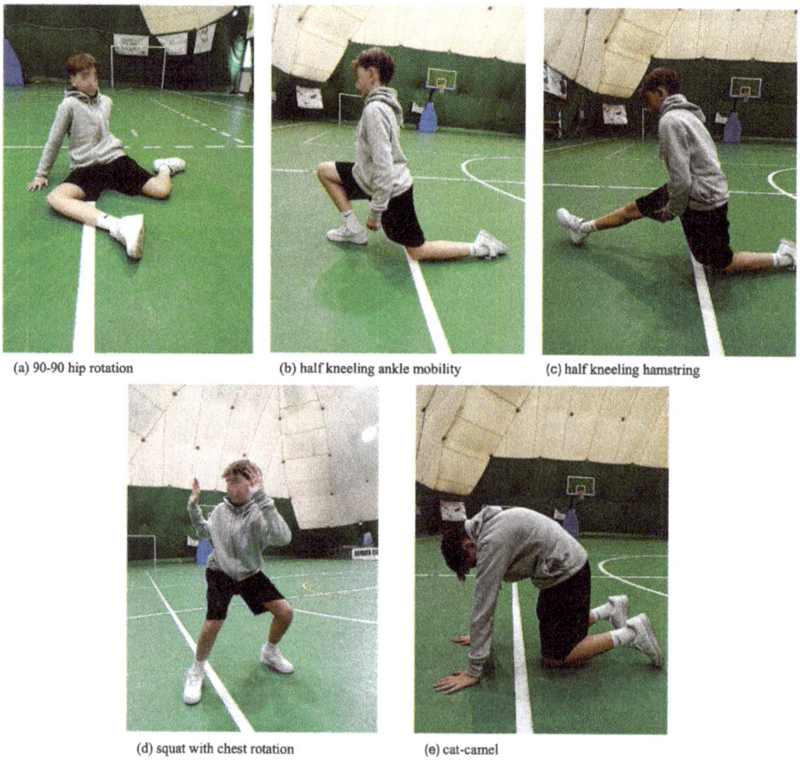

Figure 2. Mobility training exercises. The figure shows pictures of the Participant performing each exercise of the Mobility training protocol: (**a**) 90–90 hip rotation; (**b**) half-kneeling ankle mobility; (**c**) half-kneeling hamstring; (**d**) squat with chest rotation; (**e**) cat-camel.

The fourth exercise was the squat with chest rotation. The athletes performed a squat starting from a standing position with the shoulders abducted at 90° and the elbows also flexed at 90°. At the maximum squat phase, they twisted their torso in both directions, ensuring that the pelvis does not rotate towards the side of the twist (Figure 2d). A set of 12 repetitions was performed on each side. The last exercise was the cat-camel. The athletes started in a quadruped position, with hands at shoulder height and knees at hip height. From this position, creating an anteversion of the pelvis, they brought the abdominal area towards the ground, keeping the shoulders and knees fixed. After holding the position for two seconds, they did the opposite, arching their back toward the ceiling, thus causing a retroversion of the pelvis. The exercise was repeated once for one minute (Figure 2e).

2.4. Load Progression and Session Structure

To ensure a progressive and comparable internal load to the CTG, the progression criteria for the mobility exercises were based on the controlled increase in the range of motion (ROM) and movement quality. For the static exercises (90–90 hip rotation and half-kneeling ankle mobilization), participants were instructed to gradually increase the stretching intensity week by week, aiming for mild discomfort without pain. For the dynamic exercises (half-kneeling hamstring stretch, squat with thoracic rotation, and cat-camel), the progression focused on achieving a greater ROM and superior motor control with each repetition, while the execution time and repetition count remained fixed. Both training protocols were designed to be matched for total time under tension. Excluding one exercise per protocol where repetitions were the metric (NHE for core training; squat with thoracic rotation for mobility training), both sessions had an identical total duration of 6 min and used consistent 30 s rest intervals between sets and exercises.

2.5. Statistical Analysis

A priori power analysis was conducted using G*Power software (G*Power, 2007, version 3.1, Düsseldorf, Germany) to estimate the required sample size for a repeated measures ANOVA with a mixed design. Based on effect sizes observed in the previous literature involving similar athletic populations and interventions, a medium effect size (f = 0.25) was selected. With an alpha level of 0.05, power set at 0.80, and an assumed correlation of 0.5 between repeated measures, the analysis indicated that a minimum total sample size of 34 participants (17 per group) would be required to detect a statistically significant interaction effect. The analysis used two primary statistical approaches: Linear Mixed-Effects Models (LMMs) with random intercepts for participants, and traditional repeated-measures Analysis of Variance (ANOVA) (2 conditions × 2-time intervals) used to analyze the differences within and between MTG and CTG for each dependent variable. The LMM was estimated via maximum likelihood with robust (clustered) standard errors, serving as a sensitivity analysis to confirm the robustness of the ANOVA findings. The significance threshold was set at $\alpha = 0.05$ (two-tailed). To address multiple comparisons, False Discovery Rate (FDR) correction was applied within the YBT (six directions) and Functional Hop Test (eight measures) families. The normality of the data was checked by the Shapiro–Wilk test. An independent *t*-test was conducted to assess baseline differences among the participants' characteristics between the groups. Post hoc pairwise comparisons were conducted with a Bonferroni adjustment to control for Type I error. The assumption of homogeneity of variance was assessed using Levene's Test for each variable at each time point. Effect sizes for within-group changes over time are reported as Hedges' g_av with 95% confidence intervals, calculated using a standard formula to correct for small sample bias. Between-group effect sizes were reported as Cohen's d with their 95% confidence intervals for all outcome measures. The SPSS® (IBM®, Chicago, IL, USA) version 29.0.2.0 software and the Jamovi (jamovi project, 2022, Version 2.3, Sydney, Australia) software were used for statistical analysis.

3. Results

Five participants were excluded from data analysis because they had stopped practicing basketball and did not participate in the evaluation sessions. Thirty-one participants (age: 14.8 ± 2.04 years, weight: 70 ± 11.8 kg, BMI: 22.9 ± 3.07 kg·m^{-2}) completed both the T0 and T1 evaluations and were included in the data analysis, comprising CTG (n = 17) and MTG (n = 14). The overall mean training sessions adherence was 86.96 ± 10.02%. Table S1 (Supplementary Materials) reports adherence for each participant as the percentage of sessions attended. The participant flow through the study is summarized in the CONSORT diagram (Figure 3).

The independent *t*-test showed no significant differences between groups at baseline ($p > 0.05$). Table 1 summarizes baseline participants' characteristics per group.

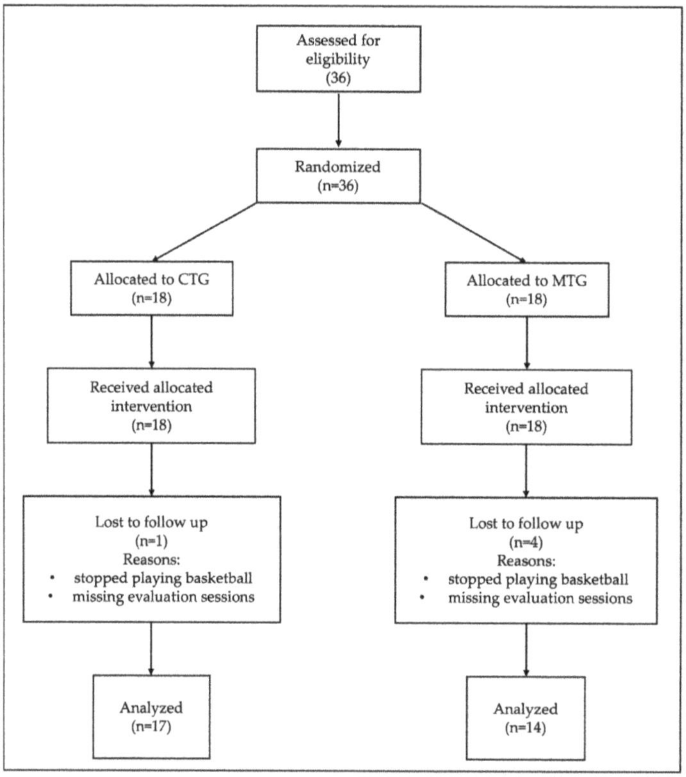

Figure 3. CONSORT flow diagram of the study. The diagram shows participant recruitment, allocation, and analysis through the phases of the randomized trial. Control group (CTG); mobility group (MTG). Thirty-six male basketball players were randomized into two intervention groups. Five participants were lost to follow-up due to discontinuation of basketball practice and non-participation in evaluation sessions (partially at T0 and completely at T1). Thirty-one participants were included in the final data analysis.

Table 1. Participants' characteristics at the baseline were divided by group.

Variables	Mobility Training (M ± SD)	Core Training (M ± SD)	T Student's	*p*-Value
age (years)	14.71 ± 2.27	14.88 ± 1.90	0.2890	0.824
height (cm)	174.73 ± 7.44	174.87 ± 10.29	−0.0381	0.970
weight (kg)	71.09 ± 10.99	69.14 ± 12.81	0.4012	0.692
BMI (kg/m^2)	23.17 ± 2.30	22.63 ± 3.60	0.4388	0.665
basketball experience (years)	4.82 ± 2.71	3.80 ± 2.14	1.0695	0.295

Mean (M) and standard deviation (SD).

A violation was found for T0 posterior lateral YBT for the D (p = 0.018) and ND limb YBT anterior (p = 0.042). For all other variables, the assumption was met (all $p > 0.05$). Table S2 in the Supplementary Materials shows Levene's Test of equality of error variances for all outcome measures.

3.1. Main Effect Analysis

Mixed ANOVA showed a significant main effect of time, for the OST F (1, 29) = 155.86, $p < 0.001$, partial η^2 = 0.843 (very large), the Agility T-test F (1, 29) = 12.13, p = 0.002, partial

$\eta^2 = 0.295$ (large), the YBT ND PL F (1, 29) = 20.18, $p < 0.001$, partial $\eta^2 = 0.410$ (large), the YBT ND PM F (1, 29) = 16.39, $p < 0.001$, partial $\eta^2 = 0.361$ (large), the YBT D PM F (1, 29) = 35.40, $p = 0.001$, partial $\eta^2 = 0.550$ (large), and the YBT D PL F (1, 29) = 18.24, $p < 0.001$, partial $\eta^2 = 0.386$ (large), the ND Hop Test 6 m F (1, 29) = 4.53, $p = 0.042$, partial $\eta^2 = 0.135$. The main effect of group was significant, only for the OST F (1, 29) = 4.36, $p = 0.046$, partial $\eta^2 = 0.131$ (medium-to-large). The time × group interaction was not significant for any of the variables considered. Table S3 (Supplementary Materials) presents the F-value, degrees of freedom, *p*-value, and partial η^2 for the main effect for each variable from ANOVA analysis.

LMM showed a significant main effect of time in the YBT PL for both the D limb (F (1, 58) = 14.203, $p < 0.001$) and the ND limb (F (1, 58) = 16.843, $p < 0.001$), without a significant group effect or group × time interaction being observed. A significant main effect of time was also found for YBT in the PM direction. This was true for the D limb (F (1, 58) = 6.557, $p = 0.013$) and the ND limb (F (1, 58) = 10.691, $p = 0.002$). For the OST total score, significant main effects were found for both group (F (1, 58) = 7.001, $p = 0.010$) and time (F (1, 58) = 90.900, $p < 0.001$).

No significant effects of group ($p = 0.496$) or time ($p = 0.109$) were found for the Agility T-Test performance. For both the D and ND limbs, the analyses of single-leg hop distance showed no significant main effects for Group or Time (all $p > 0.05$). No significant main effects of group or time were found for the triple hop distance on either limb (all $p > 0.05$). No significant effects of group or time were found for the crossover triple hop performance on either the D or ND limbs (all $p > 0.05$). The time to complete the six-meter hop test showed no significant changes for either group or time on both the D and ND limbs (all $p > 0.05$). The time × group interaction was not significant for any of the variables considered. Table S4 compares the main effect of time across statistical methods.

3.2. Within-Group Pairwise Comparison

Mixed ANOVA

The within-group changes, effect sizes, and between-group differences in change are detailed in Table S5 (Supplementary Materials). In addition to significant time effects, both groups demonstrated substantial absolute and relative improvements in key performance metrics.

Within-group analysis revealed a statistically significant improvement in the squat test for both CTG (MD [95% CIs] = −3.059 [−3.797, −2.321]; $p = 0.001$) and MTG (MD [95% CIs]= −3.643 [−4.456, −2.830]; $p = 0.001$). These changes corresponded to large relative improvements of 115.5% and 254.9%, respectively, with very large effect sizes (Hedges' g > 2.8), indicating a robust intervention effect. In the CTG, significant gains were also observed in the ND Hop Single-Leg Test (MD [95% CIs] = −8.294 [−16.162, −0.426]; $p = 0.040$), representing a 7.2% improvement, which was greater than the non-significant 1.2% change observed in the MTG. The between-group difference in change for this variable was −6.94 cm [95% CI: −17.69, 3.82]. To investigate the effects of the interventions on functional lower-limb asymmetry, we calculated the Limb Symmetry Index (LSI) for the single-leg hop test (ND Hop Single-Leg ÷ D Hop Single-Leg × 100), and we performed a mixed ANOVA on LSI. An LSI of 100% indicates perfect symmetry. At baseline, there was no significant difference in LSI between groups ($p = 0.674$). A mixed-model ANOVA revealed no significant time × group interaction (F (1, 29) = 0.036, $p = 0.851$), indicating that the changes in symmetry over time did not differ significantly between the CTG and MTG. The main effect of time was also non-significant (F (1, 29) = 0.298, $p = 0.589$). Descriptively, the mean LSI increased by 1.95% in the CTG (from 101.16% to 103.11%) and by 0.95% in the MTG (from 103.30% to 104.25%).

Furthermore, the number of athletes with a clinically relevant asymmetry (LSI < 90%) in the CTG was reduced from 4/17 at T0 to 2/17 at T1. No such reduction was observed in the MTG (3/14 at both T0 and T1).

For dynamic balance, CTG improved ND YBT PM (MD [95% CIs] = −9.309 [−17.093, −1.526]; p = 0.021) and PL reaches (MD [95% CIs] = −9.110 [−16.150, −2.070]; p = 0.013), D YBT PM (MD [95% CIs] = −17.279 [−26.364, −8.194]; p = 0.001) and PL reaches (MD [95% CIs] = −8.108 [−15.620, −0.595]; p = 0.035). Similarly, the MTG showed significant improvements in ND YBT posteromedial (MD [95% CIs] = −13.614 [−22.190, −5.037]; p = 0.003) and PL reaches (MD [95% CIs] = −13.899 [−21.657, −6.141]; p = 0.001), D PL reaches (MD [95% CIs] = −15.234 [−23.512, −6.956]; p = 0.02) and PM reach (MD [95% CIs] = −22.050 [−32.061, −12.039]; p = 0.03). The MTG consistently showed larger relative improvements across all these YBT directions (D PL: MTG +16.7% vs. CTG +8.5%). Both groups significantly improved in the Agility T-Test CTG (MD [95% CIs] = 0.572 [0.072, 1.073]; p = 0.026), MTG (MD [95% CIs] = 0.696 [0.145, 1.248]; p = 0.02). The magnitude of change was similar, with mean time reductions of 0.57 s (−4.0%) and 0.70 s (−4.8%) for the CTG and MTG, respectively. The between-group difference in change was minimal (−0.12 s [95% CI: −0.87, 0.62]), indicating comparable effects on agility.

3.3. Between-Group Pairwise Comparison

Between-group comparisons at T0 and T1 showed no statistically significant differences between CTG and MTG for most variables. However, the ANOVA mixed model showed a significant difference in the ND YBT posterolateral reach (MD [95% Cis = 8.019 [1.327, 14.712], p = 0.021; Cohen's d = 0.66, 95% CI for d: −0.06 to 1.38) and squat test (MD [95% Cis = 1.218 [0.128, 2.309], p = 0.030; Cohen's d = 0.63, 95% CI for d: −0.09 to 1.35) between groups at T0. However, since this difference was observed only at baseline, it is reasonable to assume that it was a random occurrence. Table S5 (Supplementary Materials) shows between-group comparisons (CTG vs. MTG) for all outcome measures at T0 and post-intervention T1 by mean difference (CTG—MTG) with standard error, p-value, and 95% confidence intervals (95% CIs). However, the analysis of between-group differences in change scores (Table S6, Supplementary Materials) revealed specific areas where the interventions may have diverged. While the time × group interaction in the ANOVA was not significant, the between-group difference in change for the Sit-and-Reach test was 2.72 cm [95% CI: 1.08, 4.36], indicating a significantly greater improvement in flexibility for the MTG. A similar, statistically significant difference in change was observed for the YBT ND ANT (4.65% [95% CI: 0.06, 9.24]), favoring the MTG.

Table 2 shows descriptive statistics (means and standard errors) for all outcome measures.

Table 2. Descriptive statistics (means and standard errors) for all outcome measures by group and time point.

Variable	Groups	Time	Mean	Std. Error	IC 95% (Lower)	IC 95% (Upper)
DYBT ANT (%)	CTG	T0	84.178	2.985	78.072	90.283
	CTG	T1	82.381	2.662	76.936	87.826
	MTG	T0	80.752	3.290	74.024	87.480
	MTG	T1	79.890	2.934	73.890	85.890
DYBT PL (%)	CTG	T0	95.295	2.218	90.760	99.831
	CTG	T1	103.403	3.627	95.985	110.821
	MTG	T0	91.406	2.444	86.408	96.405
	MTG	T1	106.640	3.997	98.466	114.814

Table 2. *Cont.*

Variable	Groups	Time	Mean	Std. Error	IC 95% (Lower)	IC 95% (Upper)
DYBT PM (%)	CTG	T0	86.124	3.081	79.823	92.426
	CTG	T1	103.403	3.627	95.985	110.821
	MTG	T0	84.590	3.395	77.646	91.534
	MTG	T1	106.640	3.997	98.466	114.814
NDYBT ANT (%)	CTG	T0	83.430	3.649	75.966	90.893
	CTG	T1	81.970	3.194	75.438	88.502
	MTG	T0	78.544	4.021	70.320	86.768
	MTG	T1	81.732	3.519	74.534	88.930
NDYBT PL (%)	CTG	T0	98.161	2.199	93.664	102.659
	CTG	T1	107.271	3.203	100.720	113.822
	MTG	T0	90.142	2.423	85.186	95.098
	MTG	T1	104.040	3.530	96.821	111.259
NDYBT PM (%)	CTG	T0	87.210	2.744	81.598	92.821
	CTG	T1	96.519	4.022	88.294	104.744
	MTG	T0	88.167	3.023	81.984	94.351
	MTG	T1	101.781	4.432	92.717	110.845
BESS	CTG	T0	2.882	0.172	2.530	3.235
	CTG	T1	2.765	0.197	2.363	3.167
	MTG	T0	3.286	0.190	2.898	3.674
	MTG	T1	3.000	0.217	2.557	3.443
OST Total Score	CTG	T0	2.647	0.358	1.914	3.380
	CTG	T1	5.706	0.338	5.014	6.398
	MTG	T0	1.429	0.395	0.621	2.236
	MTG	T1	5.071	0.373	4.309	5.834
D Back Scratch (cm)	CTG	T0	7.447	1.596	4.182	10.712
	CTG	T1	8.324	1.750	4.744	11.903
	MTG	T0	8.079	1.759	4.481	11.676
	MTG	T1	7.350	1.929	3.405	11.295
ND Back Scratch (cm)	CTG	T0	1.694	2.360	−3.140	6.528
	CTG	T1	3.381	2.112	−0.945	7.707
	MTG	T0	0.964	2.523	−4.204	6.132
	MTG	T1	2.643	2.258	−1.982	7.268
Sit-and-Reach (cm)	CTG	T0	4.153	1.958	0.149	8.157
	CTG	T1	4.088	1.707	0.597	7.580
	MTG	T0	−1.236	2.157	−5.648	3.176
	MTG	T1	1.421	1.881	−2.426	5.269
Agility T-Test (s)	CTG	T0	14.192	0.421	13.331	15.052
	CTG	T1	13.619	0.349	12.905	14.334
	MTG	T0	14.520	0.464	13.572	15.468
	MTG	T1	13.824	0.385	13.036	14.611
D Hop Single Leg (cm)	CTG	T0	113.529	6.909	99.398	127.661
	CTG	T1	121.765	8.109	105.181	138.349
	MTG	T0	111.571	7.614	96.000	127.143
	MTG	T1	113.214	8.935	94.939	131.489
ND Hop Single Leg (cm)	CTG	T0	115.471	7.342	100.454	130.487
	CTC	T1	123.765	7.586	108.250	139.279
	MTG	T0	114.143	8.091	97.596	130.690
	MTG	T1	115.500	8.359	98.404	132.596

Table 2. *Cont.*

Variable	Groups	Time	Mean	Std. Error	IC 95% (Lower)	IC 95% (Upper)
D Hop Triple (cm)	CTG	T0	402.706	21.908	357.898	447.513
	CTG	T1	399.176	20.975	356.277	442.076
	MTG	T0	362.500	24.142	313.125	411.875
	MTG	T1	364.714	23.114	317.442	411.987
ND Hop Triple (cm)	CTG	T0	395.941	19.042	356.996	434.886
	CTG	T1	407.176	18.452	369.438	444.915
	MTG	T0	362.643	20.983	319.728	405.558
	MTG	T1	366.571	20.333	324.985	408.157
D Crossover Triple (cm)	CTG	T0	318.412	24.574	268.152	368.672
	CTG	T1	322.235	25.035	271.034	373.437
	MTG	T0	294.000	27.079	238.616	349.384
	MTG	T1	307.786	27.587	251.364	364.207
ND Crossover Triple (cm)	CTG	T0	322.176	19.693	281.900	362.453
	CTG	T1	345.176	21.418	301.372	388.981
	MTG	T0	297.286	21.700	252.904	341.668
	MTG	T1	311.214	23.601	262.944	359.484
D Hop Test 6 m (s)	CTG	T0	3.089	0.104	2.877	3.302
	CTG	T1	2.999	0.107	2.780	3.217
	MTG	T0	3.184	0.114	2.950	3.418
	MTG	T1	3.071	0.118	2.830	3.311
ND Hop Test 6 m (s)	CTG	T0	3.022	0.116	2.785	3.258
	CTG	T1	2.999	0.107	2.780	3.217
	MTG	T0	3.208	0.127	2.947	3.469
	MTG	T1	3.071	0.118	2.830	3.311

Core Training Group (CTG); Mobility Training Group (MTG); baseline (T0); post-intervention (T1); dominant (D); non-dominant (ND); Y-Balance Test (YBT); anterior (ANT); posterolateral (PL); posteromedial (PM); Balance Error Scoring System (BESS); Overhead Squat Test (OST). Data are presented as estimated marginal means ± standard error, with the corresponding 95% confidence interval (CI). The CTG included $n = 17$ participants; the MTG included $n = 14$ participants.

3.4. Sensitivity Analysis: Methodological Convergence Mixed ANOVA vs. LMM Comparison

The results demonstrated strong methodological convergence, identified significant time effects from T0 to T1 for YBT ND PM (mixed ANOVA: $p < 0.001$, LMM: $p = 0.002$), YBT ND PM (both $p < 0.001$), YBT D PM (mixed ANOVA: $p = 0.001$, LMM: $p = 0.014$), YBT D PL (both $p < 0.001$), and OST (LMM: $p < 0.001$; mixed ANOVA: $p < 0.001$). All methods agreed on the lack of significant time × group interactions (all $p > 0.50$). All approaches consistently found no improvements in hop tests, static balance, or flexibility. The Agility T-Test and the 6 m hop test showed methodological dependence, with significant improvement in ANOVA ($p = 0.002$) but not in LMM ($p = 0.114$). The 6 m timed hop approached was significant in ANOVA ($p = 0.042$) but not in LMM ($p = 0.342$) Figure 4 shows individual variation for the variable, resulting in statistically significant improvements in all methods.

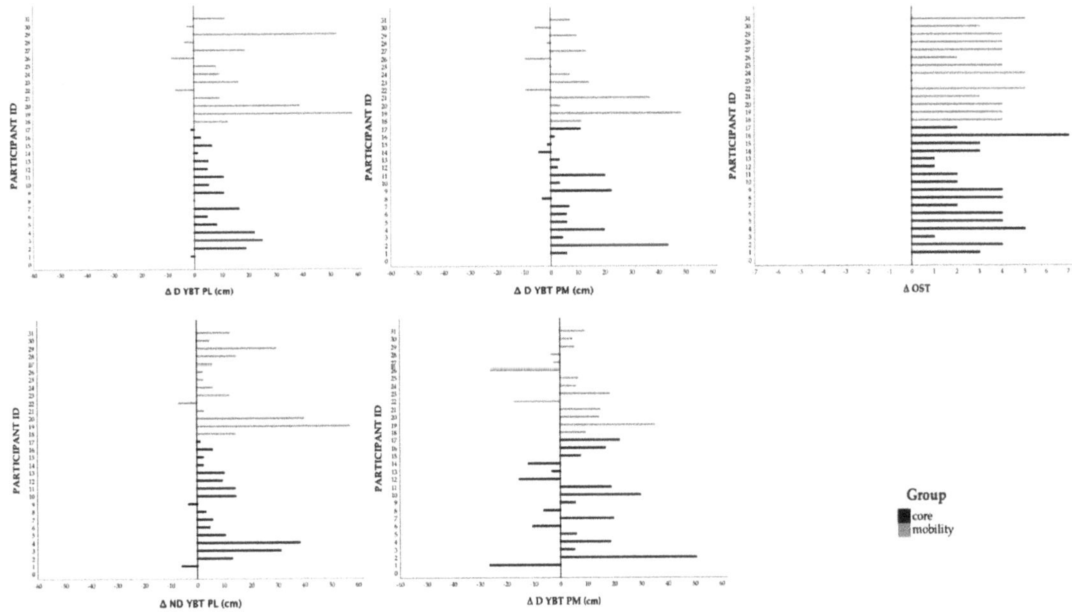

Figure 4. Individual variation (T0–T1) for Y-Balance Test (YBT) posterolateral reach (PL), posteromedial reach (PM) for dominant (D) and non-dominant (ND) limb, and Overhead Squat Test (OST) scores that showed statistically significant improvements. Lines represent change over time for each participant, stratified by intervention group.

4. Discussion

This study aimed to analyze the influence of core or mobility training programs on the development of specific physical abilities in young basketball players. The primary finding of this study, confirmed through LMM with hierarchical FDR correction, is that both training protocols elicited significant improvements in specific domains of dynamic balance in the PL and PM directions of the YBT, our primary outcomes, and functional mobility as measured by the OST (all pFDR < 0.05). Critically, the absence of significant time × group interactions across all statistical approaches provides robust evidence that the rate and magnitude of improvement did not differ between interventions. However, the analysis of the estimated changes and their variability provides deeper insights. CTG led to significant improvements in the Functional Hop Test single leg for the ND limb (7.2% vs. 1.2% in MTG). This finding did not survive FDR correction when considered within the broader context of the eight hop test measures (pFDR = 0.819). This suggests that what appeared to be a potential advantage in dynamic trunk control and lower-limb power transmission may represent a Type I error rather than a robust training effect. The hop test single leg is predictive for lower limb strength, explosive power, and dynamic stability [51]. A previous study showed improvement in an exercise with similar biomechanics to the hop test, the single-leg squat, after 8 weeks of core-muscle training, resulting in better neuromuscular control [10].

Core strengthening changes trunk kinematics in the coronal and sagittal planes, and sagittal plane trunk control significantly influences knee biomechanics. Kulas et al. showed that hamstring activation and anterior shear at the knee are affected by trunk posture [48], while other authors observed that greater trunk flexion during landing and cutting is associated with increased hip and knee flexion angles [52,53]. Core stability training has been shown to improve single-leg hop performance and reduce asymmetry between limbs [54], and similar effects have been observed in the upper limb [55]. However, in Mohammadi's study [54], symmetry was assessed between the injured and uninjured limb, with the performance of the injured limb approaching that of the uninjured one after the training period. We observed improvement only in the ND limb. It may be reasonable to draw a parallel between the disadvantaged condition of the limb and the similar gains reported in both studies in response to core stability training. The greater improvements in the ND limb's reach further underscore the asymmetrical adaptations that can occur due to habitual dominance in limb use. ND limbs are often less efficient in neuromuscular control, making them more responsive to proprioceptive and mobility stimuli [56]. Therefore, incorporating exercises such as the plank, particularly those involving a single-leg position (Figure 1b,d), may have enhanced limb stability. However, the functional asymmetries calculated through the LSI revealed no significant time × group interaction. This indicates that both training protocols had similar effects on inter-limb symmetry over the 8 week intervention period. The CTG showed a slightly greater numerical improvement in symmetry (+1.95%) compared to the MTG (+0.95%). While this pattern aligns with the observed improvement in ND limb performance in the CTG, the lack of statistical significance suggests this was not a consistent effect across all athletes. The unilateral components of the core training protocol may provide a stimulus for addressing asymmetries, but our study might have lacked the statistical power to possibly detect such an effect. Future studies with larger samples specifically targeting athletes with pre-existing asymmetries are needed to clarify this potential relationship. The lack of clear differential effects between the two training modalities, despite both groups showing significant improvements, has already been observed in youth athletic populations [57,58]. Several factors may explain this finding. First, the intervention duration of 8 weeks might have been sufficient to elicit general neuromuscular adaptations but insufficient for more specific, modality-dependent adaptations to fully manifest. Second, the outcome measures used are global performance tests, and they may not be sensitive enough to detect differences in the neuromuscular mechanisms targeted by core versus mobility training. While core training might enhance trunk stiffness, and mobility training might improve joint kinematics, both pathways could lead to a similar enhancement in overall dynamic performance during a complex task like the YBT or Agility T-Test. The principle of training specificity suggests that transfer to sport-specific skills is complex, and the relationship between isolated physical qualities like core strength or mobility and integrated athletic performance is not always direct [49]. Finally, in adolescent populations, who are highly responsive to any structured training stimulus, the mere introduction of a novel, supervised training regimen can produce significant gains, potentially overshadowing more subtle inter-modal differences.

Significant OST improvements were observed in both groups and remained robust after multiple comparisons correction. The MTG demonstrated a remarkably large relative improvement of 254.9%, compared to 115.5% in the CTG, though the between-group difference in change was not significant (0.58 points [−0.54, 1.71]). This is particularly relevant in athletic populations, such as basketball players, where optimal joint mobility is critical for performance and injury prevention. These findings are consistent with previous literature suggesting that dynamic and targeted mobility exercises can enhance functional movement patterns [59]. Furthermore, the OST, often used as a screening tool for movement quality and functional deficits, showed improvements aligned with increased neuromuscular control and joint mobility. This test is especially sensitive to limitations in thoracic spine extension, hip and ankle dorsiflexion, and core stability, all of which are crucial for the explosive and multidirectional movements required in basketball [19,21,22]. Moreover, squatting ability is essential to the biomechanics of an effective defensive stance or triple-threat position in basketball. Several studies have emphasized the relationship between OST performance and functional athletic outcomes. Sever et al. (2023) [60] demonstrated that the overhead deep squat was one of the most informative components of the Functional Movement Screen tool in assessing global movement quality in athletes. Athletes with higher OST scores demonstrated better biomechanical efficiency during sport-specific tasks. Also, Tee and colleagues supported the use of the Overhead Squat as a diagnostic tool for identifying mobility restrictions and movement compensation patterns [61]. The observed improvements in OST performance following the interventions may be attributed to enhanced neuromuscular coordination, which promotes more efficient motor unit recruitment and synchronization. This neuromuscular adaptation not only contributes to greater movement economy but also reinforces joint stability, which is essential in mitigating the risk of common sports injuries such as anterior cruciate ligament tears and ankle sprains [62]. Proprioceptive input and sensorimotor integration are enhanced through dynamic mobility training, fostering improved postural control and reflexive stability during complex athletic tasks [63]. Therefore, our findings reinforce the growing body of evidence that both traditional strength-based protocols and mobility-oriented training can positively influence lower-limb muscular function, joint integrity, and movement control. YBT posteromedial and posterolateral directions performance improved significantly in both groups under investigation. Notably, the MTG showed consistently larger relative improvements across all YBT directions (e.g., D PL: MTG +16.7% vs. CTG +8.5%), and the individual response plots (Figure 4) confirmed a highly consistent positive trend across nearly all participants in both groups. The YBT is a validated clinical tool and has been widely employed in both athletic and rehabilitative settings to identify deficits and predict injury risk. Specifically, the posteromedial and posterolateral directions are considered more challenging due to the diagonal movement patterns that require greater motor control, core activation, and proprioceptive integration than the anterior direction [36] and were utilized to assess neuromuscular characteristics, including dynamic balance and flexibility [47]. The improvement observed in both groups may be attributable to the focus on joint range of motion and neuromuscular facilitation that such exercises typically emphasize. Enhanced joint mobility, particularly at the hip, ankle, and thoracic spine segments directly stimulated in our mobility exercises, has been associated with improved sensorimotor control, which is critical for maintaining balance during dynamic tasks [51]. Hip mobility plays a central role in allowing the body to shift weight efficiently during single-leg stance tasks, while ankle dorsiflexion is essential for effective forward progression and stabilization [50]. Moreover, mobility exercises may stimulate proprioceptive mechanisms by involving end-range joint positions and controlled oscillatory movements that challenge the somatosensory and vestibular systems. Studies have shown that proprioceptive enhancement through mobility-focused training can significantly improve dynamic balance and reduce the risk of falls or injury, both in athletic [64] and pathological populations [65], and rebounding workouts have also been reported to induce rapid balance adaptations [66]. Data suggests that mobility and core training, stimulating proprioceptive pathways, and engaging complex motor patterns, may confer a functional advantage in tasks demanding multidirectional balance control, particularly in posterolateral and posteromedial movements, such as the frequent split stance during a basketball game, optimizing dynamic postural control. The Agility T-Test also showed significant improvement in both groups (mean differences CTG: 0.57, MTG: 0.70), corresponding to relative improvements of −4.0% and −4.8%, respectively. The between-group difference in change was minimal (−0.12 s [−0.87, 0.62]), indicating identical effects on agility and suggesting that enhancements in core stability or joint mobility may translate into faster and more coordinated changes in direction. Given that agility is a composite skill involving strength, coordination, and balance, the improvements across both interventions reinforce the idea that such training modalities can benefit athletic movement efficiency. In addition, given that previous studies have identified agility, assessed via the *t*-test, as a reliable predictor of playing time in comparable populations, the inclusion of such protocols may directly influence athletes' game performance [67,68]. Conversely, no significant changes were observed in any of the eight Functional Hop Test measures after FDR correction (all pFDR > 0.34), nor in static balance (BESS) or flexibility measures. This specificity of training effects suggests that 8 weeks of either core or mobility training provides sufficient stimulus for neuromuscular control adaptations but insufficient load or specificity for measurable improvements in explosive strength and power. This lack of improvement may be attributed to several interrelated factors, including the duration, intensity, and specificity of the intervention. Static balance is a multifaceted neuromuscular ability that involves the integration of sensory input from the visual, vestibular, and proprioceptive systems. Evidence suggests that improving balance, especially under static conditions, may require either a longer intervention period or training protocols specifically designed to challenge the postural control system. For example, Lesinski et al. performed a meta-analysis on balance training and highlighted that balance improvements are strongly moderated by the duration and intensity of the training, with interventions lasting between 11 and 12 weeks showing significantly larger effects on balance performance [69]. Thus, the 8 weeks of training in our study were probably not enough. Furthermore, BESS may not be sensitive enough to detect subtle changes over short timeframes, particularly in healthy individuals or athletic populations with already well-developed postural abilities. In this context, dynamic balance assessments, such as the YBT may offer greater sensitivity to neuromuscular adaptations induced by general training protocols like those mentioned previously. Improvements in tests such as SRT and Back Scratch are often more evident when the intervention includes regular and targeted stretching routines. According to Samson et al., flexibility (Sit-and-Reach performance) gains are best elicited through static stretching protocols lasting at least 30 s per muscle group, repeated 3 times, compared to the dynamic protocols [70]. If the intervention in question lacked dedicated stretching components or was of insufficient duration, it is unsurprising that no significant gains were detected. Similarly, horizontal jumping performance (hop tests) requires high levels of muscular strength, neuromuscular coordination, and explosive power. Significant improvements in such tests typically follow plyometric training regimens specifically tailored to the lower extremities. Markovic et al. underscore that plyometric training induces marked improvements in hopping ability, but only after sport-specific interventions [71]. Indeed, according to the principle of training specificity [72], athletes whose performance depends on generating force in the horizontal direction, such as sprinters and long jumpers, typically focus on plyometric training. In contrast, sports like basketball and volleyball demand vertical force production, primarily engaging in vertical jumping exercises. In the absence of such targeted exercises, global training interventions may not yield measurable changes in short-term hop performance. Moreover, plyometric exercise on an elastic surface has been shown to acutely decrease reactive power while maintaining leg stiffness [73], highlighting modality-specific adaptations of the stretch-shortening cycle.

Despite the meaningful findings, this study has limitations that must be acknowledged when interpreting the results. First and foremost, the absence of a true control group limits the ability to attribute observed improvements solely to the interventions applied. Including a control group in future studies would provide a more robust framework for causal inference. Secondly, the limited sample size, and the considerable inter-individual variability in responses, could indicate that the study may have been underpowered to reliably detect more subtle, modality-dependent effects even if supported by an a priori sample size calculation ($n = 34$ participants), the final analyzed sample (31 participants) was lower than the a priori sample size calculation required to adequately power the detection of a group-by-time interaction. This reduction in statistical power could increase the uncertainty of our null findings and limit definitive conclusions regarding the equivalence of the two interventions. For a transparent discussion of statistical power, between-group effect sizes (Cohen's d) with 95% confidence intervals were calculated for all outcomes. In addition, as demonstrated by comparable studies [5] in a highly similar population (20 basketball players, age: 15.70 ± 0.75 years) and intervention (core stability training group or the traditional strength training group), sample sizes around $n = 30$ are often sufficient to detect significant effects in this research domain. Our use of hierarchical FDR correction, while methodologically rigorous, may have been overly conservative for detecting subtle between-group differences. However, the complete absence of even nominal time × group interactions (all $p > 0.24$) across all outcome measures suggests that any undetected differential effects would likely be small and of limited practical significance. However, a small cohort raises concerns about the representativeness of the findings, particularly in populations as heterogeneous as youth athletes, where biological age, training history, and sport specialization may vary significantly. Larger, adequately powered studies are needed to confirm the findings and establish normative data across different sports and age groups. Another limitation is the short duration of the intervention and the lack of long-term follow-up. Without post-intervention monitoring over time, it is unclear whether the improvements observed are transient adaptations or reflect durable neuromuscular changes. Incorporating longitudinal designs and delayed retention testing in future research would help clarify the sustainability of training effects and their potential role in long-term athletic development.

5. Conclusions

Based on the consistent lack of significant time × group interactions across all statistical methods and the application of rigorous multiple comparisons correction, we conclude that both training programs were similarly effective at improving dynamic balance and functional movement quality in young basketball players. Therefore, the choice between these two training modalities can be based on practical considerations rather than presumed efficacy differences, such as athlete preference, equipment availability, or their specific integration into the overall training schedule. This study aims to inform coaches, strength and conditioning professionals, and sports scientists on the relative effectiveness of adding core and mobility interventions, thereby helping optimize training protocols for performance enhancement and injury prevention in youth basketball. By focusing on adolescents, a population in a crucial stage of motor development and injury vulnerability, this work contributes to the body of evidence supporting early intervention with functional training modalities. Future studies should explore combined interventions using a larger sample, a longer training period, and standardized outcomes to find possible differences between the effects of the two training modalities and improve comparability and better define their role in sports performance enhancement.

Supplementary Materials: The following supporting information can be downloaded at: https://www.mdpi.com/article/10.3390/sports13110398/s1, Table S1: Session completion and adherence rates for each participant ($n = 31$). Adherence was calculated as the percentage of completed sessions out of 24 scheduled sessions; Table S2: Homogeneity of Variances (Levene's Test) for All Outcome Measures at T0 and T1; Table S3: Results for the Group × Time Interaction and Main Effect of Time from Repeated Measures ANOVA; Table S4: Main Effect of Time Across Statistical Methods: Linear Mixed Models (LMM) and ANOVA with False Discovery Rate (FDR) Correction; Table S5: Within-subjects analysis. Pre- to Post-Intervention (T0–T1) Change Scores and Effect Sizes (Hedges' g_av) for Outcome Measures in the CTG and MTG Groups; Table S6: Between-Group Comparisons (CTG vs. MTG) for All Outcome Measures at Baseline (T0) and post-intervention (T1).

Author Contributions: Conceptualization, A.A., A.F. and C.C.; methodology, A.A., A.F. and C.C.; formal analysis, A.A.; investigation, M.T., M.P. and A.A.; writing—original draft preparation, A.A.; writing—review and editing, G.M., A.F. and C.C.; supervision, G.M. and C.C.; project administration, A.A., G.M. and C.C.; funding acquisition, A.A., A.F., C.C. and G.M. All authors have read and agreed to the published version of the manuscript.

Funding: This study was supported by the "PreRoF4 OA" project, funded by PIACERI 2024–2026, BIOMETEC, University of Catania, Italy.

Institutional Review Board Statement: The study was conducted in following the Declaration of Helsinki, and approved by the Scientific Committee of the 'Research Center on Motor Activities' at the University of Catania (Catania, Italy), protocol CRAM-57-2024, and approval date 17 July 2024.

Informed Consent Statement: Informed consent was signed by the participants' legal guardians and the adolescents themselves to participate in the study.

Data Availability Statement: Data available in a publicly accessible repository: The original data presented in the study are openly available at https://github.com/ccortis/DatayouthBB.git (accessed on 20 October 2025).

Acknowledgments: The authors would like to thank the coaches and the players of the "Sporting Club Adrano A.S.D" basketball team for participating in our study, for their dedication, professional attitude, and adherence to the protocols administered.

Conflicts of Interest: The authors declare no conflicts of interest.

Abbreviations

The following abbreviations are used in this manuscript:

CTG	core training group
MTG	mobility training group
BESS	balance error scoring system
YBT	y-balance test
OST	Overhead Squat test
SRT	Sit-and-Reach test
ANT	anterior reach
PL	posterolateral reach
PM	posteromedial reach
D	dominant limb
ND	non-dominant limb
M	mean
SD	standard deviation
MD	mean difference
NHE	Nordic hamstrings exercise
LSI	Limb Symmetry Index
FDR	False Discovery Rate

References

1. Petway, A.J.; Freitas, T.T.; Calleja-González, J.; Medina Leal, D.; Alcaraz, P.E. Training load and match-play demands in basketball based on competition level: A systematic review. *PLoS ONE* **2020**, *15*, e0229212. [CrossRef]
2. Amato, A.; Giustino, V.; Patti, A.; Proia, P.; Trivic, T.; Drid, P.; Obradovic, A.; Manojlovic, M.; Mondoni, M.; Paoli, A.; et al. Young basketball players have better manual dexterity performance than sportsmen and non-sportsmen of the same age: A cross-sectional study. *Sci. Rep.* **2023**, *13*, 20953. [CrossRef]

3. de Bruin, M.; Coetzee, D.; Schall, R. The relationship between core stability and athletic performance in female university athletes. *S. Afr. J. Sports Med.* **2021**, *33*, v33i31a10825. [CrossRef]
4. Hessam, M.; Fathalipour, K.; Behdarvandan, A.; Goharpey, S. The Effect of McGill Core Stability Training on Movement Patterns, Shooting Accuracy, and Throwing Performance in Male Basketball Players: A Randomized Controlled Trial. *J. Sport Rehabil.* **2023**, *32*, 296–304. [CrossRef] [PubMed]
5. Gong, J.; Gao, H.; Sui, J.; Qi, F. The effect of core stability training on the balance ability of young male basketball players. *Front. Physiol.* **2023**, *14*, 1305651. [CrossRef] [PubMed]
6. Liang, I.J.; Lin, L.L.; Huang, C.C. The Effects of Different Core Stability Training on Trunk Stability and Athletic Performance in Adolescent Female Basketball Players. *J. Sport Rehabil.* **2025**, *34*, 747–753. [CrossRef] [PubMed]
7. Sakai, Y.; Ito, H.; Egami, Y.; Ohoto, N.; Hijii, C.; Yanagawa, M.; Satoh, S.; Jingu, S. Favourable association of leg fat with cardiovascular risk factors. *J. Intern. Med.* **2005**, *257*, 194–200. [CrossRef]
8. Tazji, M.K.; Sadeghi, H.; Abbasi, A.; Aziminia, M.; Shahhosseini, A.; Marjani, M.E.; Koumantakis, G.A. The Effects of Core Stabilization Trunk Muscle Fatigue on Lower Limb Stiffness of Basketball Players. *Sports* **2023**, *11*, 200. [CrossRef]
9. Luo, S.; Soh, K.G.; Zhao, Y.; Soh, K.L.; Sun, H.; Nasiruddin, N.J.M.; Zhai, X.; Ma, L. Effect of core training on athletic and skill performance of basketball players: A systematic review. *PLoS ONE* **2023**, *18*, e0287379. [CrossRef]
10. Sasaki, S.; Tsuda, E.; Yamamoto, Y.; Maeda, S.; Kimura, Y.; Fujita, Y.; Ishibashi, Y. Core-Muscle Training and Neuromuscular Control of the Lower Limb and Trunk. *J. Athl. Train.* **2019**, *54*, 959–969. [CrossRef]
11. Spencer, S.; Wolf, A.; Rushton, A. Spinal-Exercise Prescription in Sport: Classifying Physical Training and Rehabilitation by Intention and Outcome. *J. Athl. Train.* **2016**, *51*, 613–628. [CrossRef]
12. Cook, G.; Burton, L.; Hoogenboom, B.J.; Voight, M. Functional movement screening: The use of fundamental movements as an assessment of function—Part 1. *Int. J. Sports Phys. Ther.* **2014**, *9*, 396–409. [PubMed]
13. Myer, G.D.; Kushner, A.M.; Brent, J.L.; Schoenfeld, B.J.; Hugentobler, J.; Lloyd, R.S.; Vermeil, A.; Chu, D.A.; Harbin, J.; McGill, S.M. The back squat: A proposed assessment of functional deficits and technical factors that limit performance. *Strength Cond. J.* **2014**, *36*, 4–27. [CrossRef] [PubMed]
14. Sople, D.; Wilcox, R.B. 3rd. Dynamic Warm-ups Play Pivotal Role in Athletic Performance and Injury Prevention. *Arthrosc. Sports Med. Rehabil.* **2025**, *7*, 101023. [CrossRef] [PubMed]
15. Antoranz, Y.; Sáez de Villarreal, E.; Del Campo Vecino, J.; Jiménez-Saiz, S.L. Sure Steps: Key Strategies for Protecting Basketball Players from Injuries-A Systematic Review. *J. Clin. Med.* **2024**, *13*, 4912. [CrossRef]
16. McGuine, T.A.; Greene, J.J.; Best, T.; Leverson, G. Balance as a predictor of ankle injuries in high school basketball players. *Clin. J. Sport Med.* **2000**, *10*, 239–244. [CrossRef]
17. Elias, L.J.; Bryden, M.P.; Bulman-Fleming, M.B. Footedness is a better predictor than is handedness of emotional lateralization. *Neuropsychologia* **1998**, *36*, 37–43. [CrossRef]
18. Efird, J. Blocked randomization with randomly selected block sizes. *Int. J. Environ. Res. Public Health* **2011**, *8*, 15–20. [CrossRef]
19. Read, P.J.; Hughes, J.; Stewart, P.; Chavda, S.; Bishop, C.; Edwards, M.; Turner, A.N. A Needs Analysis and Field-Based Testing Battery for Basketball. *Strength Cond. J.* **2014**, *36*, 13–20. [CrossRef]
20. Bird, S.P.; Markwick, W.J. Musculoskeletal Screening and Functional Testing: Considerations for Basketball Athletes. *Int. J. Sports Phys. Ther.* **2016**, *11*, 784–802.
21. Post, E.G.; Olson, M.; Trigsted, S.; Hetzel, S.; Bell, D.R. The Reliability and Discriminative Ability of the Overhead Squat Test for Observational Screening of Medial Knee Displacement. *J. Sport Rehabil.* **2017**, *26*, 1–14. [CrossRef] [PubMed]
22. McMillian, D.J.; Rynders, Z.G.; Trudeau, T.R. Modifying the Functional Movement Screen Deep Squat Test: The Effect of Foot and Arm Positional Variations. *J. Strength Cond. Res.* **2016**, *30*, 973–979. [CrossRef] [PubMed]
23. Minick, K.I.; Kiesel, K.B.; Burton, L.; Taylor, A.; Plisky, P.; Butler, R.J. Interrater Reliability of the Functional Movement Screen. *J. Strength Cond. Res.* **2010**, *24*, 479–486. [CrossRef] [PubMed]
24. Rikli, R.E.; Jones, C.J. Development and validation of a functional fitness test for community-residing older adults. *J. Aging Phys. Act.* **1999**, *7*, 129–161. [CrossRef]
25. Aparicio, V.A.; Marín-Jiménez, N.; Castro-Piñero, J.; Flor-Alemany, M.; Coll-Risco, I.; Baena-García, L. Association between Flexibility, Measured with the Back-Scratch Test, and the Odds of Oxytocin Administration during Labour and Caesarean Section. *J. Clin. Med.* **2024**, *13*, 5245. [CrossRef]
26. Ayala, F.; Sainz de Baranda, P.; De Ste Croix, M.; Santonja, F. Reproducibility and criterion-related validity of the sit and reach test and toe touch test for estimating hamstring flexibility in recreationally active young adults. *Phys. Ther. Sport* **2012**, *13*, 219–226. [CrossRef]
27. Petrigna, L.; Trovato, B.; Roggio, F.; Zanghì, M.; Sortino, M.; Amato, A.; Musumeci, G. A standard operating procedure proposal for the warm-up of sit and reach test in young adults. *J. Sports Med. Phys. Fit.* **2025**, *65*, 729–734. [CrossRef]
28. Semenick, D. Tests and Measurements: The T-test. *Natl. Strength Cond. Assoc. J.* **1990**, *12*, 36. [CrossRef]

29. Pauole, K.; Madole, K.; Garhammer, J.; Lacourse, M.; Rozenek, R. Reliability and Validity of the T-Test as a Measure of Agility, Leg Power, and Leg Speed in College-Aged Men and Women. *J. Strength Cond. Res.* **2000**, *14*, 443–450.
30. Alemdaroğlu, U. The relationship between muscle strength, anaerobic performance, agility, sprint ability and vertical jump performance in professional basketball players. *J. Hum. Kinet.* **2012**, *31*, 149–158. [CrossRef]
31. Riemann, B.L.; Guskiewicz, K.M.; Shields, E.W. Relationship between Clinical and Forceplate Measures of Postural Stability. *J. Sport Rehabil.* **1999**, *8*, 71–82. [CrossRef]
32. Bell, D.R.; Guskiewicz, K.M.; Clark, M.A.; Padua, D.A. Systematic review of the balance error scoring system. *Sports Health* **2011**, *3*, 287–295. [CrossRef]
33. Bressel, E.; Yonker, J.C.; Kras, J.; Heath, E.M. Comparison of static and dynamic balance in female collegiate soccer, basketball, and gymnastics athletes. *J. Athl. Train.* **2007**, *42*, 42.
34. Plisky, P.J.; Gorman, P.P.; Butler, R.J.; Kiesel, K.B.; Underwood, F.B.; Elkins, B. The reliability of an instrumented device for measuring components of the star excursion balance test. *N. Am. J. Sports Phys. Ther.* **2009**, *4*, 92–99. [PubMed]
35. Fullam, K.; Caulfield, B.; Coughlan, G.F.; Delahunt, E. Kinematic analysis of selected reach directions of the Star Excursion Balance Test compared with the Y-Balance Test. *J. Sport Rehabil.* **2014**, *23*, 27–35. [CrossRef] [PubMed]
36. Plisky, P.J.; Rauh, M.J.; Kaminski, T.W.; Underwood, F.B. Star Excursion Balance Test as a predictor of lower extremity injury in high school basketball players. *J. Orthop. Sports Phys. Ther.* **2006**, *36*, 911–919. [CrossRef] [PubMed]
37. Ross, M.D.; Langford, B.; Whelan, P.J. Test-retest reliability of 4 single-leg horizontal hop tests. *J. Strength Cond. Res.* **2002**, *16*, 617–622.
38. Fitzgerald, G.K.; Lephart, S.M.; Hwang, J.H.; Wainner, M.R.S. Hop tests as predictors of dynamic knee stability. *J. Orthop. Sport Phys.* **2001**, *31*, 588–597. [CrossRef]
39. Myers, B.A.; Jenkins, W.L.; Killian, C.; Rundquist, P. Normative data for hop tests in high school and collegiate basketball and soccer players. *Int. J. Sports Phys. Ther.* **2014**, *9*, 596.
40. Kramer, J.F.; Nusca, D.; Fowler, P.; Webster-Bogaert, S. Test-retest reliability of the one-leg hop test following ACL reconstruction. *Clin. J. Sport Med.* **1992**, *2*, 240–243. [CrossRef]
41. Bolgla, L.A.; Keskula, D.R. Reliability of lower extremity functional performance tests. *J. Orthop. Sport Phys.* **1997**, *26*, 138–142. [CrossRef] [PubMed]
42. Slade, S.C.; Dionne, C.E.; Underwood, M.; Buchbinder, R. Consensus on Exercise Reporting Template (CERT): Explanation and Elaboration Statement. *Brit J. Sport Med.* **2016**, *50*, 1428–1437. [CrossRef] [PubMed]
43. Sansone, P.; Conte, D.; Tessitore, A.; Rampinini, E.; Ferioli, D. A Systematic Review on the Physical, Physiological, Perceptual, and Technical-Tactical Demands of Official 3 × 3 Basketball Games. *Int. J. Sports Physiol. Perform.* **2023**, *18*, 1233–1245. [CrossRef] [PubMed]
44. Ekstrom, R.A.; Donatelli, R.A.; Carp, K.C. Electromyographic analysis of core trunk, hip, and thigh muscles during 9 rehabilitation exercises. *J. Orthop. Sports Phys. Ther.* **2007**, *37*, 754–762. [CrossRef]
45. Narouei, S.; Imai, A.; Akuzawa, H.; Hasebe, K.; Kaneoka, K. Hip and trunk muscles activity during nordic hamstring exercise. *J. Exerc. Rehabil.* **2018**, *14*, 231–238. [CrossRef]
46. Mok, N.W.; Yeung, E.W.; Cho, J.C.; Hui, S.C.; Liu, K.C.; Pang, C.H. Core muscle activity during suspension exercises. *J. Sci. Med. Sport* **2015**, *18*, 189–194. [CrossRef]
47. Benis, R.; Bonato, M.; La Torre, A. Elite female basketball players' body-weight neuromuscular training and performance on the Y-balance test. *J. Athl. Train.* **2016**, *51*, 688–695. [CrossRef]
48. Kulas, A.S.; Hortobágyi, T.; Devita, P. The interaction of trunk-load and trunk-position adaptations on knee anterior shear and hamstrings muscle forces during landing. *J. Athl. Train.* **2010**, *45*, 5–15. [CrossRef]
49. Prieske, O.; Muehlbauer, T.; Granacher, U. The Role of Trunk Muscle Strength for Physical Fitness and Athletic Performance in Trained Individuals: A Systematic Review and Meta-Analysis. *Sports Med.* **2016**, *46*, 401–419. [CrossRef]
50. Basnett, C.R.; Hanish, M.J.; Wheeler, T.J.; Miriovsky, D.J.; Danielson, E.L.; Barr, J.B.; Grindstaff, T.L. Ankle dorsiflexion range of motion influences dynamic balance in individuals with chronic ankle instability. *Int. J. Sports Phys. Ther.* **2013**, *8*, 121–128.
51. Dominguez-Navarro, F.; Casaña, J.; Perez-Dominguez, B.; Ricart-Luna, B.; Cotolí-Suárez, P.; Calatayud, J. Dynamic balance and explosive strength appears to better explain single leg hop test results among young elite female basketball athletes. *Sci. Rep.* **2023**, *13*, 5476. [CrossRef]
52. Blackburn, J.T.; Padua, D.A. Influence of trunk flexion on hip and knee joint kinematics during a controlled drop landing. *Clin. Biomech.* **2008**, *23*, 313–319. [CrossRef]
53. Nagano, Y.; Ida, H.; Akai, M.; Fukubayashi, T. Relationship between three-dimensional kinematics of knee and trunk motion during shuttle run cutting. *J. Sports Sci.* **2011**, *29*, 1525–1534. [CrossRef]
54. Fallah Mohammadi, M.; Dashti Rostami, K.; Shabanzadeh, S.; Hosseininejad, S.E.; Ghaffari, S.; Thomas, A. Does core stability training improve hopping performance and kinetic asymmetries during single-leg landing in anterior cruciate ligament reconstructed patients? *Res. Sports Med.* **2024**, *32*, 268–278. [CrossRef] [PubMed]

55. Papale, O.; Di Rocco, F.; Festino, E.; Gammino, V.; Cortis, C.; Fusco, A. Do Hand Exercises Influence Physiological Hand Tremor? An Observational Cohort Study on Healthy Young Adults. *Appl. Sci.* **2024**, *14*, 4467. [CrossRef]
56. Han, J.; Anson, J.; Waddington, G.; Adams, R. Proprioceptive performance of bilateral upper and lower limb joints: Side-general and site-specific effects. *Exp. Brain Res.* **2013**, *226*, 313–323. [CrossRef] [PubMed]
57. Moran, J.; Sandercock, G.; Ramirez-Campillo, R.; Clark, C.C.T.; Fernandes, J.F.T.; Drury, B. A Meta-Analysis of Resistance Training in Female Youth: Its Effect on Muscular Strength, and Shortcomings in the Literature. *Sports Med.* **2018**, *48*, 1661–1671. [CrossRef]
58. Barker, A.; Lloyd, R.S.; Buchheit, M.; Williams, C.; Oliver, J. The BASES expert statement on trainability during childhood and adolescence. *Sport Exerc. Sci.* **2014**, *41*, 22–23.
59. Page, P. Current concepts in muscle stretching for exercise and rehabilitation. *Int. J. Sports Phys. Ther.* **2012**, *7*, 109–119.
60. Sever, O.; Kır, R.; Baykal, C.; Akyildiz, Z.; Nobari, H. Overhead squat assessment reflects treadmill running kinematics. *BMC Sports Sci. Med. Rehabil.* **2023**, *15*, 118. [CrossRef]
61. Tee, J.C.; Klingbiel, J.F.; Collins, R.; Lambert, M.I.; Coopoo, Y. Preseason Functional Movement Screen component tests predict severe contact injuries in professional rugby union players. *J. Strength Cond. Res.* **2016**, *30*, 3194–3203. [CrossRef]
62. Hibbs, A.E.; Thompson, K.G.; French, D.; Wrigley, A.; Spears, I. Optimizing performance by improving core stability and core strength. *Sports Med.* **2008**, *38*, 995–1008. [CrossRef] [PubMed]
63. Paillard, T. Effects of general and local fatigue on postural control: A review. *Neurosci. Biobehav. Rev.* **2012**, *36*, 162–176. [CrossRef] [PubMed]
64. Wang, P.; Liu, Y.; Chen, C. Effects of neuromuscular training on dynamic balance ability in athletes: A systematic review and meta-analysis. *Heliyon* **2024**, *10*, e35823. [CrossRef] [PubMed]
65. Proia, P.; Amato, A.; Puleo, R.; Arnetta, F.; Rizzo, F.; Di Grigoli, L.; Zangla, D.; Schirò, G.; Ragonese, P.; Messina, G. Efficacy of 12 weeks of proprioceptive training in patients with multiple sclerosis. *J. Hum. Sport Exerc.* **2019**, *14*, S1986–S1992. [CrossRef]
66. De Maio, M.; Di Rocco, F.; Papale, O.; Festino, E.; Fusco, A.; Cortis, C. Could Mini-Trampoline Training Be Considered as a New Strategy to Reduce Asymmetries? *Appl. Sci.* **2023**, *13*, 3193. [CrossRef]
67. Hoare, D.G. Predicting success in junior elite basketball players--the contribution of anthropometic and physiological attributes. *J. Sci. Med. Sport* **2000**, *3*, 391–405. [CrossRef]
68. Ben Abdelkrim, N.; Castagna, C.; Jabri, I.; Battikh, T.; El Fazaa, S.; Ati, J.E. Activity Profile and Physiological Requirements of Junior Elite Basketball Players in Relation to Aerobic-Anaerobic Fitness. *J. Strength Cond. Res.* **2010**, *24*, 2330–2342. [CrossRef]
69. Lesinski, M.; Hortobágyi, T.; Muehlbauer, T.; Gollhofer, A.; Granacher, U. Effects of Balance Training on Balance Performance in Healthy Older Adults: A Systematic Review and Meta-analysis. *Sports Med.* **2015**, *45*, 1721–1738. [CrossRef]
70. Samson, M.; Button, D.C.; Chaouachi, A.; Behm, D.G. Effects of dynamic and static stretching within general and activity specific warm-up protocols. *J. Sports Sci. Med.* **2012**, *11*, 279–285.
71. Markovic, G.; Mikulic, P. Neuro-musculoskeletal and performance adaptations to lower-extremity plyometric training. *Sports Med.* **2010**, *40*, 859–895. [CrossRef]
72. Sale, D.G. Neural adaptation to resistance training. *Med. Sci. Sports Exerc.* **1988**, *20*, S135–S145. [CrossRef]
73. Di Rocco, F.; Papale, O.; Festino, E.; De Maio, M.; Cortis, C.; Fusco, A. Acute Effects of Mini Trampoline Training Session on Leg Stiffness and Reactive Power. *Appl. Sci.* **2023**, *13*, 9865. [CrossRef]

sports

MDPI

Article

Warming Up for Basketball: Comparing Traditional vs. Small-Sided Game Approaches in Youth Players

Pierpaolo Sansone [1], Massimiliano Vanacore [2], Jorge Lorenzo-Calvo [3], Álvaro Bustamante-Sánchez [4], Alejandro Vaquera [5] and Daniele Conte [2,6,*]

1 Department of Education and Sport Sciences, Pegaso Telematic University, Centro Direzionale Isola F2, 80143 Naples, Italy; pierpaolo.sansone@unipegaso.it
2 Department of Movement Human and Health Sciences, University of Rome "Foro Italico", 00135 Rome, Italy; massimiliano.vanacore00@gmail.com
3 Deporte y Entrenamiento Research Group, Facultad de Ciencias de la Actividad Física y del Deporte, Universidad Politécnica de Madrid, 28040 Madrid, Spain; jorge.lorenzo@upm.es
4 Department of Sports Sciences, Faculty of Medicine, Health and Sports, Universidad Europea de Madrid, C/Tajo, s/n, Villaviciosa de Odón, 28670 Madrid, Spain; alvaro.bustamante@universidadeuropea.es
5 VALFIS Research Group, Institute of Biomedicine (IBIOMED), Faculty of Sciences of Physical Activity and Sports, University of León, 24007 León, Spain; avaqj@unileon.es
6 Department of Coaching Science, Lithuanian Sports University, 44221 Kaunas, Lithuania
* Correspondence: daniele.conte@uniroma4.it

Abstract: This study compared the external [movement load (ML)] and internal [rating of perceived exertion (RPE), mean and peak heart rate (HRmean, HRpeak)] loads, performance and enjoyment between time-matched (~12 min) traditional (TRAD) and small-sided game (SSG) warm-ups in youth basketball players. Using a counterbalanced crossover design, 24 male players (16.0 $\pm$ 0.1 years) performed both warm-up types after reporting fatigue (ROF) and completing an 8 min standardized pre-warm-up. Before and after each warm-up, players completed 20 m sprint and countermovement jump (CMJ) tests; enjoyment (ENJ) was assessed post-warm-up. No significant differences were found between warm-ups for ROF ($p = 0.053$), RPE ($p = 0.259$), or HRmean ($p = 0.053$). However, SSG induced a higher HRpeak than TRAD ($p = 0.001$), while ML was greater in TRAD ($p < 0.001$). No interaction, time effect, or typology effect emerged for performance in sprinting and change of direction, although CMJ was higher after TRAD ($p = 0.047$). Enjoyment did not differ significantly ($p = 0.066$), although with a large effect size (r = 0.612). The greater ML in TRAD may reflect more dynamic basketball actions compared with SSG, which emphasized static tasks (e.g., screening, boxing out) yet produced higher HRpeak. Coaches may consider SSG warm-ups to replicate game-specific conditions while controlling the external load and maintaining adequate physiological preparation.

Keywords: basketball performance; internal load; external load; youth athletes

1. Introduction

Basketball is a high-intensity, stochastic, court-based team sport with considerable physical and physiological demands [1]. During competition, basketball players are required to perform a variety of multiplanar movements, including sprints, jumps, decelerations, and static exertions, while also scanning the dynamic technical–tactical scenario and controlling the ball [1–3]. It is therefore evident that the demands of basketball games posit significant physical, physiological, technical–tactical and perceptual–cognitive demands on players.

In order to appropriately prepare basketball players for training and competition, warm-up procedures are an essential step [4,5]. Warm-up activities encompass a variety of training modalities, including general and specific mobility drills, injury prevention exercises, neuromuscular activation and strength, basketball-specific actions such as jumping, shuffling and changes of direction, technical actions such as dribbling, passing and shooting, and reactive, open-skill drills [4]. The progressive implementation of these varied exercises aims at closely replicating the diversified demands of the subsequent performance environment (i.e., training and games), optimizing players' readiness and minimizing injury risk [6,7]. These benefits are obtained through a variety of mechanisms, including increased core temperature, improved oxygen uptake kinetics, post-activation performance enhancement and cognitive priming [6,8].

Previous basketball studies have described the effectiveness of warm up strategies on subsequent player's performance, showing that the inclusion of mobility, strength, plyometrics and reactive agility exercise can improve the players' jumping and sprinting capacities [9,10]. While basketball literature is abundant on physical-oriented warm-up procedures, less is known about the effects of more sport-specific warm-ups. In fact, basketball games are a dynamic, open-skill environment in which players' performance is not solely determined by physical qualities. Basketball games require players to perform around 200 ball possessions requiring continuous assessment of the technical–tactical scenarios, decision-making and response inhibition to optimally perform and avoid errors [2,11]. In fact, a recent survey on basketball warm-up practices evidenced how basketball-specific drills are the most used activities in pre-game warm-ups at national and international competitive levels [4]. Among the available training modalities, small-sided games (SSGs) might be a quite valuable choice for basketball warm-up. SSGs are typically implemented because they closely replicate the competitive scenarios from several perspectives: physical, physiological, technical–tactical and cognitive [12]. During SSGs, team sport players are immersed in an environment that is closely resemblant of the real games, therefore requiring them to perform specific movements at high intensity while also performing technical–tactical actions which are characteristic of the sport. While basketball studies have described the demands of different SSGs, demonstrating their high relevance and specificity [12,13], little is known on the effectiveness of SSGs as a warm-up procedure to appropriately prepare basketball players to compete. While previous studies have shown that SSGs induce improvements in jumping, sprinting and change of direction in soccer [14,15] and handball [16] players, which suggest their efficacy as a warm-up strategy, to the best of the author's knowledge no study has examined SSG warm-ups in basketball settings. Therefore, the aim of this study was to compare the effects of traditional (TRAD) and small-sided game (SSG) warm-up protocols on external and internal loads, physical performance and enjoyment levels in youth basketball players.

2. Materials and Methods

2.1. Participants

Twenty-four male basketball players from two under-17 teams (twelve per team) competing in the top-tier Italian Basketball Federation (FIP) championship took part in the study (age: 16.0 ± 0.1 years; stature: 1.82 ± 0.07 m; body mass: 73.8 ± 9.1 kg; playing experience: 8.6 ± 3.1 years). An a priori power analysis determined a minimum sample size of 11 players (α = 0.05, β = 0.95, effect size = 1.23), based on previous research comparing warm-up protocols in elite handball players [16]. All players were free from injuries affecting performance in the month before testing. The study was approved by the University of Rome "Foro Italico" ethics committee (CAR. 192/2024).

2.2. Design

This study encompassed a randomized cross-over design, in which participants performed physical tests before and after two different warm-up typologies: traditional (TRAD) and small-sided games (SSG). The full experimental protocol was carried out one to two weeks after the completion of the in-season period. The 24 players were divided into groups of 6 based on coaching staff's suggestions to create balanced teams for the SSGs. Each group was composed of four guards, as well as small forward (positions 1-2 and 3) and two power forward and/or center (positions 4-5). The two protocols were completed on two separate testing days, approximately one week apart. The order of warm-up strategies was randomized and counterbalanced. Furthermore, a familiarization session was conducted during the preceding week, in which players were introduced to the testing procedures, rating scales, and both warm-up protocols.

The structure of each experimental session (TRAD and SSG) is displayed in Figure 1. The experimental sessions were preceded by an 8 min introductory warm-up, performed without the use of the ball and supervised by a strength and conditioning coach accredited by the Italian Basketball Federation. Following this, after ~2.5 min of recovery, players completed countermovement jump (CMJ) and 20 m sprint tests, which served as baseline values. They then performed one of the two warm-up protocols, each lasting approximately 12 min. At the conclusion of these protocols, and after ~2.5 min of recovery, players were re-assessed using the CMJ test, the 20 m sprint test, and the change of direction test (5-0-5). The recovery period of 2.5 min was selected based on a detailed analysis of basketball competition, which demonstrated that this interval typically corresponds to the time between the conclusion of the warm-up and the commencement of official matches.

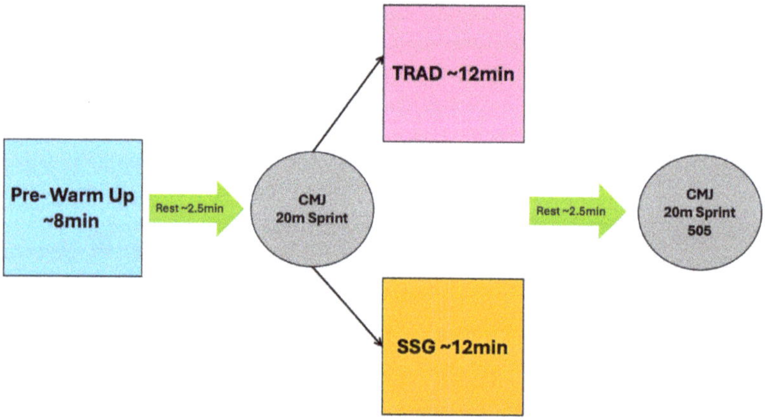

Figure 1. Study design. Note: TRAD = traditional warm-up; SSG = small-sided game warm-up; CMJ = Countermovement Jump Test; 505 = 505 test.

2.3. Procedures

2.3.1. Warm-Up Typologies

The pre-warm-up was structured to follow a progressive sequence of movements, commencing with ground-based exercises and subsequently advancing to upright activities (Supplementary Tables S1 and S2). The proposed exercises were designed in accordance with evidence-based recommendations for warm-up protocols reported in the literature [6,17,18]. The session was divided into two primary components: Pillar Preparation, including as a series of exercises aimed at enhancing joint mobility and stability of the major kinetic segments, and Movement Preparation, consisting of dynamic stretching drills and sport-specific locomotor patterns. Collectively, these exercises were intended to elicit neuromuscular readiness and to prepare athletes for acceleration, jumping, and change-of-direction demands typically observed during competitive play or, in this case, during motor performance testing.

The traditional warm-up (Figure 2) was designed to reflect the activity commonly performed by youth basketball teams during pre-game routines. It was performed on a half-court by one of the two groups of six players and consisted of four drills:

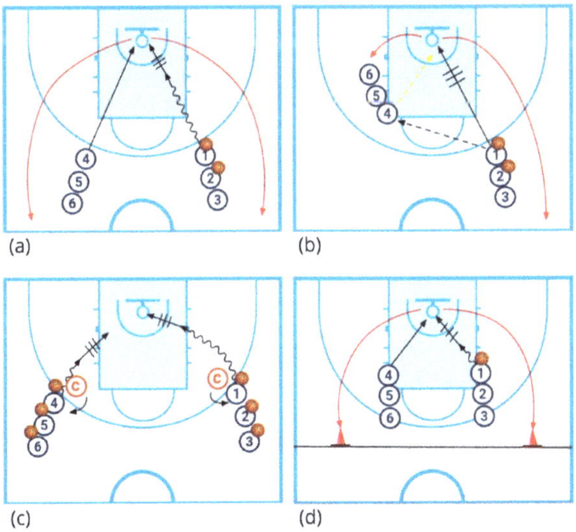

Figure 2. Exercises performed during the traditional warm-up: (**a**) lay-up drill; (**b**) "give-and-go" drill; (**c**) dribble and shot decision drill; (**d**) fast lay-up drill without dribbling. Symbols ⟶: off-ball run; - - ➜: ball pass; — — ➜: give-and-go pass; ∿➜: movements while dribbling the ball; ⟶: shooting; ↘: switch lines; Ⓒ: coach; ① players without ball; ① players with ball.

(1) Lay-up drill: Players are divided into two lines at the wing positions, with three players on the right wing and three on the left wing. The first player in the right-hand line begins by dribbling the ball and finishing with a layup. Simultaneously, the corresponding player from the left line collects the rebound, passes the ball to the next player in the right-hand line, and joins that line. The shooter rotates to the opposite line. The drill lasts a total of 4 min, 1 min and 30 s per side, with 30 s allocated for switching sides.

(2) Give-and-go drill: Three players line up at the right-wing position and three at the left elbow. The first player on the right wing passes the ball to the first player at the left elbow and then cuts toward the basket. The cutter receives a return pass and completes the action with either a layup or a mid-range jump shot. The passer at the elbow grabs the rebound and joins the right-wing line after passing the ball to the next player in that line. The shooter rotates to the elbow line. The drill lasts three minutes in total, with approximately 1 min and 20 s per side and 20 s for switching sides.

(3) Dribble and shot decision drill: Each player has a ball and positions themselves at the extended elbow, with three players per side. Two staff members act as passive defenders, standing in front of the first player in each line. Players initiate their move based on the space left open by the staff member, selecting the appropriate finishing option. If the area near the basket is occupied, the player executes a mid-range shot; if it is free, the

player drives to the basket and finishes with a layup or another solution. The drill lasts 3 min in total, divided into 1 min and 20 s per side, plus time for switching lines.

(4) Fast lay-up drill without dribbling: The initial setup of the first drill is reused for this final drill. In this variation, players are not permitted to dribble before executing the layup, making it a faster-paced activity typically performed immediately before tip-off. The rebounder passes the ball to the next player for the layup, then sprints to the sideline near the bench area before returning to perform another layup. This drill lasts two minutes in total, divided into one minute per side.

The SSG warm-up (Figure 3) was structured to provide a situational progression, moving from 1v1 to 3v3. This warm-up was performed on a half-court by one of the two groups of six players, simultaneously with the TRAD warm-up conducted on the opposite half-court. It consisted of three drills with a total duration of approximately twelve minutes:

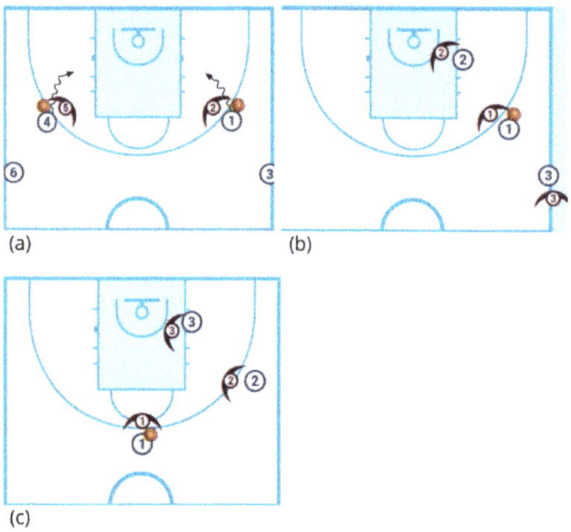

Figure 3. Exercises included in the SSG (small-sided game) warm-up: (**a**) 1v1; (**b**) 2v2; (**c**) 3v3. Symbols ①: offensive player without ball; ① offensive player with ball. ①: defensive player; : movements while dribbling the ball.

(1) 1v1: The six players are divided into two groups of three on each wing. The first pairs on each side begin playing 1v1 from the wing position simultaneously. After the initial possession, the offensive player becomes the defender, while the waiting player (the third in line) rotates in as the new offensive player. The defender from the first possession rests until the second possession concludes, at which point they become the offensive player in the subsequent sequence. Two constraints were imposed on the offense: (1) ball handling was limited to a maximum of four dribbles to regulate the duration of each 1v1 action, and (2) players were forbidden from crossing the imaginary midline extending from the basket to midcourt. This rotation continues for two minutes per side before switching wings for an additional two minutes.

(2) 2v2: Players are paired according to playing positions, forming three balanced pairs by role. The first team begins on offense against the second team, with the offensive setup consisting of a ball-handler at the wing and a teammate positioned at the low post. Following the first possession, the defensive team rests until the conclusion of the next possession, while the third team (waiting during the first possession) becomes the offensive team in the second sequence. The initial offensive team switches to defense in the second possession. This offense–defense rotation continues for four minutes, with the low-post position alternating sides whenever teams return on offense. Players were encouraged to

incorporate pick-and-roll actions during this SSG drill and were free to include any type of defense.

(3) 3v3: The six players are divided into two teams of three, competing in 3v3 with offense and defense alternating after each possession. Play begins with the offensive players positioned at the top (point guard), wing, and low post on the same side. In the following offensive sequence, the alignment shifts to the opposite wing and low-post side. If no basket is scored, play continues through both offensive and defensive rebounding. The drill lasts a total of five minutes, consisting of two minutes of play and one minute of passive rest, followed by another two minutes of play. After each scored basket, teams are allowed a five-second recovery, included within the total drill duration.

2.3.2. Load Monitoring

Each warm-up protocol was monitored using both external and internal load measures. For the assessment of external load, Firstbeat Sport Sensors (Firstbeat, Yliothispistonkatu, Finland) equipped with a triaxial accelerometer sampling at 50 Hz were employed. Specifically, values for Movement Load and Movement Intensity (both expressed in arbitrary units [A.U.]) were calculated over the duration of each warm-up protocol (TRAD and SSG). Movement Load was derived using a previously described formula, which accounts for accelerations across the three axes [19]. Movement Intensity was defined as the mean Movement Load per minute.

For the evaluation of internal load, the same devices were used with a sampling frequency of 1 s. The collected data were subsequently downloaded and processed via the proprietary software. Objective measures of internal load included average heart rate (average HR) and peak heart rate (peak HR), as recorded by the Firstbeat system. In addition, subjective internal load was assessed using the Rating of Perceived Exertion (RPE), based on the modified CR10 scale proposed by Foster et al. (2001) [20]. RPE data were collected at the conclusion of each warm-up protocol, with participants individually reporting their values in the presence of the research team, ensuring that responses were provided without influence from other athletes.

2.3.3. Performance Tests

The CMJ test with arm swing was used to assess jumping performance through the Optojump system (Optojump, Microgate, Bolzano, Italy). Players started in the erect standing position (with feet placed hip-width to shoulder-width apart) and were instructed to jump "as high and as fast as possible" [21] using a self-selected countermovement depth. Players performed two trials, separated by ~2 min of passive rest, with the highest jump achieved at each time point being used for analysis [21]. Excellent test–retest reliability has been previously shown for this procedure [22]. Furthermore, maximal sprint performance over 10 m and 20 m was assessed using a 20 m sprint test with a 10 m split using three sets of timing gates (Racetime 2 Light Radio Kit, Microgate, Bolzano, Italy) positioned 0, 10, and 20 m from the start line [23]. Moreover, change of direction (COD) ability was assessed using the 505 test employing the same timing gate system described above positioned 10 m from the starting line, with cones placed at the 15 m mark [24]. Participants sprinted from the start, passed through the timing gates, continued to the cones, executed a 180° turn, and then sprinted back through the timing gates [24]. The time taken to cover the distance from the 10 m gate to the 15 m cones and back to the 10 m gate was recorded as the 505 COD performance.

2.3.4. Perceived Fatigue and Enjoyment

The overall perception of fatigue was asked to each player before each experimental session using the previously validated Rating-of-Fatigue (ROF) scale [25], ranging between

0 ("not fatigued at all") and 10 ("total fatigue and exhaustion—nothing left"). This scale was also previously used with basketball athletes [26]. Additionally, a previously validated scale was adopted to assess players' enjoyment levels on a 1–7 Likert scale [27] at the end of each warm-up typology. This scale was previously used in basketball athletes [28].

2.4. Statistical Analysis

For each dependent variable analyzed with parametric statistics, means and standard deviations were calculated as descriptive statistics. Successively, linear mixed models were employed to analyze jump (CMJ) and sprint (10 and 20 m) performance, with two independent variables: (1) warm-up type (TRAD vs. SSG) and (2) time (pre- vs. post-warm-up). Due to technical sampling issues, sprint data were available for only 12 players (one team). For the 505 test results and for external and internal workload measures (movement load, movement intensity, average HR, peak HR), linear mixed models were also applied, but including only one independent variable (warm-up type). In all models, "player" was specified as a random effect. The LMM analyses were run using the Jamovi software (version 2.3.21, retrieved from https://www.jamovi.org accessed on 28 August 2025). The t statistics calculated from the LMM were then converted into Cohen d effect sizes and associated 95% CI using the RStudio software (version 4.2.1). Effect sizes were interpreted as follows: <0.2, trivial; 0.20 to 0.59, small; 0.60 to 1.19, moderate; 1.2 to 1.99, large; and ≥2.0, very large [29].

For the perceptual measures RPE, ROF, and ENJ, differences between the two warm-up types were analyzed using the Wilcoxon signed-rank test (non-parametric analysis) and descriptive statistics were calculated with median and interquartile range. The non-parametric analysis was calculated using the Jamovi software previously described. Moreover, effect sizes for pairwise comparison were calculated using the r-value [30] and were interpreted according to Cohen's benchmarks as no effect (0–0.09); small (0.10–0.29); medium (0.30–0.49); and large (≥0.5) [31]. For all statistical tests, the significance level was set at $p < 0.05$.

3. Results

TRAD warm-up showed higher movement load [$p < 0.001$; ES(95%CI) = 1.54 (0.88; 2.20); large] and movement intensity [$p < 0.001$; ES(95%CI) = 1.80 (1.11; 2.48); large] compared to SSG warm-up (Figure 4).

Conversely, higher HRpeak [$p = 0.001$; ES(95%CI) = −1.07; (−1.69; −0.46); moderate] was found in SSG compared to TRAD warm-up. Moreover, moderately higher HRmean [ES(95%CI) = −0.61 (−1.20; −0.01)] was found also in SSG compared to TRAD warm-up, although with no statistical difference ($p = 0.053$) (Figure 5).

The analysis of RPE showed no significant difference between the two warm-up typologies ($p = 0.259$; r = 0.270; small) (Figure 6).

Considering performance tests, no differences were evident between conditions for each physical test, except for higher CMJ values [$p = 0.047$; ES(95%CI) = −0.58 (−1.16; −0.01), small] found in TRAD compared to SSG warm-up (Table 1).

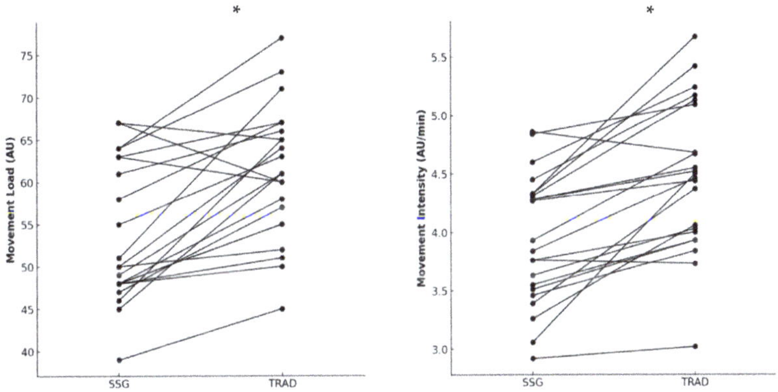

Figure 4. Differences in movement load and movement intensity between small-sided game (SSG) and traditional (TRAD) warm-up. Note: * indicates $p < 0.001$.

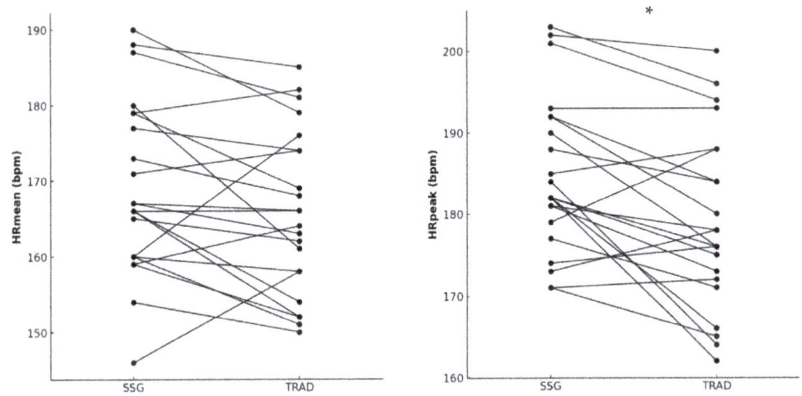

Figure 5. Differences in mean heart rate (HRmean) and peak heart rate (HRpeak) between small-sided game (SSG) and traditional (TRAD) warm-up. Note: * indicates $p = 0.001$.

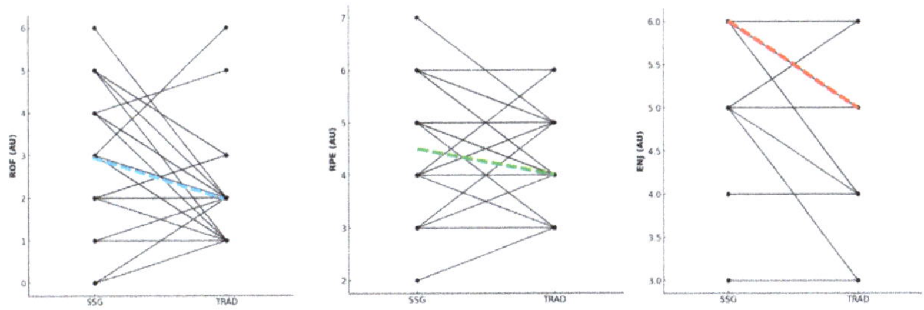

Figure 6. Differences in rate of fatigue (ROF), rating of perceived exertion (RPE) and enjoyment (ENJ) between small-sided game (SSG) and traditional (TRAD) warm-up. Note: dashed lines indicate the connection between the median values.

Table 1. Mean SD for jumping and sprinting performances before and after each warm-up typology.

Dependent Variable	TRAD PRE	TRAD POST	SSG PRE	SSG POST	P Interaction	P WU Typology	P Time
CMJ (cm)	47.5 ± 11.4	47.4 ± 11.6	46.6 ± 11.3	46.7 ± 11.6	0.804	0.047	0.996
20 m (s)	3.18 ± 0.90	2.91 ± 0.89	2.93 ± 0.89	2.93 ± 0.89	0.459	0.680	0.592
10 m (s)	1.86 ± 0.12	1.70 ± 0.51	1.72 ± 0.52	1.69 ± 0.51	0.959	0.796	0.140

Note: CMJ = Countermovement Jump; 20 m = 20 m sprint time; 10 m sprint time; TRAD = traditional warm-up; SSG = small-sided game warm-up; WU = warm-up.

Finally, SSG warm-up showed a moderately higher ROF (r = 0.443) and a largely (r = 0.612) higher enjoyment compared to TRAD warm-up, although both results showed non-statistically significant differences (p = 0.053 and p = 0.066 for ROF and enjoyment, respectively) (Figure 6).

4. Discussion

The aim of this study was to compare the demands of a traditional basketball warm-up with those of an SSG of equated duration. The main findings of this study were that (i) TRAD had higher external load and intensities, likely due to higher distances covered and more jumps performed; (ii) HR responses were higher in SSG, possibly induced by more static exertions alongside heightened psychological and cognitive demands; (iii) similar performance improvements were induced for sprinting and COD, while CMJ height was higher after TRAD, possibly because of minor variations in the athlete's conditions across experimental days; and (iv) players expressed higher ROF after SSG than TRAD, while RPE was similar across conditions.

Between the two warm-ups, TRAD had higher external loads and intensities compared to SSGs while inducing similar performance improvements. This fact should be well considered by basketball practitioners since accumulating excessive external loads before an official game might not be desirable. This is particularly true for starting players, who are exposed to greater external loads during games and might develop fatigue earlier [32]. Differently, HRmean and HRpeak were moderately higher in SSG. This contrasting result between external and internal load outcomes is critical for basketball coaches and practitioners. It is possible that the actions performed during SSGs reflect typical basketball scenarios in which players fight for their position on the court—such as boxing out, setting picks, or post moves. These actions involve more static exertions, which are typically executed during basketball game-play (1.5 occurrences per minute) [33]. While these quasi-isometric actions do not feature positional displacement, and therefore do not impact external loads, they increase the player's HR [1]. Since SSGs were played on half-courts and with opposition, it is plausible that players had higher HR responses under this condition because of increased static exertions, which were not featured in the TRAD warm-up. Furthermore, previous research has shown that increased cognitive demands lead to heightened HR responses [34]. During the SSGs, players likely experienced greater mental demands, induced by the greater complexity of the scenario in which they had to continuously evaluate the opponents' and teammates' actions, while on the other hand, the TRAD warm-up required only internally paced activities. Therefore, the higher mental demands of SSGs might have also contributed to the higher HR responses found.

One of the main goals of a warm-up is to enhance the player's physical capacities [4]. In the current study, none of the protocols led to significant improvement in performance tests. A possible explanation is the 8 min pre-warm-up performed before each condition, which may have masked the effects of the subsequent TRAD and SSG warm-ups. While a pre-warm-up is necessary to prepare players for baseline assessments (e.g., CMJ, sprint) and is commonly included in similar studies investigating warm-up strategies (REF), it is possible that its execution had already primed the players for simple actions such as jumping and sprinting. Consequently, the additional TRAD and SSG warm-ups may not have elicited further post-activation potentiation effects. This is one of the key outcomes of this study and it should be considered also when designing future research with similar aims.

Comparing the effects of TRAD and SSG warm-ups on performance outcomes, no prominent differences were found. While a small significant difference was found across warm-ups, this might be due to minor variations in the athletes' conditions across experimental days. This hypothesis is supported by the absence of time effects in either condition, and the higher ROF reported by players in the SSG day, while perception of effort was similar. It appears therefore that SSGs can be used as a warm-up strategy in youth basketball players as they do not differ from TRAD warm-ups in terms of physical preparation of players. Furthermore, SSGs might be preferred over TRAD as they stimulate technical–tactical and cognitive abilities while preparing players physically and physiologically [12], thus being a more effective and efficient training choice.

From the perceptual standpoint, TRAD and SSG warm-ups induced similar perceptions of effort (i.e., RPE scores), while ENJ was largely higher for SSGs. Our findings corroborate previous studies which demonstrated that the ball content of SSGs elicits positive affective responses in team sport players [35,36]. Thus, while perceived demands were similar, the SSG warm-up was preferred by players, making it an optimal choice for youth basketball coaches who want to keep their players in good spirit and well motivated.

Although this study provides important insights for basketball coaches and practitioners, some limitations should be acknowledged. Firstly, the external load was monitored only with proxy variables, while more details might have been obtained using different technologies which provide specific activity profiles (i.e., accelerations, jumps, changes of direction). Secondly, player's readiness following the warm-up conditions was measured only by means of a physical performance test, without considering the mental and technical–tactical readiness, which are essential for team sports [37]. Additionally, the outcomes of our study are referred only to youth male players, limiting the generalizations to other basketball populations. Finally, our players were only tested on two occasions, highlighting the short-term effects of the two warm-up protocols, with no information available about the long-term responses (i.e., during the actual training sessions or official match). Therefore, future studies should (i) compare basketball warm-up procedures evaluating their activity profiles in more detail; (ii) evaluate the effects of different warm-ups on the psychological and technical–tactical readiness of players; (iii) replicate this study in other basketball populations (i.e., female and/or adult players) to better generalize the results; and (iv) include a long-term analysis to verify the effect of different warm-up strategies on the post-warm-up activities.

5. Conclusions

Based on the outcomes of this study, basketball coaches are encouraged to adopt SSG-based warm-ups when aiming to reduce external load while eliciting higher internal demands through game-based scenarios involving static positions (e.g., picking, screening). When preceded by a pre-warm-up routine, both SSG and traditional warm-ups can be used interchangeably to prepare players for jumping, sprinting, and change-of-direction performance. Importantly, given the substantially higher enjoyment reported during SSG compared to traditional warm-ups, coaches should consider prioritizing this modality to enhance players' enjoyment and, potentially, their adherence to training across the season. Overall, SSG warm-ups not only can prepare players physically in the short term but also increase their enjoyment—both of which are important for optimal performance.

Supplementary Materials: The following supporting information can be downloaded at https://www.mdpi.com/article/10.3390/sports13120452/s1: Table S1: Pillar preparation structure: type of exercise, number of repetitions to perform, and exercise goal.; Table S2: Movement preparation structure: type of exercise, number of repetitions to perform, and exercise goal.

Author Contributions: Conceptualization, D.C. and M.V.; methodology, D.C. and M.V.; formal analysis, D.C.; writing—original draft preparation, D.C., P.S. and M.V.; writing—review and editing, P.S., M.V., Á.B.-S., J.L.-C., A.V. and D.C.; visualization, D.C. and M.V.; supervision, D.C.; project administration, D.C. All authors have read and agreed to the published version of the manuscript.

Funding: This research received no external funding.

Institutional Review Board Statement: The study was conducted in accordance with the Declaration of Helsinki, and approved by the Institutional Review Board of the University of Rome "Foro Italico" (protocol code CAR. 192/2024 on 15 April 2024).

Informed Consent Statement: All participants, and a parent/guardian for those under 18, provided written informed consent for their data to be used for research purposes.

Data Availability Statement: The original contributions presented in this study are included in the article/Supplementary Materials. Further inquiries can be directed to the corresponding author.

Acknowledgments: The authors thank the athletes and the coaching staff of the under-17 teams Tiber Basket Roma and Virtus Roma for participating in the study.

Conflicts of Interest: The authors declare no conflicts of interest.

References

1. Stojanović, E.; Stojiljković, N.; Scanlan, A.T.; Dalbo, V.J.; Berkelmans, D.M.; Milanović, Z. The activity demands and physiological responses encountered during basketball match-play: A systematic review. *Sports Med.* **2018**, *48*, 111–135. [CrossRef] [PubMed]
2. Mann, D.T.; Williams, A.M.; Ward, P.; Janelle, C.M. Perceptual-cognitive expertise in sport: A meta-analysis. *J. Sport Exerc. Psychol.* **2007**, *29*, 457–478. [CrossRef]
3. Ferioli, D.; Rampinini, E.; Martin, M.; Rucco, D.; Torre, A.; Petway, A.; Scanlan, A. Influence of ball possession and playing position on the physical demands encountered during professional basketball games. *Biol. Sport* **2020**, *37*, 269–276. [CrossRef] [PubMed]
4. Flórez-Gil, E.; Boullosa, D.; Calleja-González, J.; Vaquera, A. A cross-national survey of basketball strength and conditioning coaches' warm-up practices. *Int. J. Sports Physiol. Perform.* **2025**, *20*, 1501–1508. [CrossRef]
5. Schelling, X.; Fernández, J.; Ward, P.; Fernández, J.; Robertson, S. Decision support system applications for scheduling in professional team sport: The team's perspective. *Front. Sports Act. Living* **2021**, *3*, 678489. [CrossRef] [PubMed]
6. McGowan, C.J.; Pyne, D.B.; Thompson, K.G.; Rattray, B. Warm-up strategies for sport and exercise: Mechanisms and applications. *Sports Med.* **2015**, *45*, 1523–1546. [CrossRef] [PubMed]
7. Aerts, I.; Cumps, E.; Verhagen, E.; Wuyts, B.; Van De Gucht, S.; Meeusen, R. The effect of a 3-month prevention program on the jump-landing technique in basketball: A randomized controlled trial. *J. Sport Rehabil.* **2015**, *24*, 21–30. [CrossRef] [PubMed]
8. Díaz-García, J.; Rubio-Morales, A.; Manzano-Rodríguez, D.; García-Calvo, T.; Ring, C. Cognitive priming during warmup enhances sport and exercise performance: A Goldilocks effect. *Brain Sci.* **2025**, *15*, 235. [CrossRef]
9. De Sousa Fortes, L.; Paes, P.P.; Mortatti, A.L.; Perez, A.J.; Cyrino, E.S.; de Lima-Júnior, D.R.A.A.; Moreira, A. Effect of different warm-up strategies on countermovement jump and sprint performance in basketball players. *Isokinet. Exerc. Sci.* **2018**, *26*, 219–225. [CrossRef]
10. Cerrillo-Sanchis, J.; Muñoz-Criado, I.; Pérez-Puchades, V.; Palmero-Martín, I.; Galcerán-Ruiz, J.; Portes-Sanchez, R.; Chulvi-Medrano, I.; Domínguez-Navarro, F.; Morales-Hilario, E.; Mur-Gomar, B.; et al. Applying a specific warm-up on basketball performance: The Basket-Up approach. *Appl. Sci.* **2024**, *14*, 5969. [CrossRef]
11. National Basketball Association. Advanced Stats. 2020. Available online: https://www.nba.com/stats/teams/advanced/ (accessed on 20 December 2020).
12. Sansone, P.; Gasperi, L.; Makivic, B.; Gomez-Ruano, M.A.; Tessitore, A.; Conte, D. An ecological investigation of average and peak external load intensities of basketball skills and game-based training drills. *Biol. Sport* **2023**, *40*, 649–656. [CrossRef] [PubMed]

13. Bredt, S.G.; de Souza Camargo, D.; Vidigal Borges Mortoza, B.; Pereira de Andrade, A.G.; Paolucci, L.A.; Lemos Nascimento Rosso, T.; Moreira Praça, G.; Chagas, M.H. Additional players and half-court areas enhance group tactical-technical behavior and decrease physical and physiological responses in basketball small-sided games. *Int. J. Sports Sci. Coach.* **2022**, *17*, 1079–1088. [CrossRef]
14. Zois, J.; Bishop, D.; Aughey, R. High-intensity warm-ups: Effects during subsequent intermittent exercise. *Int. J. Sports Physiol. Perform.* **2015**, *10*, 498–503. [CrossRef]
15. Thapa, R.K.; Clemente, F.M.; Moran, J.; Garcia-Pinillos, F.; Scanlan, A.T.; Ramirez-Campillo, R. Warm-up optimization in amateur male soccer players: A comparison of small-sided games and traditional warm-up routines on physical fitness qualities. *Biol. Sport* **2023**, *40*, 321–329. [CrossRef]
16. Dello Iacono, A.; Vigotsky, A.D.; Laver, L.; Halperin, I. Beneficial effects of small-sided games as a conclusive part of warm-up routines in young elite handball players. *J. Strength Cond. Res.* **2021**, *35*, 1724–1731. [CrossRef]
17. Bompa, T.O.; Haff, G.G. *Periodization*; Human Kinetics: Champaign, IL, USA, 2009.
18. Bishop, D. Warm up II: Performance changes following active warm up and how to structure the warm up. *Sports Med.* **2003**, *33*, 483–498. [CrossRef] [PubMed]
19. Conte, D.; Rampinini, E.; Trimarchi, F.; Ferioli, D. Interunit reliability of Firstbeat Sport sensors as accelerometer-based tracking devices in basketball. *Int. J. Sports Physiol. Perform.* **2025**, *20*, 727–730. [CrossRef] [PubMed]
20. Foster, C.; Florhaug, J.A.; Franklin, J.; Gottschall, L. A new approach to monitoring exercise training. *J. Strength Cond. Res.* **2001**, *15*, 109–115. [CrossRef]
21. Pernigoni, M.; Calleja-González, J.; Lukonaitienė, I.; Tessitore, A.; Stanislovaitienė, J.; Kamarauskas, P.; Conte, D. Comparative effectiveness of active recovery and static stretching during post-exercise recovery in elite youth basketball. *Res. Q. Exerc. Sport* **2024**, *95*, 272–280. [CrossRef]
22. Attia, A.; Dhahbi, W.; Chaouachi, A.; Padulo, J.; Wong, D.P.; Chamari, K. Measurement errors when estimating the vertical jump height with flight time using photocell devices: The example of Optojump. *Biol. Sport* **2017**, *34*, 63–70. [CrossRef]
23. Pernigoni, M.; Perazzetti, A.; Digno, M.; Tessitore, A.; Kamandulis, S.; Conte, D. Chill without thrill: A crossover study on whole-body cryotherapy and postmatch recovery in high-level youth basketball players. *Int. J. Sports Physiol. Perform.* **2024**, *19*, 1218–1226. [CrossRef]
24. Nimphius, S.; McGuigan, M.R.; Newton, R.U. Relationship between strength, power, speed, and change of direction performance of female softball players. *J. Strength Cond. Res.* **2010**, *24*, 885–895. [CrossRef] [PubMed]
25. Micklewright, D.; St Clair Gibson, A.; Gladwell, V.; Al Salman, A. Development and validity of the rating-of-fatigue scale. *Sports Med.* **2017**, *47*, 2375–2393. [CrossRef]
26. Pernigoni, M.; Kreivytė, R.; Lukonaitienė, I.; Toper, C.R.; Kamandulis, S.; Conte, D. Is foam rolling as effective as its popularity suggests? A randomised crossover study exploring post-match recovery in female basketball. *J. Sports Sci.* **2023**, *41*, 1718–1725. [CrossRef]
27. Kendzierski, D.; DeCarlo, K.J. Physical activity enjoyment scale: Two validation studies. *J. Sport Exerc. Psychol.* **1991**, *13*, 50–64. [CrossRef]
28. Golluceli, B.; Kamandulis, S.; Pernigoni, M.; Lukonaitiene, I.; Kreivyte, R.; Conte, D. Physiological, perceived, and physical demands of recreational 3×3 basketball and high-intensity interval training in sedentary adult women. *Biol. Sport* **2025**, *42*, 89–96. [CrossRef]
29. Hopkins, W.G.; Marshall, S.W.; Batterham, A.M.; Hanin, J. Progressive statistics for studies in sports medicine and exercise science. *Med. Sci. Sports Exerc.* **2009**, *41*, 3–13. [CrossRef] [PubMed]
30. Fritz, C.O.; Morris, P.E.; Richler, J.J. Effect size estimates: Current use, calculations, and interpretation. *J. Exp. Psychol. Gen.* **2012**, *141*, 2–18. [CrossRef]
31. Cohen, J. *Statistical Power Analysis for the Behavioral Sciences*, rev. ed.; Lawrence Erlbaum Associates: Mahwah, NJ, USA, 1988. [CrossRef]
32. Gonzalez, A.M.; Hoffman, J.R.; Rogowski, J.P.; Burgos, W.; Manalo, E.; Weise, K.; Fragala, M.S.; Stout, J.R. Performance changes in NBA basketball players vary in starters vs. nonstarters over a competitive season. *J. Strength Cond. Res.* **2013**, *27*, 611–615. [CrossRef]
33. Delextrat, A.; Badiella, A.; Saavedra, V.; Matthew, D.; Schelling, X.; Torres-Ronda, L. Match activity demands of elite Spanish female basketball players by playing position. *Int. J. Perform. Anal. Sport* **2015**, *15*, 687–703. [CrossRef]
34. Heine, T.; Lenis, G.; Reichensperger, P.; Beran, T.; Doessel, O.; Deml, B. Electrocardiographic features for the measurement of drivers' mental workload. *Appl. Ergon.* **2017**, *61*, 31–43. [CrossRef] [PubMed]
35. Selmi, O.; Haddad, M.; Majed, L.; Ben Khalifa, W.; Hamza, M.; Chamari, K. Soccer training: High-intensity interval training is mood disturbing while small sided games ensure mood balance. *J. Sports Med. Phys. Fit.* **2018**, *58*, 1163–1170. [CrossRef] [PubMed]

36. Los Arcos, A.; Vázquez, J.S.; Martín, J.; Lerga, J.; Sánchez, F.; Villagra, F.; Zulueta, J.J. Effects of small-sided games vs. interval training in aerobic fitness and physical enjoyment in young elite soccer players. *PLoS ONE* **2015**, *10*, e0137224. [CrossRef] [PubMed]
37. Beato, M.; Madsen, E.E.; Clubb, J.; Emmonds, S.; Krustrup, P. Monitoring readiness to train and perform in female football: Current evidence and recommendations for practitioners. *Int. J. Sports Physiol. Perform.* **2024**, *19*, 223–231. [CrossRef] [PubMed]

sports

MDPI

Article

Effects of After-School Basketball Program on Physical Fitness and Cardiometabolic Health in Prepubertal Boys

Cristina Castro-Collado [1], Jose Manuel Jurado-Castro [1,2,3], Mercedes Gil-Campos [1,2,*], Belén Pastor-Villaescusa [1,4,5], Gracia María Quintana-Navarro [1] and Francisco Jesús Llorente-Cantarero [1,2,6]

1 University of Cordoba, Maimonides Biomedical Research Institute of Cordoba (IMIBIC), Reina Sofia University Hospital, Avda Menéndez Pidal sn, 14004 Córdoba, Spain; colladocac@gmail.com (C.C.-C.); juradox@gmail.com (J.M.J.-C.); mbpastor.ugr@gmail.com (B.P.-V.); g.quintana.navarro@gmail.com (G.M.Q.-N.); fllorente@uco.es (F.J.L.-C.)

2 Consorcio CIBER, M.P. Fisiopatología de la Obesidad y Nutrición (CIBEROBN), Instituto de Salud Carlos III (ISCIII), 28029 Madrid, Spain

3 Ciencias de la Actividad Física y El Deporte, Escuela Universitaria de Osuna (Centro Adscrito a la Universidad de Sevilla), 41640 Osuna, Spain

4 Primary Care Interventions to Prevent Maternal and Child Chronic Diseases of Perinatal and Developmental Origin (RICORS), RD21/0012/0008, Instituto de Salud Carlos III (ISCIII), 28029 Madrid, Spain

5 Spanish Network in Maternal, Neonatal, Child and Developmental Health Research (RICORS-SAMID, RD24/0013/0007), Instituto de Salud Carlos III (ISCIII), 28029 Madrid, Spain

6 Department of Specific Didactics, Faculty of Education, University of Cordoba, 14071 Córdoba, Spain

* Correspondence: mercedes_gil_campos@yahoo.es

Abstract: Objectives: This study aimed to assess changes in anthropometric measures, cardiometabolic markers, and physical fitness following a structured basketball training program in healthy prepubertal boys. Methods: The intervention consisted of a 6-week pre-season phase followed by a 32-week basketball training season conducted during the academic year. Training sessions were held three times per week at moderate to vigorous intensity, along with a weekly match. The participants were assessed at baseline, 6, 9, and 12 months. A reference group was evaluated at baseline for comparison. The study was registered at ClinicalTrials.gov (identifier: NCT07007624). Results: Seventeen boys completed the program. Anthropometric assessments revealed increases in fat-free mass in the trunk and lower limbs, along with maintenance of an adequate BMI. After nine months, participants in the intervention showed significant improvements in fitness tests, including a 45% increase in Course Navette performance ($p < 0.001$), a 21% increase in horizontal jump performance ($p = 0.001$), and a 13% increase in abdominal test performance ($p < 0.001$). Conclusion: These findings suggest that a structured, school-based basketball program may enhance physical fitness and support healthy body composition maintenance in healthy-weight prepubertal boys.

Keywords: child; physical activity; body composition; exercise; cardiovascular diseases

1. Introduction

The participation of children in group or organized physical activities plays a fundamental role in their holistic development [1]. Beyond promoting physical health, participation in such activities also fosters emotional well-being, enhances social skills, and supports cognitive development by encouraging cooperation, discipline, and problem-solving abilities within a structured environment [2]. However, there is a concerning trend, as many children are not regularly involved in such activities. This lack of participation can be attributed to various factors, including the increasing dependence on technology and the limited access to suitable sports programs [3]. Understanding the causes and seeking solutions to encourage active participation of children in group physical activities are crucial for promoting a healthy lifestyle and an optimal development of social skills from an early age [4].

Regular physical activity improves physical fitness, including cardiovascular endurance, muscular strength, flexibility, lung capacity, body composition, and metabolic health [5,6]. Team sports are highly effective in improving youth health by enhancing strength, flexibility, balance, and coordination, while also reducing body fat and boosting cardiorespiratory endurance [7]. Basketball, in particular, is a comprehensive sport that involves sprinting, jumping, and feints, engaging both the upper and lower limbs [8,9]. As a team-based activity, it maintains active participation and high levels of physical activity [10]. Its high-intensity training and regular practice have been shown to produce significant improvements in physical fitness, even in children [11].

Intensive and frequent physical training can significantly influence cardiovascular health in children and adolescents [12]. While some studies focus exclusively on cardiovascular adaptations to training, there is limited research considering the effects of physical fitness on metabolism and body composition. Therefore, the objective of this study was to evaluate changes in physical fitness, cardiometabolic health, and body composition in boys participating in a regular after-school basketball training.

2. Materials and Methods

2.1. Study Design and Participants

A prospective, non-randomized controlled intervention study was conducted. The protocol was registered at ClinicalTrials.gov (NCT07007624). The study was designed and reported following the TREND statement guidelines (Supplementary Materials S1).

An after-school basketball program was offered to students from middle socioeconomic backgrounds in Córdoba (Spain). The inclusion criteria were age between 7 and 12 years, normal weight, and good health, with Tanner stage I (prepuberal). Exclusion criteria included any clinical or analytical sign of puberty, presence of disease, or use of medication that could affect blood pressure (BP), glucose, or lipid metabolism. The study was designed in accordance with the ethical principles for human research of the Declaration of Helsinki. It was approved by the local ethics and research committee at University Reina Sofia Hospital (Code: 1866). All participants and their families were informed about the study and voluntarily agreed to participate. Informed consent from their parents or legal guardians was obtained. All measurements and data collection were performed across the school year, from September to June.

A non-randomized convenience sample was selected due to ethical and logistical limitations that prevented the random assignment of children to a structured, year-long training program. First, 20 boys of the same age and gender were chosen to form a basketball team (group B), in accordance with federal recommendations. Their training sessions were monitored by a highly qualified basketball trainer. These boys were selected based on their interest in participating in basketball activities, which may have contributed to higher baseline levels of physical fitness. Three participants from the intervention group withdrew from the study due to scheduling conflicts. Their baseline anthropometric and physical fitness values were within the same range as the other interventions. Therefore, no relevant differences were identified that would suggest a systematic bias resulting from dropout. These participants were not included in the statistical analysis.

Second, a cohort of 74 boys from the same schools and social background was selected to serve as a healthy reference group (HRG), at baseline time. The purpose of including this group was to confirm that participants in the intervention group were comparable, at baseline, to a larger population of healthy prepubertal boys. All participants were healthy prepubertal boys of similar age and socioeconomic background. Although no formal matching was performed, both groups shared a common educational and social context. This healthy reference group (HRG) participated in a single assessment visit, as only one-time permission was granted.

2.2. Intervention

The basketball training program, supervised by a qualified trainer, was divided into two periods: a pre-season period at the beginning of the school year, during the first 6 weeks, and immediately afterward, a 32-week season lasting until the end of the school year. After the program concluded, recommendations to be active were provided for the summer holidays, and a follow-up assessment was conducted 3 months after the end of the intervention.

The pre-season included 5 training sessions (Monday to Friday) per week of 2 h each. This intervention was focused on dribbling, defending, and shooting skills. The season included 3 training sessions per week of 2 h each (after school) and a match during the weekend. Each session was divided into two periods separated by a break of 10 min: the first period focused on individual skills with moderate- to high-intensity (60–85% of heart rate (HR)) exercises, and the second period focused on game tactics and strategy.

2.3. Outcomes

At baseline (B_0), clinical examination, body composition, physical fitness tests, BP, and blood draws to assess biochemical parameters related to metabolism and cardiovascular health were performed in all boys included in the study. Follow-up visits were conducted at 6 months (B_6), 9 months (B_9), and 12 months (B_{12}) during which anthropometric and other measurements were repeated. No training sessions took place between B_9 and B_{12} (Figure 1). All measurements were performed under standardized conditions: after bladder emptying, 3 h after rising and eating, and without previous intensive exercise.

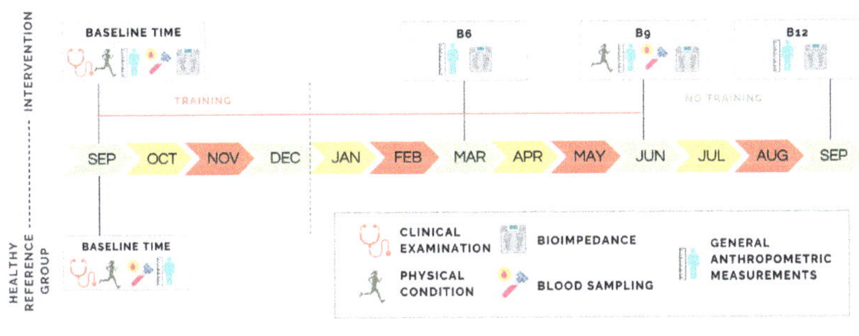

Figure 1. Activity schedule across the different time points of the study (basal B_0, and at 6, 9, and 12 months (B_6, B_9, B_{12}) in boys participating in a basketball program.

2.3.1. Clinical Examination

A comprehensive clinical evaluation was performed by trained healthcare professionals, including a structured anamnesis to collect medical and family history (particularly regarding metabolic or cardiovascular diseases), current health status, and medication use. Sexual maturity was assessed using Tanner's five-stage scale [13] through a physical examination conducted in a private setting by a pediatrician. In boys, this included the evaluation of genital development and pubic hair distribution.

2.3.2. Body Composition

Body weight and height were measured using standard techniques, a beam balance, and a precision stadiometer SECA 213 (Scale 20–205 cm; SECA, Hamburg, Germany), with the participants lightly dressed and barefoot. BMI was calculated as weight (kg)/height (m^2) and compared to growth charts for Spanish children; percentiles were calculated to determine the relative standing of each value within the data distribution [14]. The z-score was calculated to determine how far each value deviates from the mean in terms of standard deviations. Body composition components such as fat-free mass and fat mass were obtained by bioelectrical impedance analysis using a Tanita BC 418 MA Segmental Body Composition Analyser® (TANITA™, Tokyo, Japan).

2.3.3. Blood Pressure

Systolic and diastolic BP and HR were measured in the right arm in a sitting position, using a random-zero sphygmomanometer (Dinamap V-100, GE HealthCare, Chicago, IL, USA) after the participants had rested without changing position for at least 5 min. Each measurement was taken three times non-consecutively. Total systolic blood pressure (SBP) and diastolic blood pressure (DBP) values were calculated as the average of all available data from both groups.

2.3.4. Blood Biomarkers

Fasting blood samples were collected and analyzed for complete blood count, glucose, insulin, lipids, and the homeostatic model assessment for insulin resistance (HOMA-IR). Blood samples were obtained from the antecubital vein between 08.00 and 09.30 h after an overnight fast of at least 12 h. Samples collected in EDTA tubes were centrifuged and immediately stored at −80 °C. They were drawn. The blood count and general biochemical parameters were analyzed at the laboratory in the reference hospital. Glucose (coefficient of variation (CV) = 1.0%) was analyzed using the glucose oxidase method in an automatic analyzer (Roche-Hitachi Modular P and D Autoanalyser; Roche Laboratory Systems, Mannheim, Germany), and plasma insulin was analyzed by radioimmunoassay (RIA) (CV = 2.6%) using an automatic microparticle analyzer (AxSYM; Abbott Laboratories, Chicago, IL, US). Insulin resistance (IR) was calculated by the HOMA-IR. Serum triacylglycerides (TAG) (CV = 1.5%), total cholesterol (CV = 0.9%), high density lipoprotein cholesterol (HDL-c) (CV = 0.8%), and low-density lipoprotein cholesterol (LDL-c) (CV = 1.5%) were measured using an automatic analyzer (Roche-Hitachi Modular P and D Autoanalyser; Roche Laboratory Systems, Mannheim, Germany).

2.3.5. Cardiorespiratory Fitness (Course Navette Test)

The Course Navette test was employed to evaluate cardiorespiratory fitness. Participants were required to run for the maximum possible time in a continuous 20 m shuttle run at a progressively increasing speed. The test is structured in periods or stages called *paliers*, each lasting approximately one minute, during which the running speed remains constant. At the end of each period, the speed increases slightly, requiring greater physical effort. The test ends when the participant fails to reach the line at the time of the beep on two consecutive occasions. The number of completed stages allows for an indirect estimation of maximal oxygen consumption (VO_2 max) and enables the classification of aerobic performance into different levels [15].

2.3.6. Lower Body Explosive Strength (Horizontal Jump Test)

Lower-body muscular strength is evaluated through the horizontal jump test [16]. Participants performed three maximal jumps with feet together; the longest was recorded. A take-off mark ensured correct foot placement and prevented invalid attempts.

2.3.7. Core Strength (Abdominal Test)

Core strength was assessed using a 30 s sit-up test. From a supine position, participants performed as many correctly executed sit-ups as possible within the time limit, touching elbows to thighs and returning shoulders to the mat.

2.4. Sample Size

As the horizontal jump is one of the main outcomes for this study, the sample size was determined by calculating the statistical power based on a previous study [17], using G*Power software (version 3.1, Düsseldorf, Germany) for a repeated-measures ANOVA (within-subjects) design, with an expected effect size of f = 0.25, $\alpha = 0.05$, power = 0.80 and four measurements. Based on this parameter, the minimum sample size required to detect an 8% difference in horizontal jump performance was estimated to be 17 participants. The horizontal jump was selected as the basis for the power calculation due to its high responsiveness to lower-body training and suitability for assessing neuromuscular adaptations in prepubertal children. Other parameters, such as metabolic markers, were considered exploratory and were not used for sample size determination because of their greater interindividual variability and lower sensitivity to exercise in a healthy pediatric population [18]. The aim was to assess the effectiveness of the intervention in improving physical fitness, which is why the horizontal jump test was chosen.

2.5. Statistical Analysis

Data are expressed as the mean ± standard deviation. The Shapiro–Wilk test was used to assess whether the variables followed a normal distribution. To compare physical fitness, anthropometric, and biochemical parameters at different time points within the intervention group, repeated-measures ANOVA was used for variables following a normal distribution, with Bonferroni-corrected post hoc tests applied when the main effect was significant. For variables that did not meet normality assumptions, the Wilcoxon test was used for within-group comparisons (e.g., B_0 vs. B_{12}). To compare baseline values between the HRG and the intervention group, the Mann–Whitney U test was applied, as the data did not follow a normal distribution and the sample sizes were unequal. Pearson correlation coefficients were employed to examine the bivariate correlations among the variables. Correlation models were fitted to assess relationships between physical fitness, anthropometry, and biochemical parameters at different times. All statistical analyses were performed using SPSS Statistics 25 software (IBM SPSS, New York, NY, US). In all analyses, statistical significance was set at a 2-tailed p-value < 0.05. A per-protocol analysis approach was used, and therefore, no imputation was applied for missing data. Only data from participants who completed the entire intervention, and all follow-up measurements were included in the analyses.

3. Results

A total of 91 children participated in the study: 74 in the HRC and 20 in the intervention group (B), of whom 17 completed the study (Figure 2). No significant differences observed between groups (HRG)—(B_0) at baseline in weight, height, weight percentile, height percentile, BMI, and BMI z-scores. However, there was an increase in weight and height from B_0 to B_{12} in trained boys. Additionally, lower levels in both SBP and DBP were noted in B_0 compared to HRG and maintained during training (Table 1). The results of the HRG in comparison with B0 of the intervention group are presented in the Supplementary Materials (Supplementary Materials, Table S1).

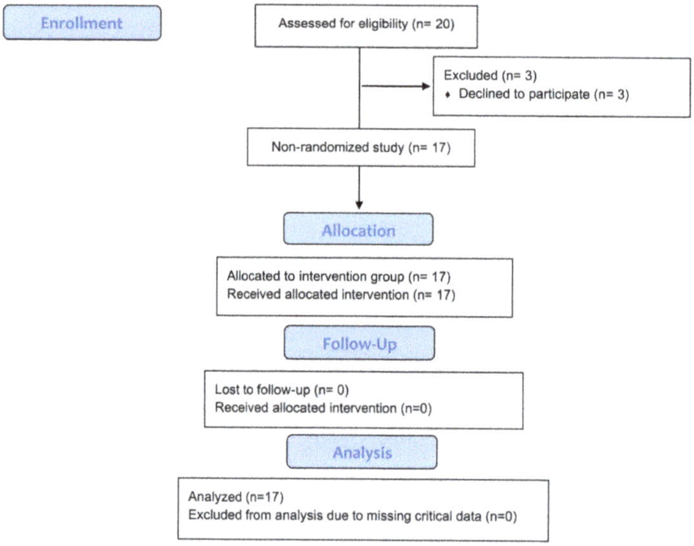

Figure 2. Flowchart of participants who completed the intervention.

Table 1. General anthropometric measurements at baseline (B_0) and at 12-month follow-up (B_{12}) in the intervention group after the basketball training program.

	B_0	B_{12}	Δ	*p*-Value
Age (year)	10.9 ± 1.41	11.9 ± 1.41	1.0	<0.001
Weight (kg)	43.8 ± 10.45	47.0 ± 10.80	3.2	<0.001
Weight percentile	56.8 ± 28.32	54.7 ± 28.61	2.1	0.826
Height (cm)	149.4 ± 8.67	153 ± 9.83	3.6	<0.001
Height percentile	65.2 ± 26.09	68.0 ± 9.83	2.8	0.361
BMI (kg/m^2)	19.5 ± 3.04	19 ± 2.57	0.5	0.555
BMI Z-score	0.1 ± 0.96	−0.1 ± 0.73	0.2	0.099
DBP (mmHg)	62.9 ± 8.90	55 ± 5.99	2.1	0.311
SBP (mmHg)	114.5 ± 7.68	108.2 ± 10.63	6.3	0.450
HR (bpm)	66.4 ± 11.57	69.7 ± 10.84	3.3	0.005

BMI: Body mass index; DBP: Diastolic blood pressure; SBP: Systolic blood pressure; HR: Heart rate. Data are expressed as mean ± standard deviation and differences (Δ: B_{12}–B_0); One-way ANOVA or Wilcoxon test was performed, depending on whether the variables followed a normal distribution, using repeated measures.

Significant differences in fat-free mass were observed in several body regions in boys trained at different times of measurements without differences in total fat-free mass (Figure 3A). Especially, in the trunk, a reduction in fat-free mass was found in B_{12} compared to B_9 (B_9: 57.26 ± 2.53% vs. B_{12}: 55.71 ± 2.4%; Δ: 1.55%) and B_0 (B_0: 57.1 ± 2.71% vs. B_{12}: 55.71 ± 2.4%; Δ: 1.39%) (Figure 3B). In upper limbs no significant differences were found except an increase in B_9 (B_9: 4.42 ± 0.37% vs. B_0: 4.31 ± 0.34%; Δ: 0.11%) and B_{12} (B_{12}: 4.43 ± 0.52% vs. B0: 4.31 ± 0.34%; Δ: 0.12%) respect to baseline in right limb (Figure 3C). Lower limbs showed an increase of fat-free mass from basal time to the end of the study (left (B_0: 16.72 ± 1.11% vs. B_{12}: 17.34 ± 0.97%; Δ: 0.62%); right (B_0: 17.32 ± 1.12% vs. B_{12}: 17.97 ± 1.07%; Δ: 0.65%)) (Figure 3D). Detailed data are presented in the Supplementary Materials (Supplementary Materials, Table S2).

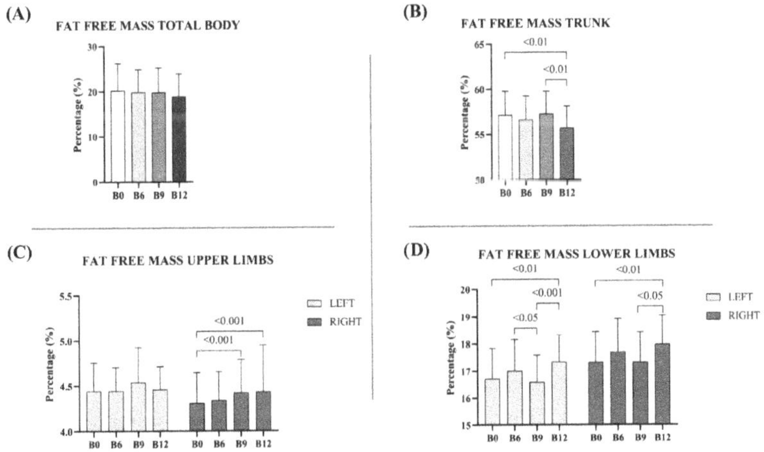

Figure 3. Percentage of fat-free mass at different times (B0, and at 6, 9, and 12 months (B6, B9, B12) in boys participating in the basketball training program. Data are expressed as mean percentages and standard deviation: (**A**) Fat-free mass total body; (**B**) Fat-free mass trunk; (**C**) Fat-free mass upper limbs; (**D**) Fat-free mass lower limbs. B0: baseline; B6: 6 months of intervention; B9: 9 months of intervention; B12: 3 months after the intervention (follow-up). Statistical significance was determined using one-way ANOVA or Wilcoxon test, depending on normality; *p*-values are reported for pairwise comparisons.

The group of basketball training showed better results in jump and abdominal tests than HRG at basal time without differences in Course Navette test (Supplementary Materials, Table S1). At B_{12}, boys improved their results in all these tests compared with their baseline data (Course Navette (B_0: 5.2 ± 2.3 min vs. B_{12}: 7.9 ± 2.2 min; Δ: 2.7 min); horizontal jump (B_0: 147.5 ± 21.3 cm vs. B_{12}: 155.2 ± 23.5 cm; Δ: 7.7 cm); abdominal test (B_0: 23.8 ± 6.6 number of repetitions vs. B_{12}: 26.3 ± 6 number of repetitions; Δ: 2.5 number of repetitions) (Figure 4). The data are presented in detail in the Supplementary Materials (Supplementary Materials, Table S3).

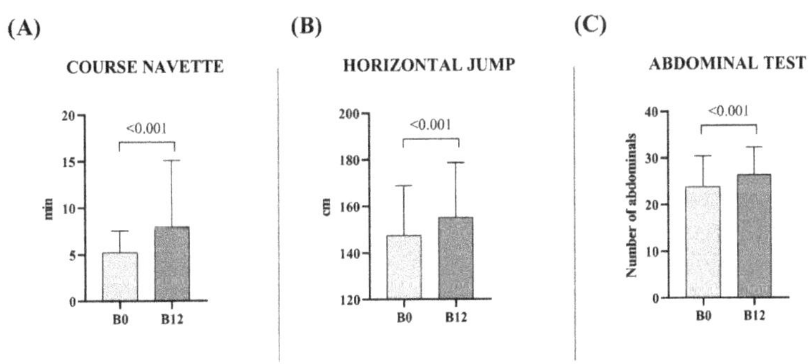

Figure 4. Physical fitness test results at baseline (B_0) and after 12 months (B_{12}) in boys participating in the basketball training program. Data are expressed as mean and standard deviation: (**A**) Course Navette; (**B**) Horizontal jump; (**C**) Abdominal test. Statistical significance was determined using one-way ANOVA or Wilcoxon test, depending on normality; *p*-values are reported for pairwise comparisons.

Blood parameters were within the normal range compared with reference values from the laboratory, indicating that all the children exhibited a state of good health at baseline (for both groups). It was maintained in the follow-up after the intervention (B_{12}) in the trained group (Table 2).

Table 2. Blood parameters at baseline (B_0) and at 12-month follow-up (B_{12}) in the intervention group after the basketball training program.

	B_0	B_{12}	Δ	*p*-Value	Reference Values
Leukocytes ($\times 10^3/\mu L$)	6.13 ± 1.56	5.49 ± 1.34	0.64	0.055	4–12.4
Hemoglobin (g/dL)	12.82 ± 2.37	13.11 ± 0.75	0.29	0.226	12–16
Iron (mg/dL)	60.50 ± 26.70	78.82 ± 21.17	18.32	0.016	50–170
Ferritin (ng/mL)	30.78 ± 12.98	30.24 ± 13.36	0.51	0.776	10–120
Glucose (mg/dL)	90.15 ± 14.46	92.29 ± 7.08	2.14	0.736	74–106
Insulin (μUI/mL)	8.09 ± 6.15	8.90 ± 3.59	0.81	0.962	3–25
HOMA-IR	1.89 ± 1.34	2.04 ± 0.86	0.15	0.981	0–2.9
Total cholesterol (mg/dL)	169.40 ± 27.83	166.18 ± 26.61	3.22	0.434	140–220
HDL-c (mg/dL)	64.15 ± 11.18	52.82 ± 11.49	11.33	<0.001	40–80
LDL-c (mg/dL)	91.75 ± 24.11	99.18 ± 23.42	7.43	0.077	50–130
Apolipoprotein a (mg/dL)	148.26 ± 23.07	129.88 ± 19.31	18.38	<0.001	105–220
Apolipoprotein b (mg/dL)	60.37 ± 14.66	61.06 ± 12.92	0.69	0.966	65–130
Triglycerides (mg/dL)	65.25 ± 20.30	68.88 ± 31.00	3.63	0.467	20–250
Aspartate Transaminase (U/L)	26.10 ± 5.31	22.82 ± 3.15	3.28	0.003	5–34
Alanine transaminase (U/L)	20.20 ± 11.15	17.35 ± 5.58	2.85	0.115	10–49
C-reactive protein (mg/dL)	2.55 ± 4.35	0.92 ± 1.25	1.63	0.017	0–10

HOMA-IR: Homeostasis model assessment of insulin resistance; HDL-c: High density lipoprotein cholesterol; LDL-c: Low density lipoprotein cholesterol. Data are expressed as mean ± standard deviation and differences (Δ: B_{12}–B_0); one-way ANOVA or Wilcoxon test was performed, depending on whether the variables followed a normal distribution, using repeated measures.

The Course Navette test was negatively correlated with BMI z-score at baseline ($r = -0.521$, $p = 0.046$), and this association became stronger at B_{12} ($r = -0.738$, $p = 0.010$), indicating that higher aerobic fitness was linked to lower BMI z-scores. At B_{12} follow-up, the Course Navette test also showed a significant inverse correlation with C-reactive protein (CRP) levels ($r = -0.714$, $p = 0.009$). In addition, at B_{12} follow-up, both horizontal jump performance ($r = -0.651$, $p = 0.022$) and abdominal test performance ($r = -0.659$, $p = 0.020$) were negatively correlated with CRP.

4. Discussion

An after-school program of basketball training conducted during the school year led to improvements in body composition and physical fitness in a group of prepubertal boys, compared with a similar group that did not receive the intervention.

While few studies have explored anthropometric and performance adaptations specifically in preadolescent basketball players, most have involved shorter interventions, heterogeneous samples, or lacked follow-up assessments. In contrast, the present study adds novel evidence from a 9-month structured basketball program in healthy-weight prepubertal boys, including data from a post-intervention training period. This approach provides a clearer understanding of both the benefits and the potential reversibility of such interventions during a critical stage of development. Some limitations in evaluating the effects of basketball training are associated with small teams with a controlled number of participants [19] or teams solely comprised of individuals of one sex [20]. However, in this study, comparison with an HRG at baseline ensured that all participants began from similar conditions with comparable health statuses prior to training. Furthermore, the intervention was conducted by expert trainers who specifically prepared this group of prepubertal boys to compete under real conditions against similar counterparts.

Previous studies have consistently demonstrated a general increase in all anthropometric traits during the training period in children who practice basketball, coupled with a decrease in fat mass [21–23]. This reduction in fat mass has been attributed to both the rapid growth of fat-free mass and a slower accumulation of fat. Excessive fat mass not only hampers mobility in sports but also adversely affects physical performance [24]. Decreasing body fat reduces strain on both the musculoskeletal and cardiovascular systems, thereby enhancing movement efficiency and the capacity for physical exercise, which leads to improved strength, endurance, and overall functional capability [25]. In the children participating in this study, a decrease in BMI z-scores and fat mass was observed, while normal-weight status was maintained. These results were accompanied by improved performance in the Course Navette test. These findings are consistent with those of a previous study in children of similar age, where participants with higher BMI achieved worse results in fitness tests [26].

Basketball emerges as an excellent candidate for enhancing body composition and bone mineral density due to its high-impact nature [27]. Sports like basketball are characterized by their impact and required actions, such as jumping, similar to volleyball [28], handball [29], or dance [30]. Furthermore, full-body sports such as swimming involve both the upper and lower limbs but lack impact on the body, as they take place in a microgravity environment where the body is not subjected to impact forces [31]. In this study, a general improvement in fat-free mass was observed in both the lower and upper limbs throughout the training period. Participation in comprehensive sports that involve both lower and upper body training has been associated with a decrease in fat mass and an improvement in fitness levels among prepubertal and early pubescent children [32].

The Course Navette test is a widely used tool to assess physical fitness, providing valuable information on maximal effort and aerobic capacity [33]. It also reflects cardiovascular and respiratory health through its estimation of maximal oxygen consumption [34]. This improvement is attributed to their commitment to an active lifestyle, characterized by regular levels of physical activity. The systematic practice of sports also promotes cardiovascular health, which is further associated with anthropometric improvements [35]. In the present study, interesting inverse correlations have been found, especially at the end of the intervention, between physical fitness and both weight and BMI z-score, and with CRP, a well-established biomarker of inflammation. These findings suggest that improvements in physical fitness may be associated with healthier body composition and reduced systemic inflammation in children by the end of the intervention.

The frequency of sport practice has been closely linked to improvements in fitness [36]. A study involving 19 basketball players in training sessions conducted twice a week for 8 weeks resulted in enhanced cardiorespiratory fitness, explosive strength, and core strength [37]. Similarly, in another study focusing on prepubertal children who trained three times a week for 12 weeks, improvements were observed in anaerobic capacity, endurance running, and overall strength [32]. Thus, training twice a week emerges as a viable option to achieve health benefits with enhancements in jumping and running performances, along with an increase in fat-free mass, as previously reported [26]. Furthermore, higher performance in horizontal jumps has been linked to improved sprints and agility in male adolescent basketball players [38].

It is also evident that participants in the intervention group demonstrated superior performance compared to those in the HRG assessed at baseline, particularly in the abdominal and horizontal jump tests. This discrepancy may be attributed to the fact that individuals in the intervention group were generally more active and inclined to participate in sports activities compared to their HRG counterparts. This suggests a potential selection bias, as children with a greater inclination toward physical activity may have been more likely to enroll in the intervention, thereby limiting the attribution of the observed improvements solely to the training program.

Both groups showed normal biochemical values at baseline, which were maintained after the intervention in the basketball group. Regular, controlled training appears to support the maintenance of a healthy metabolic profile in children. Throughout the follow-up, no significant longitudinal changes were observed in the intervention group. Only CRP showed an inverse relationship with physical fitness outcomes, suggesting a potential link between inflammatory status and fitness. In particular, basketball benefits multiple systems and supports disease prevention during youth [39]. However, the primary health-related improvements observed in this intervention were related to physical fitness and body composition, rather than metabolic markers. These benefits seem to decline after ~12 weeks of inactivity, with reductions in lean mass evident within three months after the intervention (B_{12}). Concretely, some outcomes, such as trunk fat-free mass, declined during the three-month follow-up after the intervention ended (B_{12}), indicating that the positive effects of the program may be partially reversible. This regional decline may reflect the nature of basketball, which emphasizes lower-limb activity. Therefore, reductions in trunk fat-free mass after detraining may have occurred more rapidly compared to the legs. These findings highlight the importance of maintaining regular physical activity to sustain the benefits achieved through structured training interventions. Furthermore, future studies should continue to explore whether dynamic and high-intensity sports such as basketball might positively influence metabolic health and insulin sensitivity [40].

4.1. Practical Implications

Maintaining regular physical activity is essential for preventing sedentary behaviors that increase the risk of chronic diseases. This study supports basketball as an effective strategy to promote physical fitness and maintain healthy body composition in healthy-weight prepubertal children. These findings could help inform recommendations in pediatric healthcare settings, particularly for children at risk of excess adiposity or low fitness levels. Future public policies might consider incorporating structured after-school sports programs as part of preventive health strategies for youth populations.

The program was implemented by certified basketball coaches with extensive experience in youth sports. Rather than limiting replicability, we believe this detail strengthens the internal validity of the study and sets a benchmark for structured school-based interventions. This characteristic may serve as a model for future programs aiming to replicate similar outcomes under comparable conditions.

4.2. Limitations

This study was limited to prepubertal boys, which may reduce the generalizability of findings to girls or older adolescents. The intervention was conducted in a single setting with a relatively small sample size. Participation was voluntary, and children with greater initial motivation or physical fitness may have been more likely to participate (e.g., interest in participating in basketball activities), introducing a selection bias that could explain baseline differences in some physical fitness variables. Moreover, due to ethical and logistical constraints, it was not feasible to randomly assign children to an extracurricular training program they might not have chosen to join, which limited the possibility of randomization. Future studies should include longitudinal follow-ups to assess sustained effects and explore differences by sex, maturation stage, and training modalities. Another important limitation is the absence of a longitudinal control group. The HRG was included at baseline only to ensure a similar health status to the group that would participate in the program, but it was not followed over time. Therefore, we cannot completely rule out the influence of natural growth and development on the observed changes in the intervention group. Heart rate monitoring was not conducted because it is prohibited in basketball for safety reasons, both during competitions and training sessions, as it is a high-contact sport. Additionally, in this type of sport, it is difficult to accurately assess the intensity at which each participant is exercising. However, by using physical fitness tests to assess the participants' baseline capacity, the training intensity and volume were adjusted to approximately 60–85%, based on their age. This approach ensures that participants remain within an aerobic range, avoiding excessive intensity that could push them into an anaerobic zone. All sessions were supervised by a qualified instructor with a degree in sport sciences. However, all sessions were supervised by a certified basketball coach with a degree in sport sciences. Additionally, the study included only a single follow-up measurement after the intervention ended (B_{12}), which limited the ability to evaluate the long-term sustainability of the observed benefits.

5. Conclusions

A 32-week after-school basketball training program conducted three times per week, plus a weekend match, and performed at moderate to vigorous intensity, was associated with improvements in physical fitness and body composition in healthy-weight prepubertal boys. However, randomized controlled interventions should be conducted, and meanwhile, these changes should be interpreted with caution, as natural growth and other external factors may have contributed to the observed effects. Nevertheless, these results support the integration of structured team sports like basketball into school or community programs as an effective strategy to promote children's health and prevent the early onset of metabolic disorders.

Supplementary Materials: The following supporting information can be downloaded at: https://www.mdpi.com/article/10.3390/sports13090291/s1, Table S1: Descriptive characteristics of the reference group; Table S2: Percentage of fat free mass in different times (basal B0, and at 6, 9 and 12 months (B6, B9, B12) in boys trained in a basketball program; Table S3: Physical fitness tests data at basal time in the intervention group (B0), and after a year of follow-up in the boys trained in the basketball program (B12).

Author Contributions: Conceptualization, F.J.L.-C. and M.G.-C.; methodology, F.J.L.-C. and M.G.-C.; software, C.C.-C., M.G.-C., G.M.Q.-N. and F.J.L.-C.; validation, C.C.-C., M.G.-C., G.M.Q.-N. and F.J.L.-C.; formal analysis, C.C.-C. and J.M.J.-C.; investigation, C.C.-C., M.G.-C., G.M.Q.-N. and F.J.L.-C.; resources, M.G.-C. and F.J.L.-C.; data curation, C.C.-C. and G.M.Q.-N.; writing—original draft preparation, C.C.-C. and J.M.J.-C.; writing—review and editing, C.C.-C., J.M.J.-C., M.G.-C., B.P.-V. and F.J.L.-C.; visualization, C.C.-C. and J.M.J.-C.; supervision, J.M.J.-C., M.G.-C. and F.J.L.-C.; project administration, F.J.L.-C. and M.G.-C.; funding acquisition, F.J.L.-C. and M.G.-C. All authors have read and agreed to the published version of the manuscript.

Funding: This research received no external funding.

Institutional Review Board Statement: The study was designed following the ethical principles for human research of the Declaration of Helsinki. It was approved by the local ethics and research committee in the Reina Sofia University Hospital (Code: 1866,approval date: 26 October 2011).

Informed Consent Statement: Informed consent was obtained from all participants and their guardians involved in the study.

Data Availability Statement: The data presented in this study are available on request from the corresponding author. The data are not publicly available due to the patient privacy policy.

Acknowledgments: The authors would like to thank the children and their parents for their participation in the study.

Conflicts of Interest: The authors declare no conflict of interest.

Abbreviations

The following abbreviations are used in this manuscript:

BMI	Body mass index
DBP	Diastolic blood pressure
SBP	Systolic blood pressure
HR	Heart rate
HOMA-IR	Homeostasis model assessment of insulin resistance
HDL-c	High density lipoprotein cholesterol
LDL-c	Low density lipoprotein cholesterol

References

1. Kabiri, L.S.; Rodriguez, A.X.; Perkins-Ball, A.M.; Diep, C.S. Organized Sports and Physical Activities as Sole Influencers of Fitness: The Homeschool Population. *J. Funct. Morphol. Kinesiol.* **2019**, *4*, 13. [CrossRef]
2. Bu, X.; Gao, Y.; Liang, K.; Bao, W.; Chen, Y.; Guo, L.; Gong, Q.; Lu, H.; Caffo, B.; Mori, S.; et al. Multivariate Associations between Behavioural Dimensions and White Matter across Children and Adolescents with and without Attention-Deficit/Hyperactivity Disorder. *J. Child Psychol. Psychiatry* **2023**, *64*, 244–253. [CrossRef]
3. Chang, S.H.; Kim, K. A Review of Factors Limiting Physical Activity among Young Children from Low-Income Families. *J. Exerc. Rehabil.* **2017**, *13*, 375. [CrossRef]
4. Stea, T.H.; Solaas, S.A.; Kleppang, A.L. Association between Physical Activity, Sedentary Time, Participation in Organized Activities, Social Support, Sleep Problems and Mental Distress among Adults in Southern Norway: A Cross-Sectional Study among 28,047 Adults from the General Population. *BMC Public Health* **2022**, *22*, 384. [CrossRef] [PubMed]
5. de Oliveira, D.V.; Branco, B.H.M.; de Jesus, M.C.; Sepúlveda-Loyola, W.; Gonzáles-Caro, H.; Freire, G.L.M.; Dos Santos, N.Q.; Do Nascimento Júnior, J.R.A. Relationship between Vigorous Physical Activity and Body Composition in Older Adults. *Nutr. Hosp.* **2021**, *38*, 60–66. [CrossRef]
6. Zyriax, B.C.; Windler, E. Lifestyle Changes to Prevent Cardio- and Cerebrovascular Disease at Midlife: A Systematic Review. *Maturitas* **2023**, *167*, 60–65. [CrossRef]
7. Thivel, D.; Ring-Dimitriou, S.; Weghuber, D.; Frelut, M.L.; O'Malley, G. Muscle Strength and Fitness in Pediatric Obesity: A Systematic Review from the European Childhood Obesity Group. *Obes. Facts* **2016**, *9*, 52–63. [CrossRef]
8. Oja, P.; Titze, S.; Kokko, S.; Kujala, U.M.; Heinonen, A.; Kelly, P.; Koski, P.; Foster, C. Health Benefits of Different Sport Disciplines for Adults: Systematic Review of Observational and Intervention Studies with Meta-Analysis. *Br. J. Sports Med.* **2015**, *49*, 434–440. [CrossRef] [PubMed]
9. Jiang, D.; Xu, G. Effects of Chains Squat Training with Different Chain Load Ratio on the Explosive Strength of Young Basketball Players' Lower Limbs. *Front. Physiol.* **2022**, *13*, 979367. [CrossRef] [PubMed]
10. Tsai, C.L.; Ju, J.; Chen, Z. The Mediating Role of Prosocial and Antisocial Behaviors between Team Trust and Sport Commitment in College Basketball Players. *Eur. J. Sport Sci.* **2022**, *22*, 1418–1425. [CrossRef] [PubMed]
11. Koyama, T.; Rikukawa, A.; Nagano, Y.; Sasaki, S.; Ichikawa, H.; Hirose, N. Acceleration Profile of High-Intensity Movements in Basketball Games. *J. Strength Cond. Res.* **2022**, *36*, 1715–1719. [CrossRef] [PubMed]
12. Larsen, M.N.; Madsen, M.; Nielsen, C.M.; Manniche, V.; Hansen, L.; Bangsbo, J.; Krustrup, P.; Hansen, P.R. Cardiovascular Adaptations after 10 Months of Daily 12-Min Bouts of Intense School-Based Physical Training for 8-10-Year-Old Children. *Prog. Cardiovasc. Dis.* **2020**, *63*, 813–817. [CrossRef] [PubMed]
13. Tanner, J.M.; Whitehouse, R.H.; Marubini, E.; Resele, L.F. The Adolescent Growth Spurt of Boys and Girls of the Harpenden Growth Study. *Ann. Hum. Biol.* **1976**, *3*, 109–126. [CrossRef]
14. Sobradillo, B.; Aguirre, A.; Aresti, U.; Bilbao, A.; Fernández-Ramos, C. *Curvas y Tablas de Crecimiento (Estudios Longitudinal y Transversal)*; Ergón Creación, S.A.: Madrid, Spain, 2004.

15. Ruiz, J.R.; Castro-Piñero, J.; España-Romero, V.; Artero, E.G.; Ortega, F.B.; Cuenca, M.A.M.; Enez-Pavón, D.J.; Chillón, P.; Girela-Rejón, M.J.; Mora, J.; et al. Field-Based Fitness Assessment in Young People: The ALPHA Health-Related Fitness Test Battery for Children and Adolescents. *Br. J. Sports Med.* **2011**, *45*, 518–524. [CrossRef]
16. Cadenas-Sanchez, C.; Martinez-Tellez, B.; Sanchez-Delgado, G.; Mora-Gonzalez, J.; Castro-Piñero, J.; Löf, M.; Ruiz, J.R.; Ortega, F.B. Assessing Physical Fitness in Preschool Children: Feasibility, Reliability and Practical Recommendations for the PREFIT Battery. *J. Sci. Med. Sport.* **2016**, *19*, 910–915. [CrossRef]
17. Cengizel, E.; Cengizel, Ç.Ö.; Öz, E. Effects of 4-Month Basketball Training on Speed, Agility and Jumping in Youth Basketball Players. *Afr. Educ. Res. J.* **2020**, *8*, 417–421. [CrossRef]
18. Lesinski, M.; Herz, M.; Schmelcher, A.; Granacher, U. Effects of Resistance Training on Physical Fitness in Healthy Children and Adolescents: An Umbrella Review. *Sports Med.* **2020**, *50*, 1901–1928. [CrossRef]
19. Palma-Muñoz, I.; Ramírez-Campillo, R.; Azocar-Gallardo, J.; Álvarez, C.; Asadi, A.; Moran, J.; Chaabene, H. Effects of Progressed and Nonprogressed Volume-Based Overload Plyometric Training on Components of Physical Fitness and Body Composition Variables in Youth Male Basketball Players. *J. Strength Cond. Res.* **2021**, *35*, 1642–1649. [CrossRef]
20. Sánchez-Díaz, S.; Yanci, J.; Raya-González, J.; Scanlan, A.T.; Castillo, D. A Comparison in Physical Fitness Attributes, Physical Activity Behaviors, Nutritional Habits, and Nutritional Knowledge Between Elite Male and Female Youth Basketball Players. *Front. Psychol.* **2021**, *12*, 685203. [CrossRef]
21. Malina, R.M.; Eisenmann, J.C.; Cumming, S.P.; Ribeiro, B.; Aroso, J. Maturity-Associated Variation in the Growth and Functional Capacities of Youth Football (Soccer) Players 13-15 Years. *Eur. J. Appl. Physiol.* **2004**, *91*, 555–562. [CrossRef]
22. Rinaldo, N.; Toselli, S.; Gualdi-Russo, E.; Zedda, N.; Zaccagni, L. Effects of Anthropometric Growth and Basketball Experience on Physical Performance in Pre-Adolescent Male Players. *Int. J. Environ. Res. Public Health* **2020**, *17*, 2196. [CrossRef]
23. Temfemo, A.; Hugues, J.; Chardon, K.; Mandengue, S.H.; Ahmaidi, S. Relationship between Vertical Jumping Performance and Anthropometric Characteristics during Growth in Boys and Girls. *Eur. J. Pediatr.* **2009**, *168*, 457–464. [CrossRef] [PubMed]
24. Vaquero-Cristóbal, R.; Albaladejo-Saura, M.; Luna-Badachi, A.E.; Esparza-Ros, F. Differences in Fat Mass Estimation Formulas in Physically Active Adult Population and Relationship with Sums of Skinfolds. *Int. J. Environ. Res. Public Health* **2020**, *17*, 7777. [CrossRef]
25. Hermassi, S.; van den Tillaar, R.; Bragazzi, N.L.; Schwesig, R. The Associations Between Physical Performance and Anthropometric Characteristics in Obese and Non-Obese Schoolchild Handball Players. *Front. Physiol.* **2021**, *11*, 580991. [CrossRef]
26. Nikolaidis, P.T.; Asadi, A.; Santos, E.J.A.M.; Calleja-González, J.; Padulo, J.; Chtourou, H.; Zemkova, E. Relationship of Body Mass Status with Running and Jumping Performances in Young Basketball Players. *Muscle Ligaments Tendons J.* **2015**, *5*, 187–194. [CrossRef]
27. Castro-Collado, C.; Llorente-Cantarero, F.J.; Gil-Campos, M.; Jurado-Castro, J.M. Basketball's Improvement in Bone Mineral Density Compared to Other Sports or Free Exercise Practice in Children and Adolescents: A Systematic Review and Meta-Analysis. *Children* **2025**, *12*, 271. [CrossRef]
28. Otsuka, H.; Tabata, H.; Shi, H.; Sugimoto, M.; Kaga, H.; Someya, Y.; Naito, H.; Ito, N.; Abudurezake, A.; Umemura, F.; et al. Playing Basketball and Volleyball during Adolescence Is Associated with Higher Bone Mineral Density in Old Age: The Bunkyo Health Study. *Front. Physiol* **2023**, *14*, 1227639. [CrossRef]
29. Pereira, R.; Krustrup, P.; Castagna, C.; Coelho, E.; Santos, R.; Helge, E.W.; Jørgensen, N.R.; Magalhães, J.; Póvoas, S. Effects of Recreational Team Handball on Bone Health, Postural Balance and Body Composition in Inactive Postmenopausal Women—A Randomised Controlled Trial. *Bone* **2021**, *145*, 115847. [CrossRef]
30. Yang, Y.; Koenigstorfer, J. Determinants of Fitness App Usage and Moderating Impacts of Education-, Motivation-, and Gamification-Related App Features on Physical Activity Intentions: Cross-Sectional Survey Study. *J. Med. Int. Res.* **2021**, *23*, e26063. [CrossRef] [PubMed]
31. Gomez-Bruton, A.; Montero-Marín, J.; González-Agüero, A.; García-Campayo, J.; Moreno, L.A.; Casajús, J.A.; Vicente-Rodríguez, G. The Effect of Swimming During Childhood and Adolescence on Bone Mineral Density: A Systematic Review and Meta-Analysis. *Sports Med.* **2016**, *46*, 365–379. [CrossRef] [PubMed]
32. Ingle, L.; Sleap, M.; Tolfrey, K. The Effect of a Complex Training and Detraining Programme on Selected Strength and Power Variables in Early Pubertal Boys. *J. Sports Sci.* **2006**, *24*, 987–997. [CrossRef]
33. Ramírez-Vélez, R.; Silva-Moreno, C.; Correa-Bautista, J.E.; González-Ruíz, K.; Prieto-Benavides, D.H.; Villa-González, E.; García-Hermoso, A. Self-Rated Health Status and Cardiorespiratory Fitness in a Sample of Schoolchildren from Bogotá, Colombia. The FUPRECOL Study. *Int. J. Environ. Res. Public Health* **2017**, *14*, 952. [CrossRef]
34. Lamoneda, J.; Huertas-Delgado, F.J.; Cadenas-Sanchez, C. Feasibility and Concurrent Validity of a Cardiorespiratory Fitness Test Based on the Adaptation of the Original 20 m Shuttle Run: The 20 m Shuttle Run with Music. *J. Sports Sci.* **2021**, *39*, 57–63. [CrossRef]

35. Arnaoutis, G.; Georgoulis, M.; Psarra, G.; Milkonidou, A.; Panagiotakos, D.B.; Kyriakou, D.; Bellou, E.; Tambalis, K.D.; Sidossis, L.S. Association of Anthropometric and Lifestyle Parameters with Fitness Levels in Greek Schoolchildren: Results from the EYZHN Program. *Front. Nutr.* **2018**, *5*, 10. [CrossRef]
36. Högström, G.; Nordström, A.; Nordström, P. High Aerobic Fitness in Late Adolescence Is Associated with a Reduced Risk of Myocardial Infarction Later in Life: A Nationwide Cohort Study in Men. *Eur. Heart J.* **2014**, *35*, 3133–3140. [CrossRef] [PubMed]
37. Romarate, A.; Yanci, J.; Iturricastillo, A. Evolution of the Internal Load and Physical Condition of Wheelchair Basketball Players during the Competitive Season. *Front. Physiol* **2023**, *14*, 1106584. [CrossRef]
38. Pamuk, Ö.; Makaracı, Y.; Ceylan, L.; Küçük, H.; Kızılet, T.; Ceylan, T.; Kaya, E. Associations between Force-Time Related Single-Leg Counter Movement Jump Variables, Agility, and Linear Sprint in Competitive Youth Male Basketball Players. *Children* **2023**, *10*, 427. [CrossRef] [PubMed]
39. DiFiori, J.P.; Güllich, A.; Brenner, J.S.; Côté, J.; Hainline, B.; Ryan, E.; Malina, R.M. The NBA and Youth Basketball: Recommendations for Promoting a Healthy and Positive Experience. *Sports Med.* **2018**, *48*, 2053–2065. [CrossRef]
40. Hormazábal-Aguayo, I.; Muñoz-Pardeza, J.; Huerta-Uribe, N.; Ezzatvar, Y.; García-Hermoso, A. Evaluating the Usability of Diactive-1: MHealth for Personalized Exercise and Education in Children and Adolescents with Type 1 Diabetes. *mHealth* **2025**, *11*, 16. [CrossRef] [PubMed]

sports

MDPI

Article

Effectiveness of Specific Professional Training in Male Elite Adolescent Team Handball Players

Wagner Herbert [1,2,*], Radic Vanja [3] and Hinz Matthias [2]

1 Department of Sport and Exercise Science, University of Salzburg, 5020 Salzburg, Austria
2 Department of Sport Science, Otto von Guericke University of Magdeburg, 39106 Magdeburg, Germany; matthiashinz87@yahoo.com
3 Team Handball Club Dessau-Roßlauer HV, 06844 Dessau-Roßlau, Germany; radicvanja@hotmail.de
* Correspondence: herbert.wagner@plus.ac.at; Tel.: +43-662-8044-4887

Abstract: Professional training in elite team handball academies is key to developing top players, yet its direct impact on physical performance remains unclear. This study aimed to (1) provide professional training to elite adolescent players and (2) assess performance improvements using a team handball-specific test. Thirty elite male players (six goalkeepers, 24 field players) participated in an 11-week program, with nine under-19 (17.2 $\pm$ 1.3 years) and nine under-17 (15.6 $\pm$ 0.9 years) field players completing at least 80% of sessions. All underwent pre- and post-testing using the game-based performance test. A two-way ANOVA analyzed differences between tests and age groups as well as playing positions. Significant improvements ($p < 0.05$) were found in defense and offense time and body weight for both groups. Under-17 players also showed a significant increase in peak oxygen uptake (+9%), ball velocity (+7%), and jump height (+20%). Agility in defense and offense improved in under-19 (+3%) and under-17 (+6%) players, aligning with training goals. Positional differences were observed between backcourt players and wings ($p < 0.01$) in the ball velocity, while all players showed improvements in both defense and offense performance. We suggest that professional and targeted specific training at this age has a significant impact on the long-term development of adolescent team handball players and is the basis for a professional handball career.

Keywords: training; testing; physical training; team handball match; oxygen uptake; blood lactate

1. Introduction

Team handball is an Olympic team sport played on an indoor court measuring 40 $\times$ 20 m^2. Characterized by fast-paced, intermittent defensive and offensive actions, the game's objective is to score more goals than the opposing team. A standard match consists of two 30-min halves, during which players cover distances between 3900 and 4700 m. Among elite male team handball players, relative workloads typically range from 70–80% of maximal oxygen uptake (VO2max) throughout a match, with workload reductions commonly seen in the second half. Each field player (six field players and one goalkeeper per team) undergoes numerous intensity shifts and technical demands, including direction changes (25–35 per match), jumps (10–20), throws on goal (5–10), passes (40–60), and both light (45–55) and hard (10–15) body tackles [1,2]. These high-intensity actions alternate with periods of low-intensity movement, such as walking and standing, which comprise 70–75% of total playing time. Notably, elite players spend only 1–2% of total playing time sprinting [1,3,4]. Due to their position-specific roles, backcourt players, wings, and pivots differ

https://doi.org/10.3390/sports13060193

in total playing time and total distance covered (with wings playing longer), body weight (pivots being heavier), as well as sprinting and throwing performance (wings performing more sprints, while backcourt players achieve higher ball velocities) [4–7], with these differences generally more pronounced in adult players compared to adolescents [8–11]. However, a switch between playing positions during adolescence is not uncommon, and some of the world's best wings or pivots previously played as backcourt players (backs) in their younger years. In practice, elite training in adolescent team handball tends to be less position-specific compared to the more specialized training seen at the adult elite level.

In male team handball, professional training for adolescent players is crucial for developing top-elite athletes. Such training typically involves 7–8 sessions per week, including general physical and specific team handball training, along with participation in 1–2 national or international top-level matches. Despite the rigorous frequency and intensity of this training regimen, its effectiveness is often assessed through coach observations during training and matches, as well as through general physical performance tests [10–19]. However, the aim of professional training in adolescent team handball is to enhance specific physical performance. Therefore, accurately measuring this performance is essential to assess potential improvements. A test to determine this specific physical performance is the team handball game-based performance test (GBPT), which has been validated in previous studies [20,21]. In elite adolescent team handball players, Wagner, Hinz [22] found a correlation between increasing age and specific team handball performance. Furthermore, the GBPT was used to assess the adaptation of specific performance to specific physical training in a one-year training study involving elite adult male team handball players [23]. Evaluating the effects of professional training in adolescent team handball within a controlled study can provide valuable insights into optimal training planning for this age group. In this context, it is also relevant to investigate whether players of different age groups and playing positions (backs, wings, and pivots) respond differently to the training stimulus.

Consequently, the aims of the study were (1) to provide professional training to elite adolescent team handball players, and (2) to measure their performance improvement utilizing the GBPT. We hypothesized that the professional training regimen would lead to measurable improvements in specific physical performance among elite adolescent team handball players, with significant differences in improvement between age groups (under-19 and under-17) and playing positions (backs, wings, and pivots).

2. Materials and Methods

2.1. Participants

Thirty adolescent male team handball players, consisting of six goalkeepers and 24 field players, were involved in this study. Only field players took part in the GBPT. Inclusion criteria for field players required attendance at a minimum of 80% of all training sessions during the study period. Consequently, the study included (Figure 1) nine under-19 players (age: 17.2 ± 1.3 years, body weight: 77.8 ± 6.0 kg, body height: 1.82 ± 0.04 m) and nine under-17 players (age: 15.6 ± 0.9 years, body weight: 71.5 ± 14.5 kg, body height: 1.82 ± 0.06 m).

All participants included in the study were deemed physically healthy and reported no injuries that would prevent them from participating in team handball training or matches during the study period. The Ethics Committee of the University of Salzburg approved the research protocol (reference number: GZ-44-2015) in accordance with the Declaration of Helsinki. Prior to participation, all participants signed informed consent. For players under 18 years of age, their legal guardians reviewed and signed the informed consent.

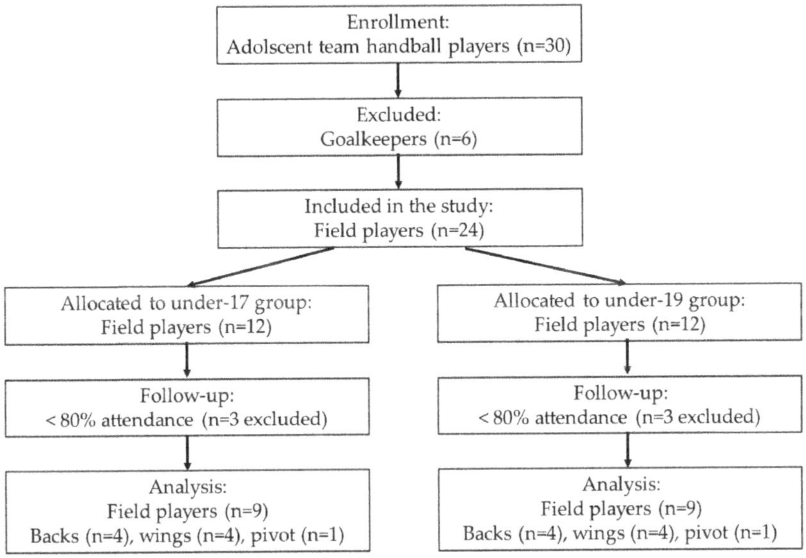

Figure 1. Consort flow allocation of the study.

2.2. *Study Design*

This study constituted a quasi-experimental study spanning an eleven-week training period, encompassing both the pre-season preparation phase and the initial three games of the highest under-19 and under-17 German Team Handball League's official season. The training regimen comprised 2–3 physical sessions and 4–5 specific team handball training sessions, amounting to a total of 7–8 sessions per week, along with 1–2 matches weekly. To assess performance improvement, all participants underwent the GBPT twice: once prior to the training period (pre-testing) and once after its completion (post-testing).

2.3. *Team Handball Game-Based Performance Test (GBPT)*

Before testing, participants completed an eight-minute general warm-up (jogging) and a fifteen-minute handball-specific warm-up involving passing, throwing, directional changes, and light contact. The GBPT began with one familiarization heat at ~70% effort, followed by eight test heats featuring handball-specific offensive and defensive actions, transitions, and active recovery phases [21].

In defense, participants sprinted three times from the 6 m to 9 m line, simulating tackles by touching padded roll mats (Figure 2) with both hands. In offense, they sprinted from the 12 m to 9 m line three times, touching 0.5 × 0.5 m floor markers with one foot while catching and passing the ball (Figure 2). In heats #2, #3, #4, #6, and #8, participants completed offensive actions with a one-legged jump shot, aiming for maximum throwing speed into the bottom corner of the goal. In heats #3 and #6, participants performed fast breaks by sprinting from defense to offense, receiving the ball at 12 m, and finishing with a jump shot at 9 m. In heats #4 and #6, they executed fast retreats from offense to defense immediately after the jump shot. A detailed description of the different movements in all heats has been published in a previous validation study of the GBPT [21].

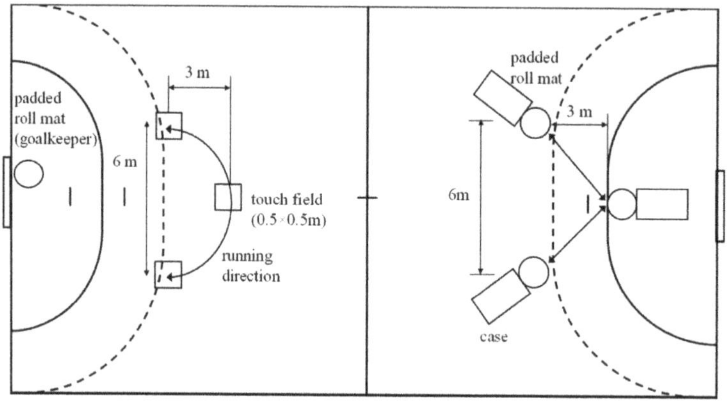

Figure 2. Schematic figure of the playing court in the team handball game-based performance test. Adapted from a previously published study [24].

Defense time (first to last contact on padded mats), offense time (contacts on floor markers), 10 m-fast break time (from 9 m defense line to midline), and 20 m-fast break time (midline to offensive floor markers) were measured using three manual stopwatches (Hanhart Stratos 2, Hanhart GmbH, Gütenbach, Germany) [20,25]. Fast retreat time was excluded due to variable acceleration after jump shots. Break durations, 20 s (between offense and defense), 15 s (between two actions), and 40 s (between heats), were controlled using Multi-Timer-Ultimate 3.1 software, with an audible countdown in the final 3 s. Jump shots were recorded at 200 fps (JVC-GC-PX100BE, Yokohama, Japan), and analyzed with Tracker 4.59 software (Douglas Brown, Aptos, CA, USA) to calculate ball velocity and jump height. Calibration used a 4-point reference from the goal (2 × 3 m). Flight time was defined as the interval between take-off and landing foot contact. Ball velocity was calculated from 2D motion over 15 frames, and jump height from flight time using gravitational acceleration. The mean values of the best three attempts were used for analysis [20].

$$h_{jump} = \frac{g}{8} \times t_{flight}^2$$

During the GBPT, heart rate and oxygen uptake were measured using a heart rate belt (Suunto T6d, Suunto, Vantaa, Finland) and a portable breath-by-breath gas analysis system (K5, Cosmed, Rome, Italy). Peak heart rate (HRpeak) and peak oxygen uptake (VO2peak) were calculated across all heats. For VO2peak, only values surrounded by two consecutive measurements above 90% of the peak were included to ensure accuracy [25].

2.4. Training Program

As outlined in the study design, the training program included an eight-week preseason preparation phase and a three-week competition phase (Figure 3), which encompassed the first three games of the official season in Germany's highest-team handball league. To structure the training effectively, seven distinct training focuses were established:

Warm-up: The warm-up phase was designed as optimal preparation for subsequent training activities, incorporating several components: individual run-in exercises, running ABC drills (e.g., heel kicks, knee lifts, step jumps, hop runs, and side-steps), ball-handling drills (e.g., bouncing, juggling, and passing), coordination exercises using ladders, rings, and benches, preparatory exercises such as complex passing drills, and/or warm-up games (e.g., small-sided games). In the competition phase, the average weekly warm-up time was 60 min, whereas, in the preparation phase, it was 80 min (Figure 4), due to the higher training volume during the preparation phase (Figure 3).

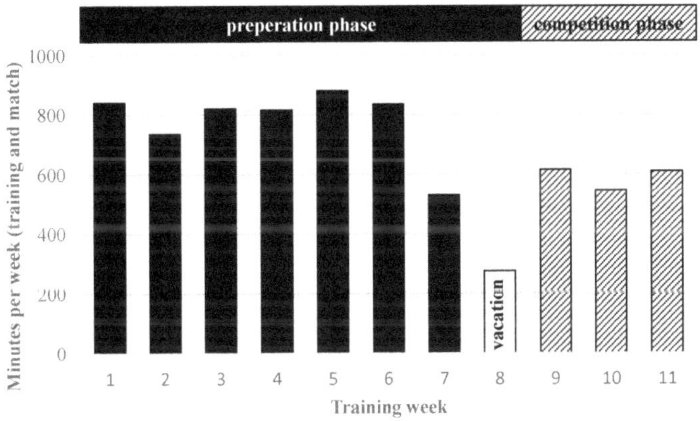

Figure 3. Total minutes per week (including training and matches) during the eleven-week training program, encompassing the preparation and competition phases as well as a vacation week, for the under-17 players.

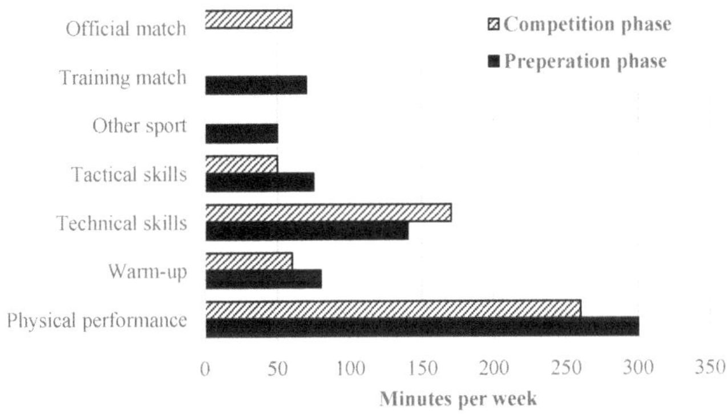

Figure 4. Mean minutes per week for the seven training focuses, separated by competition and preparation phases, in the under-17 players.

Other sport: To introduce variation into the training process, other sports such as soccer, basketball, and volleyball along with various athletic disciplines like sprinting, long jump, shot put, javelin, and swimming, were incorporated into the preparation phase.

Physical performance: Physical performance training plays a crucial role in optimizing preparation for high-performance training in elite adult team handball, particularly at this developmental stage [17,22,26]. Therefore, it was a primary focus during training sessions. This training encompassed various components, including low-intensity endurance (high volume), high-intensity interval training (both general and team handball-specific, featuring different interval lengths), sprint training, repeated sprint ability, agility training, as well as sensomotoric, mobility, and flexibility training, alongside strength and power training. Within strength and power training, particular emphasis was placed on barbell exercises such as back squats, front squats, overhead squats, split squats, deadlifts, bench presses, cleans, and power cleans. Additionally, to develop jumping and throwing power, exercises like box jumps, medicine ball drills, and elastic band exercises were incorporated. Furthermore, dumbbells and stationary strength training equipment available in the academy's gym were utilized to enhance overall strength and power. In the competition phase, the average weekly time for physical performance training was 260 min, compared to 300 min in the preparation phase (Figure 4), due to the higher training volume during the preparation phase (Figure 3). During the autumn break (vacation), the players had a week of home leave (training week #8), during which they were required to complete a home training program. This program included a 45-min warm-up and 200 min of physical performance training per week (Figure 4).

Technical skills: Team handball technical skills included basic attacking skills such as throwing, passing, faking, and feinting; complex attacking cooperations like crossing, cutting in, direct or indirect blocking, pushing, and rebounding; complex defending cooperations including closed, open, deep, or pressing defense; transitions such as fast transitions, fast breaks, fast throw-offs (defense to offense), and quick retreats (offense to defense); as well as goalkeeper training that involved drills with field players. During the preparation phase, the average training time for technical skills was 140 min per week. In the competition phase, this increased to 170 min per week due to a greater emphasis on team handball-specific training.

Tactical skills: Team handball tactical skills training included one-on-one drills and small group games (two-on-two, three-on-three, and four-on-four), attacking tactics involving all field players (six-on-six), as well as fast transition tactics. During the preparation phase, the average training time for tactical skills was 75 min per week; however, during the competition phase, it was reduced to 50 min per week. The increase in volume (+25 min) during the preparation phase was aimed at developing attacking tactics. For optimal training, team handball-specific sessions often combined warm-up, sensomotoric, mobility, and flexibility training with technical and tactical skills training. These sessions were structured with an optimal sequence of exercises, ensuring that individual drills built on one another.

The technical and tactical skills training used in the present study is typical for this age group in elite adolescent team handball. It was based on the training concept of the German Handball Federation and complemented by exercise variations from experienced coaches with the highest coaching license (Master Coach of the European Handball Federation). A detailed description of the technical and tactical training would be too extensive; however, some of these skills are described in detail (including video clips) in a book on modern methods for team handball-specific training [27].

Training match: Training matches during the preparation phase included standard training matches (50 to 60 min against rival teams), participation in national tournaments (2–3 matches over two days against other national teams), and, as a highlight, the German International Youth Championship in Düsseldorf, an international handball tournament featuring the top European teams in this age category. The average training match duration per week during the preparation phase was 70 min.

Official match: The official matches consisted of the first three games of the official season in the highest German Team Handball League, with each game having a duration of 2 × 30 min for under-19 players and 2 × 25 min for under-17 players.

External factors: All participants in the present study were athletes from a local elite team handball academy, where they followed a standardized daily schedule. This included structured training sessions, school attendance, study periods, rest, and sleep routines, with bedtimes adjusted according to age. Nutrition was consistently provided through the academy's canteen, including breakfast, mid-morning snack, lunch, afternoon snack, and dinner. No dietary supplements were consumed during the study period.

2.5. Statistical Analysis

All statistical analyses were conducted using SPSS version 29.0 (SPSS Inc., Armonk, NY, USA). Means and standard deviations were calculated for descriptive statistics. To assess differences between pre- and post-test results in the under-17 and under-19 players, a two-way repeated-measures ANOVA was employed, with "time" and "team" as well as "time" and "position" as the main factors. A Bonferroni post hoc test was used to identify significant differences between the under-17 and under-19 players as well as the playing positions, and effect size (η^2) and power ($1 - ß$) were calculated. For all statistical analyses, significance was set at $p < 0.05$, and the effect size was defined as small ($0.01 \leq \eta^2 < 0.06$), medium ($0.06 \leq \eta^2 < 0.14$), and large ($\eta^2 \geq 0.14$) [28].

3. Results

Mean values ± standard deviation and 95% confidence intervals for the under-19 and under-17 players (pre- and post-test) in the team handball game-based performance test are depicted in Table 1.

Table 1. Mean ± standard deviation (SD) and 95% confidence intervals (CI) in the under 19 and under 17 players (pre- and post-test) in the team handball game-based performance test in the peak oxygen uptake (VO2peak), peak heart rate (HRpeak), 10 and 20 m-fast break time, defense and offense time, jump height and ball velocity in the jump shot, as well as body mass and body height. F-values, *p*-values, and effect size for the factors team, time, and team × time in the two-way repeated-measures ANOVA.

	Under-19 Player		Under-17 Players				
	Pre-Test Mean ± SD (95% CI)	**Post-Test Mean ± SD (95% CI)**	**Pre-Test Mean ± SD (95% CI)**	**Post-Test mean ± SD (95% CI)**	**Team F-, *p*-Value Effect Size**	**Time F-, *p*-Value Effect Size**	**Team × Time F-, *p*-Value Effect Size**
VO_2peak (mL/kg.min)	73.9 ± 7.9 (68.1–79.8)	69.0 ± 6.6 (63.1–74.8)	65.9 ± 9.6 (60.1–71.8)	71.1 ± 10.0 (65.2–77.0)	1.03, 0.32 0.03	0.01, 0.98 0.00	3.13, 0.09 0.09
HRpeak (bpm)	192 ± 5 (189–196)	192 ± 9 (187–197)	193 ± 6 (188–198)	193 ± 7 (188–197)	0.21, 0.65 0.01	0.00, 0.98 0.00	0.05, 0.83 0.00
10 m-fast break time (s)	1.78 ± 0.08 (1.73–1.83)	1.78 ± 0.10 (1.72–1.83)	1.86 ± 0.06 (1.81–1.91)	1.85 ± 0.07 (1.79–1.90)	7.75, <0.01 ** 0.19	0.21, 0.65 0.01	0.10, 0.75 0.00
20 m-fast break time (s)	1.75 ± 0.10 (1.68–1.93)	1.79 ± 0.12 (1.71–1.86)	1.86 ± 0.10 (1.78–1.94)	1.72 ± 0.14 (1.66–1.81)	0.68, 0.41 0.02	1.26, 0.27 0.04	4.03, 0.05 0.11
Defense time (s)	5.50 ± 0.15 (5.40–5.60)	5.35 ± 0.13 (5.25–5.46)	5.77 ± 0.16 (5.67–5.88)	5.43 ± 0.18 (5.30–5.51)	10.41, <0.001 *** 0.25	25.31, <0.001 *** 0.44	4.49, 0.04 * 0.12
Offence time (s)	5.92 ± 0.29 (5.76–6.07)	5.76 ± 0.20 (5.60–5.91)	6.04 ± 0.27 (5.88–6.19)	5.61 ± 0.11 (5.45–5.76)	0.03, 0.87 0.00	15.37, <0.001 *** 0.32	3.17, 0.08 0.09
Jump height (m)	0.32 ± 0.07 (0.28–0.37)	0.38 ± 0.07 (0.34–0.42)	0.29 ± 0.05 (0.24–0.33)	0.34 ± 0.06 (0.31–0.40)	2.14, 0.15 0.06	7.97, <0.01 ** 0.20	0.07, 0.80 0.00
Ball velocity (m/s)	24.2 ± 1.3 (23.2–25.2)	24.5 ± 1.3 (23.5–25.5)	23.4 ± 1.7 (22.4–24.5)	25.0 ± 1.7 (23.8–25.8)	0.25, 0.62 0.01	2.79, 0.10 0.08	1.22, 0.28 0.04
Body mass (kg)	78 ± 6 (70–82)	80 ± 7 (72–87)	72 ± 14 (64–79)	78 ± 15 (67–82)	2.21, 0.15 0.06	0.47, 0.50 0.01	0.04, 0.83 0.00
Body height (m)	1.82 ± 0.04 (1.79–1.86)	1.83 ± 0.04 (1.80–1.86)	1.82 ± 0.06 (1.78–1.85)	1.82 ± 0.07 (1.78–1.85)	0.51, 0.48 0.02	0.06, 0.81 0.00	0.02, 0.89 0.00

(*/**/*** denotes $p < 0.05$/** $p < 0.01$/*** $p < 0.001$, respectively).

Significant differences were found between the under-19 and under-17 players in the 10 m-fast break time ($p < 0.01$) and defense time ($p < 0.001$) for the factor "team"; significant differences were also observed between pre- and post-test in defense time ($p < 0.001$), offense time ($p < 0.001$), and jump height ($p < 0.01$) for the factor "time," as well as an interaction effect between team and time ($p < 0.05$) for defense time. In addition to these significant differences in team and time with a large effect size and the interaction effect of team and time with a medium effect size, a medium effect size was also found in jump height and body mass for the factor "team," in ball velocity for the factor "time," and in VO2peak, 20 m fast-break time, and offense time for the interaction effect of team and time (Table 1).

For a detailed visualization of the results, mean values ± standard deviations for VO2peak, 10 m-fast break time, defense and offense time, jump height, and ball velocity in the jump shot are shown in Figure 5A–F. Post hoc test results are indicated with asterisks (* $p < 0.05$, ** $p < 0.01$, *** $p < 0.001$) in the figures. Among under-19 players, a decrease of 6.7% in VO2peak, a decrease of 0.2% in the 10 m-fast break time, a decrease of 2.7% in defense and offense time, along with an increase of 17.0% in jump height, and 1.1% in ball velocity, were observed. For under-17 players, we observed an increase of 8.8% in VO2peak, a decrease of 0.7% in 10 m-fast break time, a decrease of 5.9% in defense time, a decrease of 7.0% in offense time, along with an increase of 19.9% in jump height and 6.5% in ball velocity.

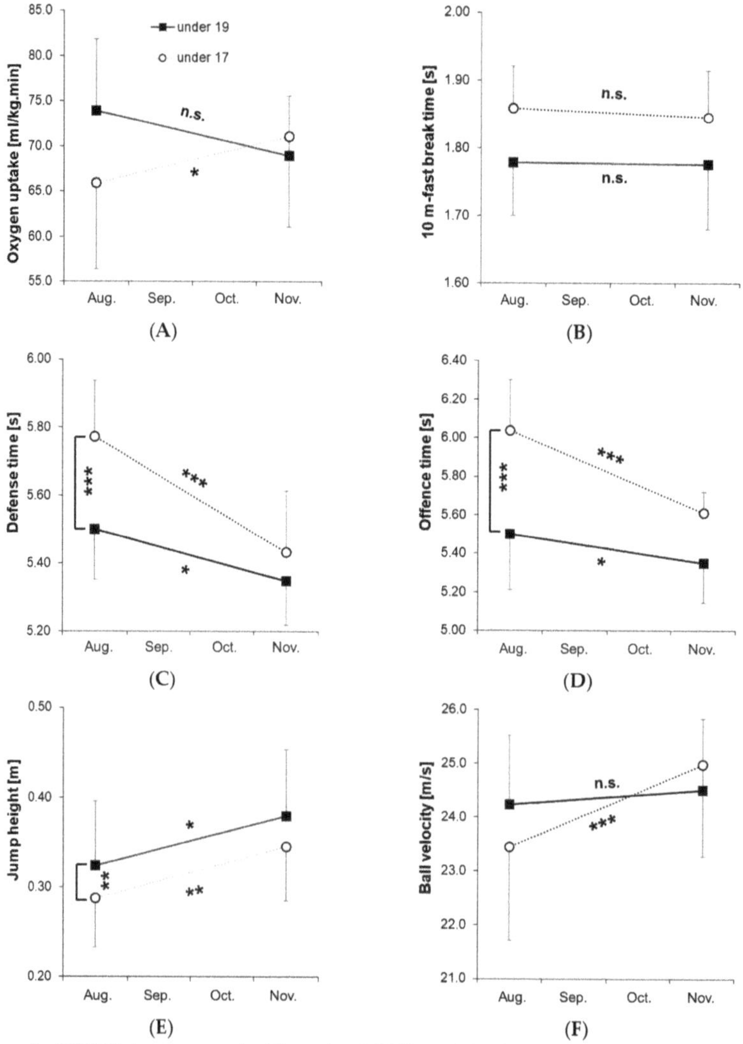

(n.s./*/**/*** denotes not significant/$p < 0.05$/** $p < 0.01$/*** $p < 0.001$, respectively)

Figure 5. Mean values ± standard deviation for under-19 and under-17 players (pre-test in August, post-test in November) in the team handball game-based performance test for peak oxygen uptake (**A**), 10 m fast-break time (**B**), defense time (**C**), offense time (**D**), jump height (**E**), and ball velocity (**F**) in the jump shot.

Due to the requirement of a minimum of 80% attendance in all training sessions, two backs and one pivot from each age group were excluded from the final analysis. As a result, data from eight backs, eight wings, and only two pivots were available to assess positional differences. Consequently, the two-way ANOVA with the factors "time" and "position" was conducted only for backs and wings. Figure 6A–D presents the mean ± standard deviation values for backs and wings in VO2peak, defense time, offense time, and ball velocity during the jump shot. For descriptive purposes, the individual values of the two pivots were also included in Figure 6A–D to illustrate potential training effects in this position.

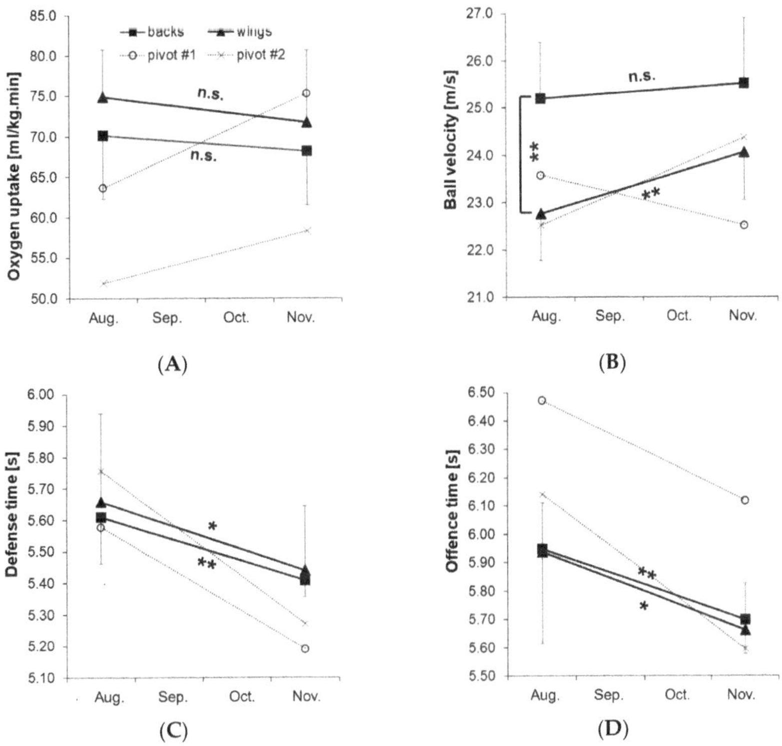

(n.s./*/** denotes not significant/$p < 0.05$/** $p < 0.01$, respectively)

Figure 6. Mean values ± standard deviation for backs and pivots (pre-test in August, post-test in November), as well as the values of the under-19 pivot (pivot #1) and under-17 pivot (pivot #2) in the team handball game-based performance test for peak oxygen uptake (**A**), ball velocity in the jump shot (**B**), defense time (**C**), and offense time (**D**).

Significant differences between backs and wings were observed in ball velocity during the jump shot (Figure 6B; F = 10.07, $p < 0.01$, $\eta^2 = 0.27$, 1-ß = 0.86), as well as in defense time (Figure 6C; F = 11.95, $p < 0.01$, $\eta^2 = 0.30$, 1-ß = 0.92) and offense time (Figure 6D; F = 13.28, $p < 0.01$, $\eta^2 = 0.32$, 1-ß = 0.94) for the factor "time." Post hoc tests revealed significant improvements in both wings ($p < 0.05$) and backs ($p < 0.01$) in defense and offense time. No significant effects for the factors "position" or "time" were found for VO2peak (Figure 6A), 10 m and 20 m fast break time, or jump height during the jump shot. Additionally, there was no significant interaction effect between "time × position" in the two-way ANOVA. Descriptive results for the two pivots showed similar trends to backs and wings in defense and offense time but differed in VO2peak (both pivots improved) and in ball velocity (Figure 5A), where the under-17 pivot improved while the under-19 pivot showed a decrease (Figure 5B).

4. Discussion

The aims of the study were to (1) provide professional training to elite adolescent team handball players and (2) measure their performance improvement using the GBPT. As expected, we found significant performance increases in both under-19 and under-17 players in defense time, offense time, and jump height during the jump shot (Table 1). Training for these age groups is designed to incorporate numerous fast movements specific to team handball scenarios (technical and tactical skills) as well as physical conditioning. At this developmental stage, enhancing offensive and defensive skills (including acceleration, deceleration, directional changes, and tackling) and jump shot performance is crucial for advancing to elite male team handball levels [22]. Interestingly, this improvement in performance was not observed in straight sprinting movements (10 m and 20 m fast-break time). However, straight sprinting is not strongly related to offense and defense in team handball [25] and has less impact on handball-specific performance [20,22,29]. Consequently, agility, speed, and power training in team handball should be tailored to enhance specific defensive, offensive, and jumping skills [26]. Notably, under-17 players showed greater improvements in defense and offense than under-19 players (Figure 5C,D). A performance gap in defense (0.31 s) and offense (0.25 s) was observed between the under-19 and under-17 players, suggesting that younger athletes may have a greater potential for performance gains.

An increase in ball velocity was observed only in under-17 players, not in under-19 players, despite the fact that post-test ball velocity was higher in under-17 players than in under-19 players (Figure 5F). This difference may be due to the smaller ball size and lighter weight used in the under-17 age group. According to the International Handball Federation (IHF) rules, ball size 3 (volume: 55–60 cm; weight: 425–475 g) is designated for adult male players and adolescent players over 16 years, while ball size 2 (volume: 54–56 cm; weight: 325–375 g) is intended for adult female players and male players aged 12 to 16. Following these guidelines, the German Handball Federation specifies ball size 3 for under-19 and ball size 2 for under-17 players. We propose that the reduced ball volume and weight for under-17 players contributed to the significant increase ($p < 0.001$) of 6.5% in ball velocity, as observed through targeted training (technical, tactical, and official matches) during the preparation and competition phases of the study.

When measuring VO2peak during the GBPT, no significant difference was found in under-19 players, but a significant increase ($p < 0.05$) was observed in under-17 players from pre-test to post-test. This increase in VO2peak among under-17 players may be attributed to high-intensity training in the preparation phase [23,26], which included (1) physical performance training, such as sprints, accelerations, decelerations, and changes of direction; (2) technical skills training, including throwing, passing, feinting, complex attacking and defending maneuvers, and fast transitions (fast breaks, throw-offs, and quick retreats); and (3) tactical skills training, including one-on-one drills, small group games, and fast transition tactics. In the elite handball academy of the present study, the long-term training approach prioritizes individual development for under-17 players (e.g., in official matches, the entire team was rotated in blocks to allow equal playing time). In contrast, for under-19 players, the focus shifts to team performance aimed at winning games and championships. We propose that this competitive focus for under-19 players may reduce high-intensity events, as it emphasizes six-on-six team skills over individualized high-intensity activities, although training intensity was not directly measured.

When analyzing positional differences, both backs ($p < 0.01$) and wings ($p < 0.05$), as well as both pivots, showed improved performance in defense and offense time. This suggests that the physical, technical, and tactical training applied in the present study effectively enhanced both defensive and offensive skills across all playing positions and age groups [10,11]. Notably, the improvement in defense time was particularly pronounced in the pivots, who outperformed their age-group peers in the post-test. Given the teams' preferred 6:0 defensive tactic, where pivots typically play in the central block requiring quick lateral movements, we attribute these gains to targeted defensive elements in the technical and tactical training [27]. As expected, backs demonstrated the highest ball velocity in the jump shot [8,9,17]. However, wings ($p < 0.01$) and the under-17 pivot showed substantial improvement, approaching the performance level of the backs from pre- to post-test. No significant changes in VO2peak were observed for backs and wings, but both pivots demonstrated improvements. These findings suggest that the specific training program not only enhances overall performance but also helps address positional or individual deficits, such as VO2peak in pivots or ball velocity in wings and under-17 players. To our knowledge, this study is the first to measure the direct impact of elite team handball training on specific physical performance, which is crucial for planning effective training in elite handball academies. However, the study also has limitations. While we documented the training as accurately as possible, we did not measure objective training intensity. For future studies, local position measurement systems and physiological metrics such as heart rate or blood lactate could provide more accurate intensity data. However, measuring load parameters such as metabolic power through local positioning systems has limited accuracy in team handball [30] and physiological metrics (e.g., heart rate, blood lactate) vary widely among individuals [20,29], making them impractical for this setting. Although training workload can also be assessed using perceived exertion, we chose not to include this measure. Instead, the team handball academy employed a long-established and proven monitoring system. Each week, the head coach, assistant coach, goalkeeper coach, physical coach, and physiotherapist collectively discussed workload, performance status, and stress levels for each player to prevent overload. This system was also applied in the present study and led to the exclusion of two players due to a heightened risk of overload. Additionally, four other players were excluded due to injuries and illness. Another limitation of the study was the small sample size, which prevented statistical evaluation of training effects for pivots. Nevertheless, the value of assessing training outcomes in elite adolescent team handball players outweighs this limitation.

5. Conclusions and Practical Implications

We conclude that the training regimen in the present study, which comprised 2–3 physical training sessions and 4–5 specific team handball sessions per week, totaling 7–8 sessions per week, along with 1–2 weekly matches, is an effective approach for enhancing the specific performance of male under-19 and under-17 players. We suggest that structured, targeted training at this developmental stage has a significant impact on the long-term development of adolescent team handball players and lays the foundation for a professional handball career. For example, the under-17 pivot showed the lowest VO2peak and was among the weakest performers across most variables in the pre-test. After receiving individualized feedback comparing his results to the mean values of the other under-17 players, he not only improved his performance by the post test but also significantly changed his training attitude. As a result, he was later selected for the national team and won a medal at the European Junior Championships. For coaches working with adolescent team handball players, we recommend implementing a well-balanced training program that integrates physical performance, technical, and tactical skills, like the training program used in the present study. To evaluate training outcomes, we advise using tests that assess team handball-specific physical performance. If the GBPT is too time- or cost-intensive, we suggest using its defense and offense components to measure defense time, offense time (requiring only a manual stopwatch), jump height, and ball velocity in the jump shot (using the free Tracker software and a video camera). For assessing specific aerobic performance, we recommend the YoYo Intermittent Recovery Test, which has shown a strong correlation (r = 0.56) with VO2peak as measured by the GBPT in elite female handball players [31].

The training program used in the present study was tailored for elite adolescent team handball players; however, the majority of adolescent players worldwide participate at a non-elite level. For these athletes, social interaction through team handball and personal fitness are often more relevant, both of which have significant implications for public health. Adapting the general structure of this training program by balancing physical conditioning with technical and tactical skills, to match the performance level of non-elite players may also improve their anaerobic and aerobic performance. Enhancing physical performance during adolescence contributes to better fitness in adulthood, even if players discontinue team handball later. Therefore, the balanced training approach presented here has the potential to help preserve and improve anaerobic performance in adolescent players more broadly, contributing to long-term health benefits and reducing performance disparities across European countries [32,33].

Supplementary Materials: The following supporting information can be downloaded at: https://www.mdpi.com/article/10.3390/sports13060193/s1, Table S1.

Author Contributions: Conceptualization, W.H. and R.V.; methodology, W.H.; software, W.H. and H.M.; validation, W.H., R.V. and H.M.; formal analysis, W.H. and H.M.; investigation, W.H., R.V. and H.M.; resources, W.H.; data curation, W.H. and H.M.; writing—original draft preparation, W.H.; writing—review and editing, W.H.; visualization, W.H.; supervision, W.H.; project administration, W.H. and R.V. All authors have read and agreed to the published version of the manuscript.

Funding: This research received no external funding.

Institutional Review Board Statement: The study was conducted in accordance with the Declaration of Helsinki and approved by the Institutional Ethics Committee of the UNIVERSITY OF SALZBURG (protocol code GZ-44-2015, approval date: 30 September 2015).

Informed Consent Statement: Informed consent was obtained from all subjects involved in the study.

Data Availability Statement: The original contributions presented in this study are included in the Supplementary Table S1. Further inquiries can be directed to the corresponding author.

Acknowledgments: We want to thank all players and coaches for their time and enthusiasm during the training and testing.

Conflicts of Interest: The authors declare no conflicts of interest.

Abbreviations

The following abbreviations are used in this manuscript:

VO2max	Maximal oxygen uptake
EHF	European Handball Federation
GBPT	Game-based performance test
HRpeak	Peak heart rate
VO2peak	Peak oxygen uptake
IHF	International Handball Federation

References

1. Michalsik, L.B.; Madsen, K.; Aagaard, P. Technical match characteristics and influence of body anthropometry on playing performance in male elite team handball. *J. Strength Cond. Res.* **2015**, *29*, 416–428. [CrossRef]
2. Michalsik, L.B.; Madsen, K.; Aagaard, P. Physiological capacity and physical testing in male elite team handball. *J. Sports Med. Phys. Fit.* **2015**, *55*, 415–429.
3. Michalsik, L.B.; Aagaard, P. Physical demands in elite team handball: Comparisons between male and female players. *J. Sports Med. Phys. Fit.* **2015**, *55*, 878–891.
4. Michalsik, L.B.; Aagaard, P.; Madsen, K. Locomotion characteristics and match-induced impairments in physical performance in male elite team handball players. *Int. J. Sports Med.* **2013**, *34*, 590–599. [CrossRef] [PubMed]
5. Manchado, C.; Pueo, B.; Chirosa-Rios, L.J.; Tortosa-Martínez, J. Time-Motion Analysis by Playing Positions of Male Handball Players during the European Championship 2020. *Int. J. Environ. Res. Public Health* **2021**, *18*, 2787. [CrossRef]
6. Manchado, C.; Martínez, J.T.; Pueo, B.; Tormo, J.M.C.; Vila, H.; Ferragut, C.; Sánchez, F.S.; Busquier, S.; Amat, S.; Ríos, L.J.C. High-Performance Handball Player's Time-Motion Analysis by Playing Positions. *Int. J. Environ. Res. Public Health* **2020**, *17*, 6768. [CrossRef]
7. Michalsik, L.B.; Aagaard, P.; Madsen, K. Technical activity profile and influence of body anthropometry on playing performance in female elite team handball. *J. Strength Cond. Res.* **2015**, *29*, 1126–1138. [CrossRef]
8. Fieseler, G.; Hermassi, S.; Hoffmeyer, B.; Schulze, S.; Irlenbusch, L.; Bartels, T.; Delank, K.-S.; Laudner, K.G.; Schwesig, R. Differences in anthropometric characteristics in relation to throwing velocity and competitive level in professional male team handball: A tool for talent profiling. *J. Sports Med. Phys. Fit.* **2017**, *57*, 985–992. [CrossRef]
9. Krüger, K.; Pilat, C.; Ückert, K.; Frech, T.; Mooren, F.C. Physical performance profile of handball players is related to playing position and playing class. *J. Strength Cond. Res.* **2014**, *28*, 117–125. [CrossRef]
10. Matthys, S.P.J.; Fransen, J.; Vaeyens, R.; Lenoir, M.; Philippaerts, R. Differences in biological maturation, anthropometry and physical performance between playing positions in youth team handball. *J. Sports Sci.* **2013**, *31*, 1344–1352. [CrossRef]
11. Mohoric, U.; Abazovic, E.; Paravlic, A.H. Morphological and Physical Performance-Related Characteristics of Elite Male Handball Players: The Influence of Age and Playing Position. *Appl. Sci.* **2022**, *12*, 11894. [CrossRef]
12. Hammami, M.; Hermassi, S.; Gaamouri, N.; Aloui, G.; Comfort, P.; Shephard, R.J.; Chelly, M.S. Field Tests of Performance and Their Relationship to Age and Anthropometric Parameters in Adolescent Handball Players. *Front. Physiol.* **2019**, *10*, 1124–1135. [CrossRef] [PubMed]
13. Ingebrigtsen, J.; Jeffreys, I.; Rodahl, S. Physical characteristics and abilities of junior elite male and female handball players. *J. Strength Cond. Res.* **2013**, *27*, 302–309. [CrossRef]
14. Lidor, R.; Falk, B.; Arnon, M.; Cohen, Y.; Segal, G.; Lander, Y. Measurement of talent in team handball: The questionable use of motor and physical tests. *J. Strength Cond. Res.* **2005**, *19*, 318–325. [CrossRef]
15. Matthys, S.P.J.; Vaeyens, R.; Fransen, J.; Deprez, D.; Pion, J.; Vandendriessche, J.; Vandorpe, B.; Lenoir, M.; Philippaerts, R. A longitudinal study of multidimensional performance characteristics related to physical capacities in youth handball. *J. Sports Sci.* **2013**, *31*, 325–334. [CrossRef] [PubMed]
16. Matthys, S.P.J.; Vaeyens, R.; Vandendriessche, J.; Vandorpe, B.; Pion, J.; Coutts, A.J.; Lenoir, M.; Philippaerts, R.M. A multidisciplinary identification model for youth handball. *Eur. J. Sport. Sci.* **2011**, *11*, 355–363. [CrossRef]
17. Rousanoglou, E.N.; Noutsos, K.S.; Bayios, I.A. Playing level and playing position differences of anthropometric and physical fitness characteristics in elite junior handball players. *J. Sports Med. Phys. Fit.* **2014**, *54*, 611–621.
18. Saavedra, J.M.; Kristjánsdóttir, H.; Einarsson, I.Þ.; Guðmundsdóttir, M.L.; Þorgeirsson, S.; Stefansson, A. Anthropometric characteristics, physical fitness and the prediction of throwing velocity in young men handball players. *Kinesiology* **2019**, *51*, 253–260. [CrossRef]
19. Visnapuu, M.; Juerimae, T. Relations of Anthropometric Parameters with Scores on Basic and Specific Motor Tasks in Young Handball Players. *Percept. Mot. Ski.* **2009**, *108*, 670–676. [CrossRef]
20. Wagner, H.; Fuchs, P.; Michalsik, L.B. On-court game-based testing in world-class, top-elite, and elite adult female team handball players. *Transl. Sports Med.* **2020**, *3*, 263–270. [CrossRef]
21. Wagner, H.; Orwat, M.; Hinz, M.; Pfusterschmied, J.; Bacharach, D.W.; Von Duvillard, S.P.; Müller, E. Testing game based performance in team-handball. *J. Strength Cond. Res.* **2016**, *30*, 2794–2801. [CrossRef] [PubMed]
22. Wagner, H.; Hinz, M.; Fuchs, P.; Bell, J.W.; von Duvillard, S.P. Specific Game-Based Performance in Elite Male Adolescent Team Handball Players. *Int. J. Sports Physiol. Perform.* **2022**, *17*, 901–907. [CrossRef] [PubMed]
23. Wagner, H.; Gierlinger, M.; Adzamija, N.; Ajayi, S.; Bacharach, D.W.; Von Duvillard, S.P. Specific physical training in male team handball. *J. Strength Cond. Res.* **2017**, *31*, 3083–3093. [CrossRef] [PubMed]
24. Wagner, H.; Hinz, M. The Relationship between Specific Game-Based and General Performance in Young Adult Elite Male Team Handball Players. *Appl. Sci.* **2023**, *13*, 2756. [CrossRef]

25. Wagner, H.; Sperl, B.; Bell, J.W.; von Duvillard, S.P. Testing Specific Physical Performance in Male Team Handball Players and the Relationship to General Tests in Team Sports. *J. Strength Cond. Res.* **2019**, *33*, 1056–1064. [CrossRef]
26. Buchheit, M.; Laursen, P.B.; Kuhnle, J.; Ruch, D.; Renaud, C.; Ahmaidi, S. Game-based Training in Young Elite Handball Players. *Int. J. Sports Med.* **2009**, *30*, 251–258. [CrossRef]
27. Wagner, H.; Radic, V. *Handball TAKT: Moderne Methoden für spielnahes Training*; Meyer & Meyer: Aachen, Germany, 2022; 294p.
28. Cohen, J. *Statistical Power Analysis for the Behavioral Sciences*; Routledge Academic: New York, NY, USA, 1988; Volume 2, 567p.
29. Weber, J.; Wegner, M.; Wagner, H. Physical performance in female handball players according to playing position. *Ger. J. Exerc. Sport. Res.* **2018**, *48*, 498–507. [CrossRef]
30. Fuchs, P.X.; Fuchs, P.; von Duvillard, S.P.; Wagner, H.; Shiang, T.Y. Critical assessment of a wide-spread method for estimating energy expenditure during accelerated running based on positioning tracking systems. *J. Sport. Health Sci.* **2022**, *11*, 641–643. [CrossRef]
31. Michalsik, L.B.; Fuchs, P.; Wagner, H. The Team Handball Game-Based Performance Test Is Better than the Yo-Yo Intermittent Recovery Test to Measure Match-Related Activities in Female Adult Top-Elite Field Team Handball Players. *Appl. Sci.* **2021**, *11*, 6551. [CrossRef]
32. Tomkinson, G.R. Global changes in anaerobic fitness test performance of children and adolescents (1958–2003). *Scand. J. Med. Sci. Sports* **2007**, *17*, 497–507. [CrossRef]
33. Tomkinson, G.R.; Olds, T.S.; Borms, J. Who are the Eurofittest? *Med. Sport. Sci.* **2007**, *50*, 104–128. [PubMed]

sports

MDPI

Article

Pairwise Comparison of Effects of Linear vs. Change of Direction Short Bout Sprint Intervals on Physical Performance of Youth Male Soccer Players

Peter Sagat

Sport Sciences and Diagnostics Research Laboratory, GSD/Health and Physical Education Department, Prince Sultan University, Riyadh 11586, Saudi Arabia; sagat@psu.edu.sa

Abstract

Our study aimed to examine and compare the effects of 12-week repeated sprint intervals with change of direction and linear sprint intervals on physical performance in young soccer players. In this randomized, parallel three-group study, we included 60 male soccer players assigned to (i) a sprint interval with change of direction group (RS–CoD; n = 20); (ii) a linear sprint interval group (RS–LiN; n = 20); and (iii) a soccer group (SOC; n = 20). Physical performance included explosive power (countermovement jump [CMJ] and squat jump [SJ]), agility (T505, 93,639, 20Y), speed (sprints over 5 m, 10 m and 20 m), anaerobic capacity (the Running-Based Anaerobic Sprint Test [RAST]) and maximal oxygen uptake (VO2max). Over the 12 weeks, the RS–CoD group displayed significantly beneficial effects in the 93639 test (effect size [ES] = 0.42), compared to the RS–LiN (ES = 0.18) and SOC (ES = 0.12) groups. The RS–CoD group also had larger improvements in their SJ (ES = 0.87; RS–LiN 0.37; SOC 0.18), CMJ (ES = 0.56; RS–LiN 0.39; SOC 0.43), 20Y test (ES = 1.05; RS–LiN 0.67; SOC 0.56) and sprints at 5 m (ES = 1.18; RS–LiN 0.50; SOC 0.21) and 20 m (ES = 1.43; RS–LiN 0.71; SOC 0.25). The RS–CoD group displayed more beneficial improvements, making the CoD interval sprints effective training stimuli.

Keywords: football; repeated sprint ability; linear sprinting; change of direction; effects

1. Introduction

High-intensity actions like sprints and vast changes of direction (CoDs) performed at maximal speeds exceeding 19.5 km*h^{-1} have become crucial for achieving an advantage over the opponent [1]. Irrespective of playing position, evidence suggests that between 4% and 18% of the total distance covered is accounted by these activities, often followed by a resting period before another action of the same intensity occurs [2]. During a top-level soccer match, a player can perform 150 to 250 high-intensity actions [3]. Although high-intensity actions require substantial physiological demands and quickly lead to fatigue [4], trends have shown that in professional soccer, the number of high-intensity actions has risen over the recent decades [5]. This would imply that such actions may adequately discriminate against soccer players at similar physical and psychological levels [6]. Along with the players' competitive level [7], high-intensity actions completed at maximal levels are associated with the repeated sprint ability (RSA), one of the key determinants in soccer [8,9].

The ability to perform repeated sprints lasting <10 s with short resting intervals between them (<60 s) is crucial for performance in soccer [10]. In practice, RSA can have beneficial effects on the enzymes of the aerobic and anaerobic systems, enhancing the level of phosphofructokinase and myokinase [11] and affecting the increased energy production. Such metabolic changes can be directly associated with explosive strength, sprints and aerobic-related adaptations [8,12]. Despite these advantages, the implementation of RSA in youth players is still lacking [13], possibly because of its specific approach and complexity [14]. Nevertheless, RSA has been constantly proven as a reliable and valid training method for improving a variety of physical performance components in adults and more elite soccer players [15,16].

In general, the RSA incorporates a methodology of linear sprints of <10 s followed by an interval of rest (<60 s) [17]. In regard to linear sprints, change of direction (CoD)-type sprints have become equally important because of their common representation during a soccer match [18]. Specifically, soccer players tend to perform >8 CoD sprint intervals in a minute [19]. Thus, the importance of performing elements with CoDs at a maximal level requires special attention, especially in young soccer players. To date, several studies have examined the effects of an RS–CoD on physical performance in male soccer players [20–24], while only a handful have differentiated between the effects of RSs in a linear direction (RS–LiN) vs. an RS–CoD [13,25–28]. Results from these studies yielded similar findings, showing no significant differences in the effects of an RS–LiN and RS–CoD in soccer players [25–27]. In a study by Sagelv et al. [25], no interaction effect (time × group) in Yo-Yo IR2 or sprint tests was found, which would suggest that both the RS–LiN and RS–CoD produced equal effects on physical performance. Similar observations have been documented in U15, U17 and U19 male soccer players, where both intervention protocols exhibited beneficial changes in the linear and slalom sprint speed, explosive power and maximal aerobic speed [26]. On the other hand, it has been noted that these types of training stimuli performed in a single session per week may not be sensitive enough to produce within-group changes over 8 weeks [27]. For an RS–LiN, unclear variations in sprinting and jumping occurred, while the RS–CoD produced somewhat larger effects, especially in sprinting activities [27]. Therefore, the effect comparison between the RS–LiN and RS–CoD remains inconclusive. Given the fact that implementing RS strategies within the training regime in youth soccer players is challenging, examining separate effects of an RS–LiN and RS–CoD on physical performance would be helpful for strength conditioning coaches to monitor and track fitness levels at individual and group levels.

The main purpose of this study was to examine the effects of a 12-week RS–LiN and RS–CoD training program on physical performance in male U17 soccer players. We hypothesized that the RS–CoD would exhibit larger effects on sprinting-, jumping- and agility-related tests and aerobic capacity in comparison to the RS–LiN.

2. Methods

Study Participants

A flow chart diagram of participants' enrolment, randomization and final analysis is presented in Figure 1. Male soccer players (age = 16.42 ± 0.21 years; height = 173.32 ± 5.80 cm; weight = 65.19 ± 6.42 kg) from three national-level competitive clubs were recruited in this randomized controlled trial. The G*power sample size calculator indicated that for the a priori analysis of variance for repeated measures (RMANOVA) with a moderate effect size of f = 0.25 [29], a statistical power of 1-β = 0.80, a *p*-value of < 0.05, 3 groups measured at two time points and hypothetical correlations between repeated measures of $r = 0.50$, the minimally required sample size would be 42. To adjust for potential follow-up loss, we increased our final sample to n = 65 soccer players. The inclusion criteria were fully active outfield male soccer players who had experienced no injury or musculoskeletal pain prior to testing and playing soccer for >8 years. The exclusion criteria included a soccer

https://doi.org/10.3390/sports14020044

player having an injury-related problem and who failed to attend >85% of training sessions during the competitive season. All data related to inclusion and exclusion criteria were collected by a questionnaire. The final sample included sixty soccer players who met the inclusion criteria and completed the study after being randomly assigned to one of three groups: a change of direction sprint group (RS-CoD; n = 20); a linear sprint group (RS-LiN; n = 20); and a soccer group performing regular training (SOC; n = 20).

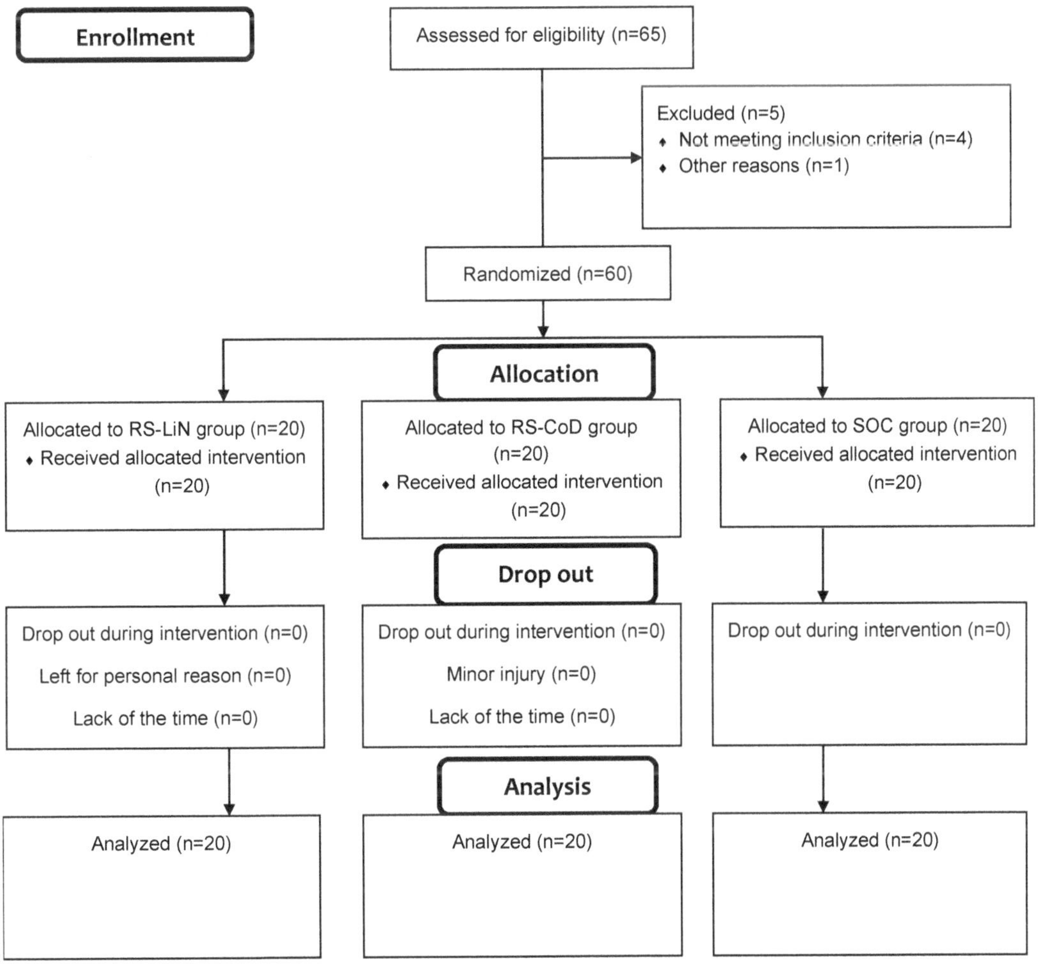

Figure 1. Flow chart diagram of participants' enrolment, randomization and final analysis.

Prior to the intervention, all participants trained regularly three days per week in the afternoon hours (between 17:00 h and 19:00 h). A common type of training consisted of a set of technical and tactical components (shooting, dribbling, passing and running with the ball) with the cooperation of the goalkeeper and other players, strength and conditioning parts consisted of small-sided games (5 vs. 5 or 10 vs. 10 soccer players including goalkeepers) and injury prevention exercises were most commonly performed at the end of a training session. For the participants who entered and completed this study, no group differences were present at baseline. The experimental protocol and potential risks were explained to all participants before they provided written consent. All the procedures

https://doi.org/10.3390/sports14020044

were anonymous and in accordance with the Declaration of Helsinki. This study was approved by the Ethical Committee Board of the Henan Polytechnic University, Henan Province (Ethical code: HPU-2024-09-4538).

3. Intervention Protocol

Based on previous studies, all the study participants completed two familiarization sessions associated with physical performance tests before an intervention in week 0 [24]. During the same week, all participants underwent laboratory and on-field testing procedures. All on-field tests and measurements were completed in a grass soccer field to mimic standardized conditions. The weather conditions were adequate, with an air temperature of 23 °C and a relative humidity of 55%. The laboratory conditions were similar to the on-field conditions, with an indoor temperature of 22 °C and a relative humidity of 53%. We followed the protocol of Sanchez-Sanchez et al. [24], where all participants were required not to eat heavily or drink caffeinated drinks for 2 h and avoid high-intensity aerobic or resistance training 48 h prior to testing. Before initiating the data collection, each participant had a warm-up period of 10 min, which included exercises for dynamic and static stretching, low and high skips and three acceleration and deceleration tasks followed by three 10 m sprints.

We followed the intervention program of Sanchez-Sanchez et al. [24] for the RS–CoD, RS–LiN and SOC groups that lasted for 12 weeks. The SOC group continued the regular soccer training routine, where the RS–CoD and RS–LiN groups completed upgraded soccer training with additional linear or change of direction sprints two times per week (Tuesday and Thursday), totaling 24 sessions. The RS–CoD group performed three sets of ten 15 m sprint intervals lasting <10 s with one CoD of 180° initiated at the end of a track, after which the participants ran at maximal speed to the starting position. Each sprint interval was followed by a recovery period of low-intensity running for <30 s. The resting period between each set was set at 4 min. In total, the weekly training volume was six sets of 10 repetitions over the first 4 weeks, with a progression of 15 repetitions in weeks 5–8 and 20 repetitions in weeks 9–12. The RS–LiN group completed the same number of sprint intervals over a 12-week intervention period, but the participants were instructed to perform linear running on a 31 m track by keeping a constant maximal pace over the entire distance. The reason for the reduced distance in the RS–CoD group is based on recommendations by Stanković et al. [29] where CoD sprints require additional energy and should be compensated for by reducing the distance by 2–3% in comparison to linear sprints.

4. Study Variables

Explosive power was assessed by two reliable and valid vertical jumps to assess the jump height (cm): (i) the countermovement jump (CMJ) and (ii) squat jump (SJ). We used the Optojump photoelectric cells (Microgate, Bolzano, Italy) to evaluate the flight time (in cm) from take-off to landing phases. The CMJ was performed with the arms on the hips, and based on a pre-recorded signal, each participant flexed their knees to approximately 90° and pushed upward as high as possible without moving the arms from the hips. The same principle was applied to the SJ, but the starting position was from the knees flexed at approximately 90°, and hands were placed on the waist area, and after holding this position for 3 s, the participant was instructed to jump upward vigorously without moving the hands from the hips. Both tests were performed three times with a 4 min rest between each trial. The reliability of all trials for tests was excellent (ICC > 0.85, coefficient of variation [CV] < 2.5%), and the best result was examined in further analyses.

https://doi.org/10.3390/sports14020044

To assess *agility*, we used the T505, 93,639 and 20Y tests. The T505 test involved sprinting to a marked point 5 m away from the starting position, touching the ground with one hand, immediately changing direction with a turn of 180° and running back to the starting point. The 93,639 test was initiated by sprinting over a course of 9 m, after which each player changed direction by 180° and started sprinting for 3 m, making another turn of 180° and running 6 m, continuing with a 180° turn and sprinting for 3 m, before making the last turn of 180° and sprinting over a 9 m course to the finish line. In total, the players covered a distance of 21 m. The final score was recorded as the time (in sec) measured by the photoelectric cell system (Witty, Microgate, Bolzano, Italy). For the 20Y test, two parallel lines were set up in the hall, 10 yards apart, with the center line located exactly halfway between them. Each line was one meter wide. A Witty photocell telemetry system was used for timing (Microgate, Bolzano, Italy), with a pair of cells placed on the center line and a starting position mark 0.5 m from the center line. The participant started from a high start position on an independent signal and repeated the test three times. The movement begins with a sprint to the sideline touched with the foot (covering 5 yards), then a sprint to the other sideline by repeating the same action (covering 10 yards) and finally a sprint back to the center line (covering 5 yards) where the time was stopped. The reliability and factorial validity properties of these tests have been previously confirmed in soccer players [30,31]. Each test included three trials (ICC > 0.80, CV < 3.0%) with a 4 min rest between the attempts, and the best result was considered for further analyses. The aforementioned tests have been illustrated and explained elsewhere [29,30].

To evaluate the *running speed*, the participants completed a set of linear sprinting tests over 5 m, 10m and 20 m [32]. In brief, a photoelectric cell system (Witty, Microgate, Bolzano, Italy) was placed at the starting and finishing lines over a distance of 20 m. Before the test began, the participant took a high standing start position approximately 40 cm behind the starting line. The time began when the participant crossed the first photocell infrared line. During the 20 m sprint section, the participants' running times at 5 m, 10 m and 20 m were recorded. Similarly to previous tests, three trials were conducted (ICC > 0.90, CV < 2.0%), with the best result being processed in further analyses.

The Running-Based Anaerobic Sprint Test (RAST) was used as a proxy for the anaerobic power output [33]. The test involved completing six 35 m sprints with 10 s rest intervals in between. From a standing start position, each participant sprinted over a course of 35 m. After crossing the 35 m line, the time stopped (and was registered), and the 10 s recovery period began. The same procedure was performed five more times, covering 210 m in total. The test was performed once. The results were presented in sec and maximal power output using the following formula: body mass (kg) * distance covered^2 * final time^{-3} [33].

The *maximal oxygen uptake* (VO2max) test was conducted using a ramp protocol on a motorized treadmill and determined by a breath-by-breath pulmonary gas exchange system (Quark b^2, COSMED, Rome, Italy). The starting speed was set at 7 km*h^{-1}, and it was increased by 1 km*h^{-1} every 1 min until volitional exhaustion. The criteria for exhaustion included the following: (i) a VO2 of <1.0 mL*kg^{-1}*min^{-1} after an increase in speed; (ii) an exchange ratio >1.1; and (iii) a peak lactate of >6 mmol*L^{-1} after exercise [34]. If the participant reported any bodily pain or discomfort, the test was stopped. The recovery period after the exercise included walking at 4.5 km*h^{-1} for 5 min. Aerobic data regarding the VO2max were averaged on a 5 s basis and included as a proxy for the cardiorespiratory capacity in further analyses.

5. Statistical Analysis

Basic descriptive statistics are presented as the mean ± standard deviation (SD). Based on previous studies [24], all data were log-transformed to omit the nonuniformity error. A

https://doi.org/10.3390/sports14020044

repeated measures analysis of variance (RMANOVA) with pre–post-measurements and the 'group' as a between-subject factor was used to examine the main effects for 'time' and an interaction term between 'time' and 'group' (time × group). If significant main effects were observed, a post hoc analysis with Bonferroni corrections was calculated. Within-group differences in pre- and post-measurements were calculated using the Student t-test for dependent samples. Cohen's D effect size statistics were used to examine the magnitude of the intervention output with the following threshold values: (i) ≥ 0.2 (small), (ii) ≥ 0.5 (moderate) and (iii) ≥ 0.8 (large) [35]. The significance was set at $\alpha < 0.05$, and it was two-sided. All analyses were calculated using the Statistical Packages for Social Sciences (SPSS) software program ver. 27 (IBM Corp., Chicago, Il, USA). The raw data of the study participants can be found in the Supplementary Material Table S1.

6. Results

The initial data suggested that no differences between the RS-CoD, RS-LiN and SOC groups were observed (p = 0.124–0.866). Table 1 shows basic descriptive statistics of the study participants, according to the RS–CoD, RS–LiN and SOC groups. No between-group differences in initial anthropometric characteristics and years of experience were found ($p > 0.05$).

Table 1. General information of the study participants, according to groups.

Variables	Total (n = 60)	RS–CoD (n = 20)	RS–LiN (n = 20)	SOC (n = 20)	p-Value
	Mean ± SD	Mean ± SD	Mean ± SD	Mean ± SD	
Age (years)	16.42 ± 0.21	16.38 ± 0.24	16.46 ± 0.20	16.41 ± 0.19	0.856
Height (cm)	173.32 ± 5.80	172.03 ± 5.48	173.95 ± 6.13	173.98 ± 5.86	0.482
Weight (kg)	65.19 ± 6.42	64.83 ± 5.01	64.44 ± 7.85	66.29 ± 6.27	0.638
BMI (kg*m^{-2})	22.29 ± 2.90	22.51 ± 1.32	21.88 ± 2.69	22.48 ± 1.41	0.501
Experience (years)	10.21 ± 1.25	10.30 ± 1.23	10.11 ± 1.31	10.22 ± 1.26	0.728

BMI: Body mass index; $p < 0.05$.

Within-group changes in physical performance are presented in Table 2. The significant and most beneficial improvements were found in the RS–CoD group. Soccer players assigned to this group displayed large increases for the T505 (mean diff. = 0.13 s, 95% CI 0.10–0.16); SJ (mean diff. = 2.03 cm, 95% CI 1.37–2.70); 20Y (mean diff. = 0.21 s, 95% CI 0.17–0.25); sprint for 5 m (mean diff. = 0.09 s, 95% CI 0.05–0.12), 10 m (mean diff. = 0.13 s, 95% CI 0.08–0.17) and 20 m (mean diff. = 0.15 s, 95% CI 0.11–0.19); and RAST (mean diff. = 0.25 s, 95% CI 0.19–0.31) and moderate increases for the 93639 (mean diff. = 0.13 s, 95% CI 0.12–0.15), CMJ (mean diff. = 1.77 cm, 95% CI 1.15–2.39), RAST power output (mean diff. = 33.17 W, 95% CI 22.21–44.12) and VO2max (mean diff. = 1.78 mL * kg^{-1} * min^{-1}, 95% CI 0.57–3.00). For the RS–LiN group, the largest improvement was observed for the 10 m sprint (mean diff. = 0.10 s, 95% CI 0.06–0.13), while 93639 displayed the least beneficial improvement (mean diff. = 0.09 s, 95% CI 0.08–0.10). In the SOC group, small to moderate ESs for physical performance were shown, where T505 (mean diff. = 0.05 s, 95% CI 0.04–0.07) and 20Y (mean diff. = 0.12 s, 95% CI 0.10–0.14) exhibited the largest increases, opposed to other variables.

https://doi.org/10.3390/sports14020044

Table 2. Physical performance in RS-CoD, RS-LIN and SOC groups before and after 12-week training intervention.

Variables	Pre	Post	Δ (%)	ES	*p*-Value
RS–CoD (*n* = 20)	Mean ± *SD*	Mean ± *SD*			
T505 (s)	2.54 ± 0.12	2.41 ± 0.10	−5.12% [b]	1.18	**<0.001**
93639 (s)	7.74 ± 0.33	7.60 ± 0.33	−1.81% [a,b]	0.42	**<0.001**
SJ (cm)	26.17 ± 2.18	28.20 ± 2.49	7.76% [a,b]	0.87	**<0.001**
CMJ (cm)	28.13 ± 3.01	29.90 ± 3.34	6.29% [a,b]	0.56	**<0.001**
20Y (s)	4.62 ± 0.20	4.41 ± 0.20	−4.55% [a,b]	1.05	<0.001
Sprint, 5 m (s)	1.23 ± 0.09	1.14 ± 0.06	−7.32% [a,b]	1.18	**<0.001**
Sprint, 10 m (s)	2.04 ± 0.11	1.92 ± 0.08	5.88% [b]	1.25	**<0.001**
Sprint, 20 m (s)	3.48 ± 0.11	3.33 ± 0.10	−4.31% [a,b]	1.43	**<0.001**
RAST (s)	6.16 ± 0.20	5.91 ± 0.18	−4.07% [b]	1.31	**<0.001**
RAST power output (W)	306.14 ± 32.30	339.31 ± 30.78	10.83% [b]	0.73	**<0.001**
VO2max (mL * kg^{-1} * min^{-1})	50.45 ± 3.15	52.23 ± 3.78	3.53% [b]	0.51	**0.006**
RS–LiN (*n* = 20)					
T505 (s)	2.47 ± 0.15	2.38 ± 0.16	−3.64%	0.58	**<0.001**
93639 (s)	7.71 ± 0.50	7.62 ± 0.49	−1.12% [c]	0.18	**<0.001**
SJ (cm)	26.44 ± 2.05	27.26 ± 2.40	3.10%	0.37	**<0.001**
CMJ (cm)	28.06 ± 2.39	29.01 ± 2.45	3.39%	0.39	**<0.001**
20Y (s)	4.62 ± 0.23	4.47 ± 0.22	−3.25%	0.67	**<0.001**
Sprint, 5 m (s)	1.23 ± 0.06	1.20 ± 0.06	−2.44%	0.50	**0.016**
Sprint, 10 m (s)	2.06 ± 0.09	1.96 ± 0.12	−4.86% [c]	0.94	**<0.001**
Sprint, 20 m (s)	3.50 ± 0.14	3.40 ± 0.14	−2.86% [c]	0.71	**<0.001**
RAST (s)	6.18 ± 0.24	6.01 ± 0.28	−2.75% [c]	0.65	**<0.001**
RAST power output (W)	343.57 ± 46.91	370.04 ± 48.51	7.70%	0.55	**<0.001**
VO2max (mL * kg^{-1} * min^{-1})	50.03 ± 2.57	51.01 ± 2.80	1.96%	0.36	**0.003**
SOC (*n* = 20)					
T505 (s)	2.49 ± 0.13	2.43 ± 0.10	−2.41%	0.52	**<0.001**
93639 (s)	7.87 ± 0.52	7.81 ± 0.52	−0.76%	0.12	**<0.001**
SJ (cm)	26.12 ± 1.91	26.46 ± 1.93	1.30%	0.18	**<0.001**
CMJ (cm)	27.45 ± 1.60	28.15 ± 1.62	2.55%	0.43	**<0.001**
20Y (s)	4.67 ± 0.22	4.55 ± 0.21	−2.57%	0.56	**<0.001**
Sprint, 5 m (s)	1.22 ± 0.10	1.20 ± 0.09	−1.64%	0.21	0.160
Sprint, 10 m (s)	2.01 ± 0.09	1.99 ± 0.07	−1.00%	0.25	0.081
Sprint, 20 m (s)	3.49 ± 0.14	3.45 ± 0.14	−1.15%	0.29	**<0.001**
RAST (s)	6.13 ± 0.22	6.05 ± 0.23	−1.31%	0.36	**<0.001**
RAST power output (W)	309.46 ± 36.26	324.93 ± 38.07	5.00%	0.42	**<0.001**
VO2max (mL * kg^{-1} * min^{-1})	50.44 ± 2.88	50.72 ± 2.89	0.56%	0.10	**<0.001**

T505: 5-0-5 agility test; 93639: agility test 93639 m; SJ: squat jump; CMJ: countermovement jump; 20Y: 20-yard agility test; RAST: running-based anaerobic sprint test; VO2max: maximal oxygen uptake; [a] denotes significant difference between the RS-LiN and RS-CoD groups ($p < 0.05$); [b] denotes significant difference between the RS-CoD and SOC groups ($p < 0.05$); [c] denotes significant difference between the RS-LiN and SOC groups ($p < 0.05$); and $p < 0.05$.

The between-group differences are presented in Table 2. The RS–CoD group exhibited significantly beneficial effects in the 93639 ($F_{2,59} = 23.79$, $p < 0.001$), SJ ($F_{2,59} = 18.12$, $p < 0.001$), CMJ ($F_{2,59} = 6.73$, $p = 0.002$), 20Y ($F_{2,59} = 10.66$, $p < 0.001$), 5 m sprint ($F_{2,59} = 8.92$, $p < 0.001$) and 20 m sprint tests ($F_{2,59} = 22.23$, $p < 0.001$), compared to the RS–LiN and SOC groups. Opposed to the SOC group, the RS–CoD group showed significantly larger changes in the T505 ($F_{2,59} = 11.10$, $p < 0.001$), 10 m sprint ($F_{2,59} = 9.21$, $p < 0.001$), RAST ($F_{2,59} = 12.58$, $p < 0.001$), RAST power output ($F_{2,59} = 5.86$, $p = 0.005$) and VO2max tests ($F_{2,59} = 3.56$, $p = 0.035$). The RS–LiN group performed better in the 93639 test, sprints at 10 and 20 m and RAST ($p < 0.05$) than the SOC group.

https://doi.org/10.3390/sports14020044

7. Discussion

The main purpose of this study was to examine whether RS–LiN and RS–CoD intervention programs would have beneficial effects on physical performance in male U17 soccer players. Findings suggest that both groups enhanced their physical performance over 12 weeks, although the RS–CoD group seemed to outpower the RS–LiN and SOC groups with more beneficial effects, especially in sprinting activities.

To date, only a handful of studies have simultaneously compared the effects in linear vs. change of direction forms in male soccer players [13,25–28]. In a 30-week intervention study, both RS–CoD and RS–LiN programs exhibited positive effects on cardiorespiratory and neuromuscular physical performance in highly trained soccer players [26]. Although the within-group differences were small to moderate, the between-group differences in pre–post-changes yielded non-significant main effects, indicating that both training interventions produced similar improvements over time [26]. Similar observations were presented in a 22-week intervention study, which compared the effects of the RS–CoD and RS–LiN for Yo–Yo IR2, sprints over 10 m and 20 m and VO2max [25]. The mentioned study showed that all male soccer players, irrespective of group, increased their Yo–Yo IR2 by 9.1%, but the 'time × group' interaction was not significant ($_{p}\eta^2 = 0.06$). Interestingly, no improvements in the sprints over 10 m and 20 m and VO2max were found [25]. In a study by Beato et al. [27], a single session of straight line vs. change of direction sprint intervals failed to lead to physical performance improvements in explosive power; RSA; or sprints over 10 m, 20 m and 40 m. Also, the main effects between RS–CoD and RS–LiN groups showed that both intervention programs exhibited no between-group differences [27]. Sanchez–Sanchez et al. [24] reported that the SOC group achieved greater improvements in aerobic capacity and sprint decrements during RS ability tests, compared with the RS-COD groups. As expected, the RSA–CoD group improved their RSA and change of direction performance, opposed to the SOC group [24]. Another study including a 6-week intervention protocol consisted of linear and change of direction sprints in female soccer players showed no significant 'time x group' main effects for aerobic, musculoskeletal and agility performance, although the group that performed change of direction sprint intervals exhibited larger improvements in sprints over 30 m, compared to the linear group [29]. In general, differences in pre–post-changes for physical performance between RS–CoD and RS–LiN groups remain non-significant, with similar improvements between the two intervention protocols, which is not in line with our study. Since we showed that the RS–CoD group exhibited greater effects in all physical performance tests in comparison to the RS–LiN and SOC groups, we could assume that the increased training stimuli with different movement patterns and volumes over 12 weeks led to larger improvements. Indeed, the training load in terms of the number of sprints was inconsistent between the studies. For example, the post-intervention number of sprints in this study was 720 over 12 weeks, while a study by Pavillon et al. [26] reported a total of 1200 sprints over 30 weeks, which would produce a different sprint/week ratio. Additionally, soccer players in the RS–CoD group were unfamiliar with CoD sprint intervals, which might have led to greater effects. This is not surprising, since evidence suggests that the CoD sprint intervals decrease with age, where younger soccer players (U15) may excel at shorter sprints and CoDs at lower speeds, while older players (U18) can demonstrate better linear sprinting abilities and power at longer distances [26]. Thus, the CoD sprint training should be initiated from an early age, but the effects are expected to be normalized by genetic predispositions [36].

The difference between CoD and linear sprints should be observed with neuromuscular and metabolic demands [19,37]. Linear sprinting primarily focuses on maximizing horizontal velocity, by changing kinematical characteristics of running through the step/stride length and pace. On the other hand, CoD sprint intervals are accompanied by

https://doi.org/10.3390/sports14020044

the acceleration–deceleration dynamics associated with a greater engagement of muscle antagonists (eccentric contraction properties) [38]. Such actions may lead to oxidative stress faster and increases in muscle damage following soccer training [39]. Opposed to linear sprinting, running with CoDs also increases energy demands, requiring greater blood lactate concentrations, heart rates and aerobic capacity [13]. As we highlighted, the more beneficial effects of CoD sprint intervals may be attributed to the high training volume across 12 weeks, as soccer players performed 720 sprint intervals, opposed to lower training volumes in other studies [26]. Unfortunately, the true energy demand of the CoD with a turn of 180° has been rarely investigated, as the speed or distance are not adjusted for the time lost during the turns, limiting the possibility of actual CoD effects on physical performance in soccer players [19].

Irrespective of a relatively high heterogeneity between the studies regarding comparisons between CoD and linear sprint intervals on physical performance, the findings of this study confirmed that sprints with a CoD of 180° may be more beneficial for physical performance improvements, as CoD movements mimic more specific movements similar to soccer. The practical implications of RSs with CoDs performed during the pre-season represent good training stimuli for physiological and performance-related outcomes. Therefore, such a training approach should be implemented within regular soccer training for additional effects, especially for sprinting activities. Because the training itself took approximately 20 min to complete, strength and conditioning coaches can consider CoD sprint intervals with a turn of 180° as a pragmatic strategy for positive increases in soccer-specific performance tests. Since these tests have been previously described as reliable and valid, the intervention protocol used in this study may be a better alternative to linear sprinting activities, due to greater changes in physical performance.

This study is not without limitations. Even though we observed significant positive effects in the RS–CoD, RS–LiN and SOC groups for physical performance, the intervention duration of 12 weeks was arbitrary chosen, and due to time restrictions, we were unable to prolong the intervention process to >20 weeks, as described in previous studies [25,26]. By performing the intervention over more weeks, it would be possible to examine the adaptation process to the RS–CoD intervention and to assume the best intervention length that would produce the greatest positive changes on physical performance. Since the research around CoD sprint intervals, training loads, durations, energy demands and effectiveness is still relatively limited, although promising, our findings should be interpreted with caution. Second, the CoD sprint interval performance has been shown to decline with age [19,26], and we were unable to examine age-related differences following RS–CoD and RS–LiN interventions. Third, no invasive methods were performed to collect blood samples, which we speculated to be correlated with changes produced by CoD or LiN sprint intervals. Nevertheless, this is one of the first studies that compares the effects of the RS–CoD and RS–LiN opposed to SOC training in U17 soccer players [40].

8. Conclusions

Based on the obtained findings, we may conclude that different types of training (RS–CoD, RS–LiN and SOC) produce beneficial and positive effects on physical performance in young soccer players. However, the largest effects are observed for the CoD sprint intervals, where the RS–CoD group exhibited more beneficial improvements in all physical performance tests, especially for sprinting activities, compared to the RS–LiN and SOC groups. Thus, this study can be considered as a good starting point to enhance or even maintain high physical performances in the pre-season period in U17 male soccer players.

https://doi.org/10.3390/sports14020044

Supplementary Materials: The following supporting information can be downloaded at https://www.mdpi.com/article/10.3390/sports14020044/s1, Table S1: Raw data of study participants.

Funding: The author would like to acknowledge the support of Prince Sultan University for paying the article processing charges (APCs) of this publication. This study was conducted by the SSDRL research lab.

Institutional Review Board Statement: All procedures performed in this study were approved by the Ethical Committee Board of the local ethical committee (ethical code: HPU-2024-09-4538), and all participants provided written informed consent prior entering this study.

Informed Consent Statement: Written informed consent was obtained.

Data Availability Statement: The datasets used and/or analyzed during the current study are available from the corresponding author on reasonable request.

Conflicts of Interest: The authors declare no conflicts of interest.

References

1. Hostrup, M.; Bangsbo, J. Performance Adaptations to Intensified Training in Top-Level Football. *Sports Med.* **2022**, *53*, 577–594. [CrossRef]
2. Carling, C.; Le Gall, F.; Dupont, G. Analysis of repeated high-intensity running performance in professional soccer. *J. Sports Sci.* **2012**, *30*, 325–336. [CrossRef]
3. Reynolds, J.; Connor, M.; Jamil, M.; Beato, M. Quantifying and Comparing the Match Demands of U18, U23, and 1ST Team English Professional Soccer Players. *Front. Physiol.* **2021**, *12*, 706451. [CrossRef] [PubMed]
4. Filter, A.; Olivares-Jabalera, J.; Dos'Santos, T.; Madruga, M.; Lozano, J.; Molina, A.; Santalla, A.; Requena, B.; Loturco, I. High-intensity Actions in Elite Soccer: Current Status and Future Perspectives. *Int. J. Sports Med.* **2023**, *44*, 535–544. [CrossRef] [PubMed]
5. Bradley, P.S.; Archer, D.T.; Hogg, B.; Schuth, G.; Bush, M.; Carling, C.; Barnes, C. Tier-specific evolution of match performance characteristics in the English Premier League: It's getting tougher at the top. *J. Sports Sci.* **2016**, *34*, 980–987. [CrossRef] [PubMed]
6. Manuel Clemente, F.; Ramirez-Campillo, R.; Nakamura, F.Y.; Sarmento, H. Effects of high-intensity interval training in men soccer player's physical fitness: A systematic review with meta-analysis of randomized-controlled and non-controlled trials. *J. Sports Sci.* **2021**, *39*, 1202–1222. [CrossRef]
7. Rampinini, E.; Sassi, A.; Morelli, A.; Mazzoni, S.; Fanchini, M.; Coutts, A.J. Repeated-sprint ability in professional and amateur soccer players. *Appl. Physiol. Nutr. Metab.* **2009**, *34*, 1048–1054. [CrossRef]
8. Chaouachi, A.; Manzi, V.; Wong, D.P.; Chaalali, A.; Laurencelle, L.; Chamari, K.; Castagna, C. Intermittent endurance and repeated sprint ability in soccer players. *J. Strength Cond. Res.* **2010**, *24*, 2663–2669. [CrossRef]
9. Baldi, M.; DA Silva, J.F.; Buzzachera, C.F.; Castagna, C.; Guglielmo, L.G. Repeated sprint ability in soccer players: Associations with physiological and neuromuscular factors. *J. Sports Med. Phys. Fit.* **2017**, *57*, 26–32. [CrossRef]
10. Michailidis, Y. The effectiveness of different training methods in soccer for repeated sprint ability: A brief review. *Appl. Sci.* **2022**, *12*, 11803. [CrossRef]
11. Ross, A.; Leveritt, M. Long-term metabolic and skeletal muscle adaptations to short-sprint training: Implications for sprint training and tapering. *Sports Med.* **2001**, *31*, 1063–1082. [CrossRef]
12. Di Mascio, M.; Ade, J.; Musham, C.; Girard, O.; Bradley, P.S. Soccer-Specific Reactive Repeated-Sprint Ability in Elite Youth Soccer Players: Maturation Trends and Association With Various Physical Performance Tests. *J. Strength Cond. Res.* **2020**, *34*, 3538–3545. [CrossRef]
13. Buchheit, M.; Mendez-Villanueva, A.; Delhomel, G.; Brughelli, M.; Ahmaidi, S. Improving repeated sprint ability in young elite soccer players: Repeated shuttle sprints vs. explosive strength training. *J. Strength Cond. Res.* **2010**, *24*, 2715–2722. [CrossRef] [PubMed]
14. Buchheit, M.; Laursen, P.B. High-intensity interval training, solutions to the programming puzzle. Part II: Anaerobic energy, neuromuscular load and practical applications. *Sports Med.* **2013**, *43*, 927–954. [CrossRef] [PubMed]
15. Spencer, M.; Bishop, D.; Dawson, B.; Goodman, C. Physiological and metabolic responses of repeated-sprint activities: Specific to field-based team sports. *Sports Med.* **2005**, *35*, 1025–1044. [CrossRef] [PubMed]
16. Asimakidis, N.D.; Bishop, C.; Beato, M.; Turner, A.N. Assessment of Aerobic Fitness and Repeated Sprint Ability in Elite Male Soccer: A Systematic Review of Test Protocols Used in Practice and Research. *Sports Med.* **2025**, *55*, 1233–1264. [CrossRef]
17. Haugen, T.; Tønnessen, E.; Hisdal, J.; Seiler, S. The role and development of sprinting speed in soccer. *Int. J. Sports Physiol. Perform.* **2014**, *9*, 432–441. [CrossRef]

https://doi.org/10.3390/sports14020044

18. Sánchez-López, S.; López-Sagarra, A.; Ortega-Becerra, M.; Jiménez-Reyes, P.; Rodríguez-Pérez, M.A. Change of direction performance in soccer players: Comparison based on horizontal force–velocity profile. *Appl. Sci.* **2023**, *13*, 12809. [CrossRef]
19. Hader, K.; Mendez-Villanueva, A.; Palazzi, D.; Ahmaidi, S.; Buchheit, M. Metabolic Power Requirement of Change of Direction Speed in Young Soccer Players: Not All Is What It Seems. *PLoS ONE* **2016**, *11*, e0149839. [CrossRef]
20. Ferrari Bravo, D.; Impellizzeri, F.M.; Rampinini, E.; Castagna, C.; Bishop, D.; Wisloff, U. Sprint vs. interval training in football. *Int. J. Sports Med.* **2008**, *29*, 668–674. [CrossRef]
21. Nedrehagen, E.S.; Saeterbakken, A.H. The Effects of in-Season Repeated Sprint Training Compared to Regular Soccer Training. *J. Hum. Kinet.* **2015**, *49*, 237–244. [CrossRef] [PubMed]
22. Chaalali, A.; Rouissi, M.; Chtara, M.; Owen, A.; Bragazzi, N.L.; Moalla, W.; Chaouachi, A.; Amri, M.; Chamari, K. Agility training in young elite soccer players: Promising results compared to change of direction drills. *Biol. Sport* **2016**, *33*, 345–351. [CrossRef] [PubMed]
23. Makhlouf, I.; Chaouachi, A.; Chaouachi, M.; Ben Othman, A.; Granacher, U.; Behm, D.G. Combination of Agility and Plyometric Training Provides Similar Training Benefits as Combined Balance and Plyometric Training in Young Soccer Players. *Front. Physiol.* **2018**, *9*, 1611. [CrossRef] [PubMed]
24. Sanchez-Sanchez, J.; Ramirez-Campillo, R.; Petisco, C.; Gonzalo-Skok, O.; Rodriguez-Fernandez, A.; Miñano, J.; Nakamura, F.Y. Effects of Repeated Sprints With Changes of Direction on Youth Soccer Player's Performance: Impact of Initial Fitness Level. *J. Strength Cond. Res.* **2019**, *33*, 2753–2759. [CrossRef]
25. Sagelv, E.H.; Selnæs, I.; Pedersen, S.; Pettersen, S.A.; Randers, M.B.; Welde, B. Effects of Linear Versus Changes of Direction Repeated Sprints on Intermittent High Intensity Running Performance in High-level Junior Football Players over an Entire Season: A Randomized Trial. *Sports* **2019**, *7*, 189. [CrossRef]
26. Pavillon, T.; Tourny, C.; Ben Aabderrahman, A.; Salhi, I.; Zouita, S.; Rouissi, M.; Hackney, A.C.; Granacher, U.; Zouhal, H. Sprint and jump performances in highly trained young soccer players of different chronological age: Effects of linear VS. CHANGE-OF-DIRECTION sprint training. *J. Exerc. Sci. Fit.* **2021**, *19*, 81–90. [CrossRef]
27. Beato, M.; Bianchi, M.; Coratella, G.; Merlini, M.; Drust, B. A Single Session of Straight Line and Change-of-Direction Sprinting per Week Does Not Lead to Different Fitness Improvements in Elite Young Soccer Players. *J. Strength Cond. Res.* **2022**, *36*, 518–524. [CrossRef]
28. Negra, Y.; Sammoud, S.; Ramirez-Campillo, R.; Bouguezzi, R.; Moran, J.; Chaabene, H. The effects of repeated sprint training with versus without change of direction on measures of physical fitness in youth male soccer players. *J. Sports Med. Phys. Fit.* **2023**, *63*, 8–15. [CrossRef]
29. Stanković, M.; Trajković, N.; Mačak, D.; Đorđević, D.; Lazić, A.; Milanović, Z. Effects of linear and change of direction high-intensity interval training on physical performance of elite female soccer players. *Biol. Sport* **2024**, *41*, 31–39. [CrossRef]
30. Sporis, G.; Jukic, I.; Milanovic, L.; Vucetic, V. Reliability and factorial validity of agility tests for soccer players. *J. Strength Cond. Res.* **2010**, *24*, 679–686. [CrossRef]
31. Mann, J.B.; Ivey, P.A.; Mayhew, J.L.; Schumacher, R.M.; Brechue, W.F. Relationship Between Agility Tests and Short Sprints: Reliability and Smallest Worthwhile Difference in National Collegiate Athletic Association Division-I Football Players. *J. Strength Cond. Res.* **2016**, *30*, 893–900. [CrossRef] [PubMed]
32. Altmann, S.; Ringhof, S.; Neumann, R.; Woll, A.; Rumpf, M.C. Validity and reliability of speed tests used in soccer: A systematic review. *PLoS ONE* **2019**, *14*, e0220982. [CrossRef]
33. De Andrade, V.L.; Santiago, P.R.; Kalva Filho, C.A.; Campos, E.Z.; Papoti, M. Reproducibility of Running Anaerobic Sprint Test for soccer players. *J. Sports Med. Phys. Fit.* **2016**, *56*, 34–38.
34. Düking, P.; Ruf, L.; Altmann, S.; Thron, M.; Kunz, P.; Sperlich, B. Assessment of Maximum Oxygen Uptake in Elite Youth Soccer Players: A Comparative Analysis of Smartwatch Technology, Yoyo Intermittent Recovery Test 2, and Respiratory Gas Analysis. *J. Sports Sci. Med.* **2024**, *23*, 351–357. [CrossRef]
35. Lakens, D. Calculating and reporting effect sizes to facilitate cumulative science: A practical primer for *t*-tests and ANOVAs. *Front. Psychol.* **2013**, *4*, 863. [CrossRef]
36. Eynon, N.; Hanson, E.D.; Lucia, A.; Houweling, P.J.; Garton, F.; North, K.N.; Bishop, D.J. Genes for elite power and sprint performance: ACTN3 leads the way. *Sports Med.* **2013**, *43*, 803–817. [CrossRef] [PubMed]
37. Lockie, R.G. The effects of linear and change-of-direction speed training on the sprint performance of young adults. In *Physical Activity Effects on the Anthropological Status of Children, Youth and Adults*; Eminivić, F., Dopsaj, M., Eds.; Nova Science Publishers: Hauppauge, NY, USA, 2016; pp. 71–116.
38. Osgnach, C.; Poser, S.; Bernardini, R.; Rinaldo, R.; di Prampero, P.E. Energy cost and metabolic power in elite soccer: A new match analysis approach. *Med. Sci. Sports Exerc.* **2010**, *42*, 170–178. [CrossRef] [PubMed]

https://doi.org/10.3390/sports14020044

39. Silva, J.R.; Rebelo, A.; Marques, F.; Pereira, L.; Seabra, A.; Ascensão, A.; Magalhães, J. Biochemical impact of soccer: An analysis of hormonal, muscle damage, and redox markers during the season. *Appl. Physiol. Nutr. Metab.* **2014**, *39*, 432–438. [CrossRef]
40. Laursen, P.; Buchheit, M. *Science and Application of High-Intensity Interval Training*; Human Kinetics: Champaign, IL, USA, 2019.

https://doi.org/10.3390/sports14020044

sports

MDPI

Article

Impact of a Congested Match Schedule on Internal Load, Recovery, Well-Being, and Enjoyment in U16 Youth Water Polo Players

Andrea Perazzetti [1,*], Arben Kaçurri [2], Masar Gjaka [3], Marco Pernigoni [4], Corrado Lupo [5] and Antonio Tessitore [1,*]

1 Department of Movement, Human and Health Sciences, University of Rome 'Foro Italico', 00135 Rome, Italy
2 Sports Research Institute, Sports University of Tirana, 1001 Tirana, Albania; akacurri@ust.edu.al
3 Department of Sport and Movement Science, University for Business and Technology, 10000 Pristina, Kosovo; masar.gjaka@ubt-uni.net
4 Department of Coaching Science, Lithuanian Sports University, 44221 Kaunas, Lithuania; marco.pernigoni@lsu.lt
5 Neuro Muscular Function Research Group, School of Exercise & Sport Sciences, Department of Medical Sciences, University of Turin, 10124 Turin, Italy; corrado.lupo@unito.it
* Correspondence: perazzettiandrea@gmail.com (A.P.); antonio.tessitore@uniroma4.it (A.T.)

Abstract: This study aimed to monitor internal load, well-being, and recovery status in U16 male water polo players during a congested competitive period. Fourteen athletes from an Italian club played 12 matches (seven friendly, five official) over 7 days. The internal match load was measured using the session-RPE method (s-RPE). Perceived enjoyment was measured with the Enjoyment Likert Scale (ENJ), while recovery and well-being were evaluated using the Perceived Recovery Scale (PRS) and the Hooper Index (HI), respectively. No significant main effects were found on s-RPE, PRS, and HI considering friendly and official matches. However, ENJ was significantly higher during official matches ($p < 0.005$). PRS values were significantly affected by daytime matches ($p < 0.005$), with better perceived recovery reported for morning matches. Linear mixed model analysis revealed significant associations between s-RPE and HI ($p = 0.001$), the fatigue item ($p = 0.001$), and the PRS ($p = 0.004$). These results suggest that as internal load increases, players experience higher fatigue and report lower recovery and well-being scores. Employing simple, non-invasive tools like the RPE, PRS, and HI can help coaches and support staff to identify early signs of overtraining or insufficient recovery, allowing for more individualized load management and injury prevention in youth water polo athletes.

Keywords: recovery status; wellbeing; youth water polo; monitoring matches

1. Introduction

In team sports, a congested match calendar has become a significant concern for practitioners, players, and sport organizations [1]. Nowadays, elite team sports players usually encounter congested schedules characterized by numerous matches within very short timeframes, both during the preseason and the competitive season. During this period, teams may also participate in multiple competitions concurrently, such as national and continental events. Research suggests that congested fixtures can impact on acute performance and well-being, limiting players' availability in various team sports [2]. The increasing frequency of fixtures has intensified discussions around effective player load management, recovery capacity, and injury risk [3]. This issue highlights the challenge posed by extended competitive schedules, which often exceed traditional periodization strategies aimed at optimizing performance and preventing overtraining [4]. To address these issues, sports teams are increasingly utilizing innovative strategies like real-time load monitoring through GPS and wearable technology, along with machine learning and artificial intelligence models [5].

In team sports, several studies have observed changes in players' training responses, through their perceived load and well-being status during regular and congested weeks. Clemente et al. [6], studying professional futsal players, observed greater session-RPE scores on matchday-3 (i.e., 3 days before a match, MD-3) in regular weeks compared to the same day in congested weeks, during which MD-3 is the day immediately after a match. Similar trends were also reported by the same author for professional handball [7], with greater scores in training loads and reduced scores in well-being during match MD-2 and MD-3 in normal weeks. Furthermore, a study on elite volleyball players [8] found greater session-RPE scores in MD-1 (i.e., 1 day before a match) in regular weeks compared to congested ones. Overall, these findings suggest that during congested weeks, coaches tend to prioritize recovery and match preparation over high training loads. Conversely, during non-congested periods, coaches are freer to adopt a tactical periodization approach to training.

The literature on team sports has highlighted the impact of congested matches on players, who often participate in over 60 official matches annually. These players often experience residual fatigue and have greater injury risks when resting for less than 3 or 4 days between matches compared to more than 6 days of recovery [9]. A longitudinal study by Chmura et al. regarding soccer found that players tended to accumulate greater fatigue in the later stages of the season, particularly when participating in additional tournaments like the national cup, the Champions League, or the Europa League [10]. In basketball, Conte et al. [11] found that players reported higher perceived fatigue and lower well-being on the second game day when playing two games per week on Friday and Saturday. In soccer, a prospective six-season study by Carling et al. [12] found a significantly greater risk of sustaining an injury in the final 15 min of play in the second match and in the first half of play in the third match during three consecutive matches played within a ≤4-day period compared to matches played outside the congested cycle.

Although a considerable amount of research has explored the effects of congested training periods in team sports, water polo has received limited attention regarding how this issue influences coaches' behavior and players' performance, recovery, and injury risk [13]. In major international water polo competitions, fixtures are typically scheduled within a few days, for example, eight matches over 15 days during the Olympic Games or national team tournaments, or three matches over four days in club competitions such as the Final Four of the Champions League and the Euro Cup. A study by Botonis et al. [14] investigated the wellness and perceived internal training load of elite Greek water polo players over four weeks leading up to the playoff phase. The period included an overloaded training phase (weeks 1 and 2), followed by a reduced training load phase (weeks 3 and 4). The results showed that the increased training load during the overloaded phase negatively affected wellness scores but did not significantly compromise sport-specific performance. Conversely, the subsequent reduction in training volume and intensity improved both wellness scores and sport-specific performance metrics by the end of the intervention, compared to the baseline and the end of the overload period. Brisola et al. [15] conducted a study on female water polo players, comparing a two-week training load intensification strategy between groups of functional and non-functional overreaching players. The findings indicate that training intensification followed by tapering can improve performance more effectively than standard training methods. Nonetheless, it may also result in functional impairment and diminished performance. Consequently, constant monitoring of performance, particularly during intensified periods, is essential to prevent negative effects. In this sense, the increased competitive commitments require frequent travel across different time zones, leading to fatigue from jet lag and reducing the time available for recovery [16]. A survey by Barrenetxea-Garcia [17] highlighted the need for tailored recovery interventions that consider the specific needs of water polo players and coaching staff. It revealed a gap between the perceived importance of recovery strategies and their actual use. Coaches play a pivotal role, but their limited understanding may lead to ineffective practices, increasing the risk of overtraining and injuries while passing on incorrect information to athletes.

In water polo, considering that preparation for significant international tournaments involves a high-volume, intensified training phase followed by a series of competitive unofficial matches designed to improve players' competitive readiness, the increased workload may impact their recovery. A study of Botonis et al. [18] examined the impact of international tournament participation on heart rate variability and perceived recovery in elite water polo athletes. Heart rate variability was assessed over five consecutive days during an intensified pre-tournament training phase and for three subsequent days while the team participated in three international matches. The results indicated that, under the accumulated fatigue and residual stress effects, perceived recovery and internal workloads were diminished on tournament days compared to the pre-tournament period (intensified training phase), suggesting that additional factors may influence the overall perception of recovery among subjects. In this context, ref. [19] examined the impact of intensified training on sleep activity, hormonal responses, and overall wellness in elite water polo players preparing for the Tokyo Olympics. Their findings revealed that substantial increases in training load during camp led to significant sleep disturbances and elevated salivary cortisol levels, both of which normalized after the camp. These results suggest that an intensified workload, coupled with insufficient recovery, may disrupt sleep patterns and potentially elevate the risk of infection. Barrenetxea-Garcia et al. [20] addressed the importance of recovery in a global survey on sleep quality, revealing that both senior and youth international water polo players reported poor sleep in terms of both quantity and quality. They frequently failed to meet recommended sleep durations and showed significant variability in sleep efficiency, especially during training camps and competitions. However, the limited research on congested fixtures in water polo primarily focuses on adult players. Except for one study examining training load distribution in a young female team, specifically its effects on upper respiratory tract infection symptoms and muscle damage markers [21], there is a lack of research on the impact of congested training periods in youth water polo. For this reason, the aim of the present study was to investigate the players' perceptions of effort, enjoyment, recovery, and well-being during a congested schedule that included both official and training matches in male youth water polo players. Based on this, we hypothesized that players' internal load (s-RPE), well-being (HI), perceived recovery (PRS), and enjoyment (ENJ) would be influenced by contextual match factors such as the time of day (morning vs. afternoon matches), the match type (friendly vs. official), and the match day sequence within the congested schedule, and that higher s-RPE would be associated with reduced PRS and HI values in the following days.

2. Materials and Methods

2.1. Subjects

Fourteen Italian U16 male water polo players (mean ± SD: age 15.4 ± 0.7 years; body mass: 67.8 ± 7.8 kg; body height: 175.6 ± 4.9 cm; body mass index: 22.0 ± 2.7; playing experience: 6.1 ± 1.2 years), all from the same club, were recruited for this study.

Informed consent was obtained from players' parents (guardians) after they were informed of the study's main objectives. This study was conducted in accordance with the ethical principles of the 1964 Declaration of Helsinki and was approved by the local ethics committee of the University of Rome 'Foro Italico' (CAR 99/2021).

Throughout the season, each player participated in regular training, matches, and tournaments, and the players belonged to the following playing positions [22]: perimetral players (*PP*, n = 8); center defenders (CD, n = 3); center forwards (CF, n = 3); and goalkeepers (GK, n = 2). Playing positions were not used for statistical analyses and are listed only to provide more detailed descriptive information regarding participant players. Furthermore, for each player, the following inclusion criteria were used for the final analysis: (i) participating in all matches during the study period for at least the mean total duration of a quarter (15 min per match) [23]; (ii) not presenting any injury or illness that could impair matches' performance; and iii) exclusion of goalkeepers from the analytical sample, as their physical demands differ significantly from those of field players.

2.2. Experimental Design

This study monitored and assessed the internal load, perceived recovery, well-being, and enjoyment of youth male water polo players during a congested match period consisting of 12 matches over 7 days. The matches were played between 18 and 29 July 2023, comprising 7 friendly matches over 4 days, followed by 1 day of rest, and then 5 official matches over the next 3 days. After each match, individual RPE scores were collected by asking players, 'How intense was your session?' using the Italian translation of the Borg category-ratio 10 scale (CR-10), as modified by Foster et al. [24]. The match internal load was then calculated using the session-RPE (s-RPE) method [25,26]. The use of the s-RPE method in youth athletes has already been validated in youth water polo players [27]. Simultaneously, players' perceived enjoyment was assessed using the Italian translation and adaptation of the Exercise Enjoyment Scale (ENJ) [23,28,29]. Every morning, the well-being status was monitored using the Hooper Index [30], while recovery was assessed using the 10-point Perceived Recovery Scale (PRS) [31] before each match. To minimize variability in individual recovery and well-being, players refrained from using any recovery interventions and were instructed to maintain consistent lifestyles and nutritional habits aligned with those of their teammates throughout the entire study period. Players' internal match load, enjoyment, perceived recovery, and well-being were analyzed in relation to (i) the playing time, defined as the total minutes played by each athlete in all matches; (ii) the match time of day, distinguished by matches played in the morning vs. matches played in the afternoon in the same day; (iii) the match type, distinguished by friendly matches (FMs) and official tournament matches (TMs); and (iv) the match day, representing the chronological days of matches played.

2.3. Procedures

Players became thoroughly familiar with the RPE, ENJ, PRS, and HI scales during the three weeks leading up to the start of this study. Throughout this period, they received both printed and digital copies (individually via WhatsApp) of the questionnaires each day, with instructions to read and interpret the scales before and after every training session, friendly match, and official match.

During the data collection period (starting 3 days before the first match and ending 3 days after the last match), players' RPE and ENJ responses were recorded within 30 min after the end of the match, before players left the swimming facility. To minimize potential post-match interference and standardize the timing of responses, players were trained to use their smartphones for online data collection, which has been shown to be a reliable tool among athletes [32]. Players completed the RPE and ENJ scales using a customized Google Forms questionnaire, which mirrored the content of the printed and digital scales provided during the familiarization period. The questionnaire was sent to their personal smartphones via WhatsApp. Using the session-RPE (s-RPE) method [26], the internal match load was calculated by multiplying each player's RPE score by the number of minutes played, with the result expressed in arbitrary units (a.u.). For the ENJ scale, players rated their match enjoyment on a 7-point scale (1 = not at all, 7 = extremely enjoyable).

Perceived recovery was assessed using the 10-point Perceived Recovery Scale [31], ranging from 0 ('very poorly recovered/extremely tired') to 10 ('very well recovered/highly energetic'). This scale has previously been used in other team sports [33,34] as well as in water polo [35]. Specifically, the PRS was administered 36 h post-match (PRS_{36h}, when there was a rest day after the last match, in the morning between 8:00 and 8:30), 12 h post-match (PRS_{12h}, in the morning between 8:00 and 8:30), and 6 h post-match (PRS_{6h}, in the afternoon between 17:30 and 18:00). Players' well-being was monitored using the Hooper Index [30], a self-assessment questionnaire based on four subjective measures, each rated on a 7-point Likert scale. These measures were administered daily at the same time as the morning PRS (between 8:00 and 8:30) and assessed the athletes' perceived levels of (i) stress, (ii) fatigue, (iii) muscle soreness (DOMS), and (iv) sleep quality. Scores for stress, fatigue, and DOMS ranged from 1 ('very, very low') to 7 ('very, very high'), while sleep was rated from 1 ('very, very bad') to 7 ('very, very good'). The overall Hooper Index score was obtained by summing up the four individual ratings.

Table 1 shows the scheduling of all matches played and the administration of the monitoring questionnaires.

Table 1. Overview of congested match schedule and timeline of monitoring questionnaire administration.

	TUE—day −1 18/07/23	WED—day 1 19/07/23	THU—day 2 20/07/23	FRI—day 3 21/07/23	SAT—day 4 22/07/23	SUN—day 5 23/07/23
a.m.		HI + PRS_{36h}	HI + PRS_{12h} FM2 RPE + ENJ	HI + PRS_{12h} FM4 RPE + ENJ	HI + PRS_{12h} FM6 RPE + ENJ	HI + PRS_{12h}
p.m.	R	FM1 RPE + ENJ	PRS_{6h} FM3 RPE + ENJ	PRS_{6h} FM5 RPE + ENJ	PRS_{6h} FM7 RPE + ENJ	R
	MON—day 6 24/07/23	TUE—day 7 25/07/23	WED—day 8 26/07/23	THU—day 9 27/07/23	FRI—day 10 28/07/23	SAT—day 11 29/07/23
a.m.	HI + PRS_{36h} TM1 RPE + ENJ	HI + PRS_{12h} TM3 RPE + ENJ	HI + PRS_{12h} TM5 RPE + ENJ	HI	HI	HI
p.m.	PRS_{6h} TM2 RPE + ENJ	PRS_{6h} TM4 RPE + ENJ		R	R	R

Note. HI = Hooper Index questionnaire; PRS = Perceived Recovery Scale questionnaire; FM = friendly match; R = Rest Day; RPE = Rated Perceived Exertion; ENJ = Enjoyment Likert Scale questionnaire; TM = tournament match.

Anthropometric measurements included body mass and height. Body mass was assessed using a Tanita SECA 762 scale (measuring range: 0–150 kg; SECA, Hamburg, Germany), while height was measured with a SECA 213 stadiometer (measuring range: 20–205 cm; SECA, Hamburg, Germany).

2.4. Statistical Analysis

Descriptive statistics for all variables are presented as the mean ± standard deviation (SD). To assess the effects of contextual factors on players' internal load, perceived recovery, well-being, and enjoyment, separate linear mixed-effects models were used. Linear mixed models were used to assess how various contextual factors affected each outcome: s-RPE, ENJ, PRS_{12h} and PRS_{6h}, HI, and its individual components (fatigue, sleep, stress, and DOMS). The fixed effects included in the models were as follows: (i) the match type (friendly match (FM) vs. tournament match (TM)); (ii) the match time of day (morning vs. afternoon, for comparison between PRS_{6h} and PRS_{12h}); and (iii) the match day (chronological progression of the congested match schedule (day 1 to day 7)). Players were included as a random factor to account for repeated measures. For each significant main effect, the effect size was calculated using Cohen's d, with the following interpretation: 0.2, trivial; 0.2–0.6, small; 0.6–1.2, moderate; 1.2–2.0, large; and 2.0, very large [36].

In addition, separate linear mixed models between continuous variables were used to assess the associations between s-RPE and PRS_{12h} and well-being indicators (HI, fatigue, sleep, stress, and DOMS). In this analysis, the intraclass correlation coefficient (ICC) was calculated to assess the consistency of the measurements.

All results of the main effect analyses are reported as F and p values. Furthermore, 95% confidence intervals (CI) were computed and reported for estimated marginal means to enhance interpretability and indicate the precision of the effects.

All statistical analyses were performed using the Jamovi software (version 2.6.44, x64; Jamovi, Sydney, Australia), and the statistical significance was set at $p < 0.05$.

3. Results

Table 2 presents the descriptive statistics (mean ± SD) for perceived exertion (RPE), enjoyment (ENJ), session-RPE (s-RPE), and players' playing time during friendly (FM) and tournament (TM) matches, respectively.

Table 2. Descriptive statistics of dependent variables (mean ± SD).

	Mean	SD
RPE_FM (a.u.)	6.72	1.70
RPE_TM (a.u.)	6.69	2.46
ENJ_FM (a.u.)	4.42	1.40
ENJ_TM (a.u.)	3.74	1.95
s-RPE_FM (a.u.)	177	80.8
s-RPE_TM (a.u.)	183	97.5
Players' playing time_a.m. (min)	25.3	8.89
Players' playing time_p.m. (min)	25.5	8.29
Players' playing time_FM (min)	25.6	8.23
Players' playing time_TM (min)	25.1	9.08

Note. RPE = Rated Perceived Exertion; FM = friendly match; TM = tournament match; ENJ = Enjoyment Likert Scale questionnaire; s-RPE = session-RPE; a.m. = morning match; p.m. = afternoon match.

The average players' PRS value was 4.5 ± 2 and 3.1 ± 2 for PRS_{12h} and PRS_{6h}, respectively, while it was 4.0 ± 2.1 for PRS_{12h} after friendly matches and 3.8 ± 2.1 for PRS_{12h} after tournament matches (Figure 1). Regarding the match time of day as a contextual factor, the linear mixed model revealed a significant main effect only on the PRS ($F = 34.7$; $p < 0.001$; estimate = −1.432; mean difference ± standard error [$PRS_{12h} - PRS_{6h}$] = 1.42 ± 0.32; 95% CI = 2.88, 4.48; ES = 0.703, moderate), while no main effects were observed for the s-RPE ($F = 0.02$; $p = 0.893$) and the ENJ ($F = 2.54$; $p = 0.113$).

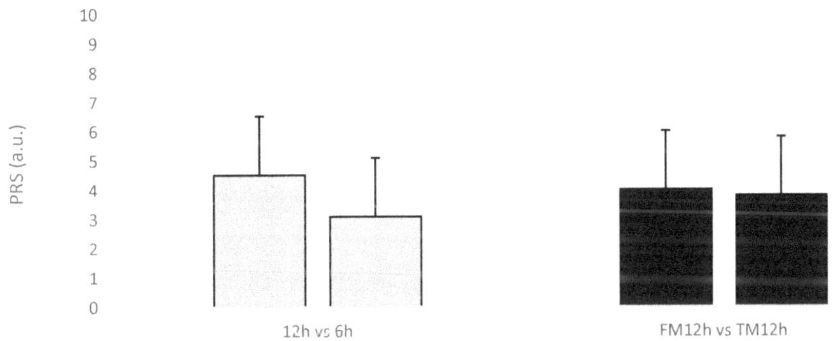

Figure 1. Comparison of PRS values between PRS_{12h} and PRS_{6h} sessions and between PRS_{12h} of friendly matches and tournament matches. Note: PRS = perceived recovery scale; 12h = PRS_{12h}; 6h = PRS_{6h}; FM12h = PRS_{12h} after friendly match; TM12h = PRS_{12h} after tournament match.

This study found no main effects on the s-RPE, PRS_{12h}, or HI when considering friendly and tournament matches. However, the ENJ was significantly influenced by the type of match (F = 9.2; $p = 0.003$, estimate = −0.742; mean difference ± standard error [ENJ_FM − EN_TM] = 0.68 ± 0.26; 95% CI = −1.22, −0.26; ES = 0.396, small) (Figure 2).

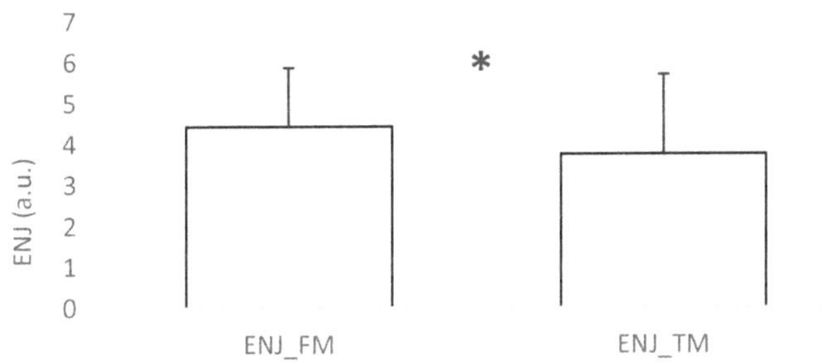

Figure 2. Comparison of ENJ values between friendly matches and tournament matches. Note. FM = friendly match; TM = tournament match; ENJ = Enjoyment Likert Scale questionnaire; * main effect showed by the linear mixed model ($p = 0.003$).

The analysis of the linear mixed model also revealed that the match-day factor had significant main effects on the HI (F = 4; $p = 0.002$; estimate = 13.89; 95% CI = 11.48, 14.79), sleep (F = 2.89; $p = 0.0014$; estimate = 3.47; 95% CI = 2.86, 3.65), PRS12h (F = 2.7; $p = 0.02$; estimate = 4.76; 95% CI = 4.30, 6.40), and the daily s-RPE (F = 16.6; $p < 0.001$; estimate = 311.1; 95% CI = 666; 865.5). In this case, given the large number of pairwise comparisons, effect sizes were not reported.

Based on the pooled match data, the linear mixed model analysis between continuous variables revealed significant relationships between s-RPE and the Hooper Index (HI) (F = 11; $p = 0.001$; estimate = 0.001; 95% CI = 11.86, 15,92; ICC = 0.798), the fatigue item (F = 11; $p = 0.001$; estimate = 0.002; 95% CI = 3.29, 4.47; ICC = 0.729), and the PRS_{12h} score (F = 9.01; $p = 0.004$; estimate = −0.003; 95% CI = 3.93, 5.59; ICC = 0.562).

Figure 3 illustrates the s-RPE and HI trends over the data collection period, starting three days before the congested match schedule and continuing until three days after its end.

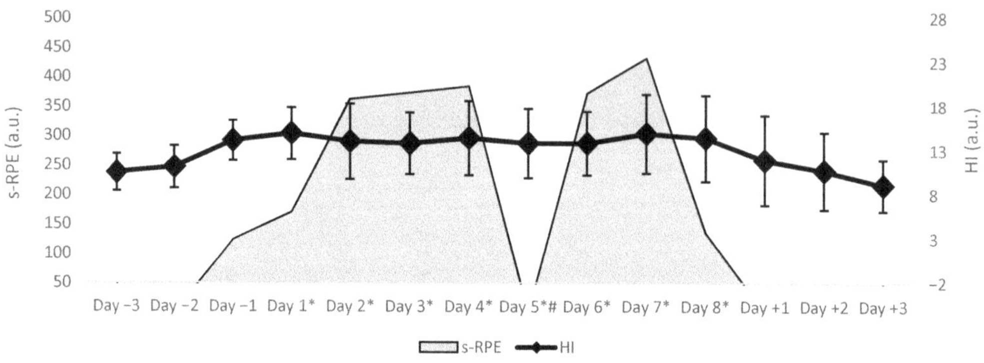

Figure 3. An overlay representation of the s-RPE and Hooper Index scale across the congested period of matches. Note: s-RPE = session-RPE; HI = Hooper Index, * = days of a congested match schedule (data collection period); # = rest day.

4. Discussion

The main purpose of this study was to examine male youth water polo players' perceptions of effort, enjoyment, recovery, and well-being factors during a congested match schedule that included both official and training matches. To the best of our knowledge, this is the first water polo study that specifically investigates matches played twice in the same day (one match in the morning and one in the afternoon) and repeatedly over consecutive days (12 matches in 7 days). This kind of scheduling provides a valuable opportunity to better understand how repeated efforts, combined with minimal recovery both on the same day and across consecutive days, affect players' perceived status.

The main findings showed that the scheduled daytime (morning vs. afternoon matches on the same day) did not significantly affect the match load as measured by the s-RPE, nor did it influence perceived enjoyment. Such findings may be attributed to the consistency in players' playing time across the two sessions. As most players participated for a similar number of minutes in both daytime matches (Table 2), their perceived exertion remained stable throughout the day. Additionally, as suggested by Botonis et al. [37], the frequent players' rotation implemented during the water polo matches likely contributed to a more even distribution of their perceived loads. With regard to enjoyment, it can be speculated that players maintained high levels due to the competitive nature of the matches and their intrinsic motivation of participating in a highly competitive event. As previously demonstrated in water polo [23], enjoyment may be more influenced by contextual factors, such as the match outcome, than by players' physical effort or well-being status.

However, the linear mixed model revealed that daytime did impact players' perceived recovery status (PRS), with values expressed before afternoon matches (PRS_{6h}) associated with scores 1.4 points lower than scores indicated before morning matches (PRS_{12h}). This difference may be attributed to the structure of the congested schedule, where afternoon matches often followed a morning fixture on the same day, without any specific post-match recovery interventions. As a result, the recovery window between matches was less than 8 h, potentially compounding fatigue and influencing players' perceptions due to the cumulative load. Our findings confirm the importance of planning recovery strategies between both congested training and matches, as previously demonstrated in the related literature [38]. In fact, as suggested by Barrenetxea-Garcia et al. [17], water polo coaches should modify their habit of underestimating recovery strategies in their periodization. Moreover, as suggested by the literature, these strategies could easily include specific nutritional interventions tailored for water polo players [39] or active recovery protocols as demonstrated in swimming settings [40]. For this reason, water polo coaches should include evidence-based recovery practices in their coaching philosophy. However, current studies suggest that many coaches still miss the habit of monitoring their athletes, highlighting a gap in the management of players' recovery [13].

Regarding the analysis of friendly and tournament matches, which presented similar s-RPE and HI values, the linear mixed model revealed a main effect for the enjoyment contextual factor, with significantly higher scores in friendly matches compared to official ones. These findings support the notion that, in water polo, the pressure to achieve results and the significance of match outcomes can negatively affect players' perceived enjoyment [23]. Specifically, the tournament matches were held at the end of a congested schedule (the last five matches within three days), under elevated stress levels and reduced motivation. By that point, players had already completed seven friendly matches, during which they could experiment with technical skills and play more freely without the burden of the competitive pressure of a tournament match.

In our group, the linear mixed model showed that the daily s-RPE was positively associated with the overall Hooper Index, especially with the fatigue sub-scale, and inversely associated with the PRS_{12h}. This result aligns with previous research regarding water polo, which found that players' perceived recovery tended to be lower due to accumulated fatigue and residual stress from consecutive matches and a preceding intensified training period [18].

Moreover, the analysis of the linear mixed model revealed that the match-day contextual factor significantly influenced the sleep sub-scale scores of Hooper Index, the perceived recovery status (PRS), and the daily session rating of perceived exertion (s-RPE). Indeed, as illustrated in Figure 3, the HI showed a gradual increase leading up to the congested match period, peaking around Day 1. This trend suggests a cumulative load effect resulting from the preparatory phase. Notably, the HI remained relatively elevated and stable throughout the central phase of the congested matches period (Day 1 to Day 7), which can be explained by a state of maintained physiological and psychological strain without full recovery between matches. A pronounced decline can be observed immediately after the final matches (from Day 8 to Day +3), indicating that players began their recovery once the intensive match schedule ended. The substantial main effect on sleep across match days aligns with the existing literature in team sport indicating that sleep quantity and quality may significantly fluctuate based on the player's daily routine [41]. Specifically, for water polo, a previous study by Botonis et al. [19] suggests that the increased workload alongside the inadequate recovery during congested period affects sleep patterns. Indeed, our results speculate that the cumulative fatigue and workload over consecutive days adversely affected players' sleep quality. Furthermore, being away from home and sleeping in an unfamiliar setting while travelling likely exacerbated their sleep disturbances [20,23]. The decline noted on specific match days in the Perceived Recovery Scale aligns with previous findings indicating that in water polo, recovery perceptions vary according to accumulated training and match load [19]. The significant rise in the daily s-RPE can be attributed to the cumulative internal load from previous days, particularly during congested schedules where players faced repeated high-intensity demands without adequate recovery time or interventions. The progressive increase in load can result in increased perceived exertion on match days, despite the external load remaining constant, as indicated by the average playing time in our study.

Limitations

This study has several limitations that should be acknowledged. The sample size was relatively small and limited to a single youth water polo team (14 players), which may affect the generalizability of the findings. Although perceived values and measures were monitored using validated questionnaires, these rely on self-reported data, which may be subject to individual bias or misinterpretation. Despite a three-week familiarization period and the athletes' regular use of these scales throughout the season, some variability in subjective responses cannot be excluded.

Furthermore, the absence of external load measures, technical–tactical analyses [42], or specific swimming tests during the data collection period [43] limits a more comprehensive understanding of the physiological demands placed on the players during the congested match schedule. Moreover, no data were collected regarding the training sessions carried out before the research period, which does not allow any comparison between a regular training period and the congested match schedule in terms of players' internal load and perceived responses.

Finally, this study focused exclusively on male youth players, and future research should aim to address these gaps and explore whether similar patterns emerge under the new 25 m rules [44], as well as among female and elite senior players.

5. Conclusions

Conducting research in real-world scenarios is essential to ensure ecological validity and practical applicability. In this regard, our study offers valuable insights into the internal match load, well-being, perceived recovery, and enjoyment of youth water polo players during a congested competition schedule. Over a seven-day period, players participated in twelve matches (averaging 1.7 matches per day), which resulted in fluctuations in s-RPE, recovery, and general well-being. Notably, perceived enjoyment was higher during official matches compared to friendly ones, suggesting that psychological factors can influence players' perception independently of physical load.

To better support youth players in such demanding contexts, coaches should consistently apply simple monitoring tools like the session-RPE method, the Hooper Index, and PRS questionnaires. These tools can provide real-time feedback to detect signs of accumulated fatigue or insufficient recovery. Coaches are also encouraged to incorporate brief psychological interventions and tailored recovery strategies, particularly when matches occur less than 6 or 12 h apart for several consecutive days. By following these guidelines, such an approach not only helps optimize short-term performance but may also contribute to safeguarding long-term players' development in youth water polo.

Author Contributions: Conceptualization, A.P. and A.T.; methodology, A.P., M.P., C.L. and A.T.; software, A.P., M.P. and A.T.; validation, A.P., A.K. and M.G.; formal analysis, A.P., A.K., M.G., M.P. and A.T.; investigation, A.P., C.L. and A.T.; resources, A.P., C.L. and A.T.; data curation, A.P., M.P. and A.T.; writing-original draft preparation, A.P., A.K. and A.T.; writing—review and editing, A.P., A.K., M.G., M.P., C.L. and A.T.; visualization, A.P., A.K., M.G., M.P., C.L. and A.T.; supervision, A.T.; project administration, A.P. All authors have read and agreed to the published version of the manuscript.

Funding: This research received no external funding.

Institutional Review Board Statement: Before the commencement of data collection, the study design was approved by the local research ethics committee of the University of Rome 'Foro Italico' (protocol code CAR 99/2021, and approval date 26 July 2021).

Informed Consent Statement: Informed consent was obtained from the parents (or legal guardians) of all players involved in the study.

Data Availability Statement: Data are contained within the article.

Acknowledgments: We deeply thank coaches Daniele Ruffelli, Andrea Esposito, and Luciano Russo for their support and the whole team players of the Italian club S. S. Lazio Nuoto for their cooperation.

Conflicts of Interest: The authors declare no conflicts of interest.

Abbreviations

The following abbreviations are used in this manuscript:

RPE	Rated Perceived Exertion
s-RPE	Session Rating of Perceived Exertion method
ENJ	Enjoyment Likert Scale
HI	Hooper Index
PRS	Perceived Recovery Scale
FM	Friendly Match
TM	Tournament Match
R	Rest Day

References

1. Kendall, G.; Lenten, L.J. When sports rules go awry. *Eur. J. Oper. Res.* **2017**, *257*, 377–394. [CrossRef]
2. Calleja-González, J.; Mallo, J.; Cos, F.; Sampaio, J.; Jones, M.T.; Marqués-Jiménez, D.; Mielgo-Ayuso, J.; Freitas, T.T.; Alcaraz, P.E.; Vilamitjana, J.; et al. A commentary of factors related to player availability and its influence on performance in elite team sports. *Front. Sports Act. Living* **2023**, *4*, 1077934. [CrossRef] [PubMed]
3. Gabbett, T.J. The training—Injury prevention paradox: Should athletes be training smarter and harder? *Br. J. Sports Med.* **2016**, *50*, 273–280. [CrossRef] [PubMed]
4. Fazackerley, L.; Minett, G.; McLaren, S.; Ward, P.; Marsh, D.; Burgess, D.; Duncan, C.; Pollard, B.; Griffith, S.; Gill, N.D.; et al. The Annual Training and Competitive Calendar in Elite Football: A Road To The Holy Grail? *Int. J. Strength Cond.* **2023**, *3*. [CrossRef]
5. Mandorino, M.; Clubb, J.; Lacome, M. Predicting soccer players' fitness status through a machine-learning approach. *Int. J. Sports Physiol. Perform.* **2024**, *19*, 443–453. [CrossRef]
6. Clemente, F.M.; Martinho, R.; Calvete, F.; Mendes, B. Training load and well-being status variations of elite futsal players across a full season: Comparisons between normal and congested weeks. *Physiol. Behav.* **2019**, *201*, 123–129. [CrossRef]
7. Clemente, F.M.; Oliveira, H.; Vaz, T.; Carriço, S.; Calvete, F.; Mendes, B. Variations of perceived load and well-being between normal and congested weeks in elite case study handball team. *Res. Sports Med.* **2019**, *27*, 412–423. [CrossRef]
8. Mendes, B.; Palao, J.M.; Silvério, A.; Owen, A.; Carriço, S.; Calvete, F.; Clemente, F.M. Daily and weekly training load and wellness status in preparatory, regular and congested weeks: A season-long study in elite volleyball players. *Res. Sports Med.* **2018**, *26*, 462–473. [CrossRef]
9. Soligard, T.; Schwellnus, M.; Alonso, J.M.; Bahr, R.; Clarsen, B.; Dijkstra, H.P.; Gabbett, T.; Gleeson, M.; Hägglund, M.; Hutchinson, M.R.; et al. How much is too much? (Part 1) International Olympic Committee consensus statement on load in sport and risk of injury. *Br. J. Sports Med.* **2016**, *50*, 1030–1041. [CrossRef]
10. Chmura, P.; Konefał, M.; Wong, D.P.; Figueiredo, A.J.; Kowalczuk, E.; Rokita, A.; Chmura, J.; Andrzejewski, M. Players' Physical Performance Decreased After Two-Thirds of the Season: Results of 3 Consecutive Seasons in the German First Bundesliga. *Int. J. Environ. Res. Public Health* **2019**, *16*, 2044. [CrossRef]
11. Conte, D.; Kamarauskas, P.; Ferioli, D.; Scanlan, A.T.; Kamandulis, S.; Paulauskas, H.; Lukonaitienė, I. Workload and well-being across games played on consecutive days during in-season phase in basketball players. *J. Sports Med. Phys. Fit.* **2020**, *61*, 534–541. [CrossRef]
12. Carling, C.; Le Gall, F.; Dupont, G. Are physical performance and injury risk in a professional soccer team in match-play affected over a prolonged period of fixture congestion? *Int. J. Sports Med.* **2012**, *33*, 36–42. [CrossRef] [PubMed]
13. Perazzetti, A.; Dopsaj, M.; Nedeljković, A.; Mazić, S.; Tessitore, A. Survey on coaching philosophies and training methodologies of water polo head coaches from three different European national schools. *Kinesiology* **2023**, *55*, 49–61. [CrossRef]
14. Botonis, P.G.; Toubekis, A.G.; Platanou, T.I. Training loads, wellness and performance before and during tapering for a Water-Polo tournament. *J. Hum. Kinet.* **2019**, *66*, 131. [CrossRef]
15. Brisola, G.M.; Dutra, Y.M.; Murias, J.M.; Zagatto, A.M. Beneficial performance effects of training load intensification can be abolished by functional overreaching: Lessons from a water polo study in female athletes. *J. Strength Cond. Res.* **2023**, *37*, e391–e402. [CrossRef] [PubMed]
16. Botonis, P.G.; Platanou, T.I.; Toubekis, A.G. Towards Olympic Games 2020: Theoretical considerations and practical implications to reduce overuse injuries in water-polo. *Med. Hypotheses* **2016**, *87*, 1–7.
17. Barrenetxea-Garcia, J.; Perazzetti, A.; Nuell, S.; Mielgo-Ayuso, J.; de Villarreal, E.S.; Calleja-González, J. Perceptions and use of recovery strategies in water polo players and coaches: A worldwide survey. *J. Exerc. Rehabil.* **2024**, *20*, 112. [CrossRef]

18. Botonis, P.G.; Smilios, I.; Platanou, T.I.; Toubekis, A.G. Effects of an international tournament on heart rate variability and perceived recovery in elite water polo players. *J. Strength Cond. Res.* **2022**, *36*, 2313–2317. [CrossRef]
19. Botonis, P.G.; Toubekis, A.G. Intensified Olympic preparation: Sleep and training-related hormonal and immune responses in water polo. *Int. J. Sports Physiol. Perform.* **2023**, *18*, 187–194. [CrossRef]
20. Barrenetxea-Garcia, J.; Perazzetti, A.; Nuell, S.; Sáez de Villarreal, E.; Mielgo-Ayuso, J.; Calleja-González, J. Poor sleep quality and quantity in water polo players and coaches: A worldwide survey. *Ger. J. Exerc. Sport Res.* **2025**, 1–9. [CrossRef]
21. Brisola, G.M.; Claus, G.M.; Dutra, Y.M.; Malta, E.S.; de Poli, R.A.; Esco, M.R.; Zagatto, A.M. Effects of seasonal training load on performance and illness symptoms in water polo. *J. Strength Cond. Res.* **2020**, *34*, 406–413. [CrossRef]
22. Perazzetti, A.; Dopsaj, M.; Mandorino, M.; Tessitore, A. Assessment of the Offensive Play in Elite Water Polo Using the Team Sport Assessment Procedure (TSAP) over an Entire Competitive Season. *J. Funct. Morphol. Kinesiol.* **2023**, *8*, 130. [CrossRef]
23. Perazzetti, A.; Dopsaj, M.; Sansone, P.; Mandorino, M.; Tessitore, A. Effects of Playing Position and Contextual Factors on Internal Match Loads, Post-Match Recovery and Well-Being Responses of Elite Male Water Polo Players. *J. Funct. Morphol. Kinesiol.* **2023**, *8*, 12. [CrossRef]
24. Foster, C. Monitoring training in athletes with reference to overtraining syndrome. *Med. Sci. Sports Exerc.* **1998**, *30*, 1164–1168. [CrossRef] [PubMed]
25. Foster, C.; Daines, E.; Hector, L.; Snyder, A.C.; Welsh, R. Athletic performance in relation to training load. *Wis. Med. J.* **1996**, *95*, 370–374.
26. Foster, C.; Florhaug, J.A.; Franklin, J.; Gottschall, L.; Hrovatin, L.A.; Parker, S.; Dodge, C. A new approach to monitoring exercise training. *J. Strength Cond. Res.* **2001**, *15*, 109–115. [PubMed]
27. Lupo, C.; Capranica, L.; Tessitore, A. The validity of the session-RPE method for quantifying training load in water polo. *Int. J. Sports Physiol. Perform.* **2014**, *9*, 656–660. [CrossRef]
28. Stanley, D.M.; Cumming, J. Are we having fun yet? Testing the effects of imagery use on the affective and enjoyment responses to acute moderate exercise. *Psychol. Sport Exerc.* **2010**, *11*, 582–590. [CrossRef]
29. Foster, C.; Farland, C.V.; Guidotti, F.; Harbin, M.; Roberts, B.; Schuette, J.; Tuuri, A.; Doberstein, S.T.; Porcari, J.P. The Effects of High Intensity Interval Training vs Steady State Training on Aerobic and Anaerobic Capacity. *J. Sports Sci. Med.* **2015**, *14*, 747–755.
30. Hooper, S.L.; Mackinnon, L.T.; Howard, A.L.F.; Gordon, R.D.; Bachmann, A.W. Markers for monitoring overtraining and recovery. *Med. Sci. Sports Exerc.* **1995**, *27*, 106–112. [CrossRef] [PubMed]
31. Laurent, C.M.; Green, J.M.; Bishop, P.A.; Sjökvist, J.; Schumacker, R.E.; Richardson, M.T.; Curtner-Smith, M. A practical approach to monitoring recovery: Development of a perceived recovery status scale. *J. Strength Cond. Res.* **2011**, *25*, 620–628. [CrossRef] [PubMed]
32. Menaspà, M.J.; Menaspà, P.; Clark, S.A.; Fanchini, M. Validity of the online athlete management system to assess training load. *Int. J. Sports Physiol. Perform.* **2018**, *13*, 750–754. [CrossRef]
33. Paul, D.J.; Tomazoli, G.; Nassis, G.P. Match-related time course of perceived recovery in youth football players. *Int. J. Sports Physiol. Perform.* **2019**, *14*, 339–342. [CrossRef] [PubMed]
34. Berriel, G.P.; Costa, R.R.; da Silva, E.S.; Schons, P.; de Vargas, G.D.; Peyré-Tartaruga, L.A.; Kruel, L.F.M. Stress and recovery perception, creatine kinase levels, and performance parameters of male volleyball athletes in a preseason for a championship. *Sports Med.—Open* **2020**, *6*, 26. [CrossRef]
35. Barrenetxea-Garcia, J.; Murua-Ruiz, A.; Mielgo-Ayuso, J.; Nuell, S.; Calleja-González, J.; de Villarreal, E.S. Recovery in water polo: How much do we have to know? A systematic review. *J. Exerc. Rehabil.* **2022**, *18*, 225. [CrossRef] [PubMed]
36. Hopkins, W.; Marshall, S.; Batterham, A.; Hanin, J. Progressive statistics for studies in sports medicine and exercise science. *Med. Sci. Sports Exerc.* **2009**, *41*, 3. [CrossRef]
37. Botonis, P.G.; Arsoniadis, G.G.; Smilios, I.; Toubekis, A.G. In-season training load variation-heart rate recovery, perceived recovery status, and performance in elite male water polo players: A pilot study. *Sports Health* **2025**, *17*, 144–149. [CrossRef]
38. Barrenetxea-Garcia, J.; Busto, N.; Calleja-González, J.; de Villarreal, E.S.; Perazzetti, A.; Nuell, S.; Garai, S.; Mielgo-Ayuso, J. The impact of foam rolling recovery tool on oxidative stress biomarkers and performance in-water polo players: A randomized controlled trial. *J. Exerc. Rehabil.* **2025**, *21*, 140–150. [CrossRef]
39. Miguel-Ortega, Á.; Barrenetxea-Garcia, J.; Rodríguez-Rodrigo, M.A.; García-Ordóñez, E.; Mielgo-Ayuso, J.; Calleja-González, J. Ergonutrition Supplementation and Recovery in Water Polo: A Systematic Review. *Nutrients* **2025**, *17*, 1319. [CrossRef]
40. Toubekis, A.G.; Tsolaki, A.; Smilios, I.; Douda, H.T.; Kourtesis, T.; Tokmakidis, S.P. Swimming performance after passive and active recovery of various durations. *Int. J. Sports Physiol. Perform.* **2008**, *3*, 375–386. [CrossRef]
41. Nedelec, M.; Aloulou, A.; Duforez, F.; Meyer, T.; Dupont, G. The variability of sleep among elite athletes. *Sports Med.—Open* **2018**, *4*, 34. [CrossRef] [PubMed]
42. Perazzetti, A.; Dopsaj, M.; Tessitore, A. Technical and tactical evaluation of ball possession in international youth water polo matches using the Team Sport Assessment Procedure (TSAP) instrument. *Monten. J. Sports Sci. Med.* **2023**, *19*, 3–9. [CrossRef]

43. Perazzetti, A.; Tessitore, A.; Özkol, M.Z.; Novoselac, N.; Dopsaj, M. Assessment of Youth Water Polo Players' Swimming Sprint Potential: A New Approach to Building an International Model. *J. Funct. Morphol. Kinesiol.* **2025**, *10*, 200. [CrossRef] [PubMed]
44. World Aquatics. World Aquatics Competition Regulations. 2025. Available online: https://www.worldaquatics.com/rules/competition-regulations (accessed on 20 June 2025).

sports

MDPI

Article

Run-Based Tests Performed on an Indoor and Outdoor Surface Are Comparable in Adolescent Rugby League Players

Michael A. Carron [1,2] and Vincent J. Dalbo [1,2,*]

[1] School of Health, Medical and Applied Sciences, Central Queensland University, Rockhampton, QLD 4702, Australia; m.carron@cqu.edu.au
[2] Health Education Lifestyle and Performance (HELP) Laboratory, St Brendan's College, Yeppoon, QLD 4703, Australia
* Correspondence: v.dalbo@cqu.edu.au

Abstract: At non-professional levels of rugby league, run-based tests are commonly performed on outdoor turfed fields and on indoor multipurpose sport surfaces, and results are monitored to gauge player performance and progression. However, test–retest reliability has not been conducted on indoor surfaces in adolescent rugby league players, and no research has examined if results obtained on outdoor and indoor surfaces are comparable for practitioners. Adolescent, male, rugby league players (N = 15; age = 17.1 ± 0.7 years) completed a 20 m linear sprint test (10- and 20 m splits), 505-Agility Test, and Multistage Fitness Test (MSFT) weekly for three consecutive weeks. Absolute (coefficient of variation (CV)) and relative (intraclass correlation coefficient (ICC)) reliability of each run-based test performed on the indoor surface was quantified. Dependent *t*-tests, Hedges *g*, and 95% confidence intervals were used to examine if differences in performance occurred between indoor and outdoor surfaces. Effect size magnitudes were determined as *Trivial*: <0.20, *Small*: 0.20–0.49, *Medium*: 0.50–0.79, and *Large*: ≥0.80. All tests were considered reliable on the indoor surface (CV < 5.0%; ICCs = *moderate-good*) except for the 505-Agility Test (CV = 4.6–5.1%; ICCs = *poor*). Non-significant ($p > 0.05$), *trivial* differences were revealed between surface types for 10 ($g = 0.15$, 95% CI = −0.41 to 0.70) and 20 m ($g = 0.06$, 95% CI = −0.49 to 0.61) sprint tests, the 505-Agility Test (Right: $g = -0.53$, 95% CI = −1.12 to 0.06; Left: $g = -0.40$, 95% CI = −0.97 to 0.17), and the MSFT ($g = 0.25$, 95% CI = −0.31 to 0.81). The 10 and 20 m linear sprint test and MSFT have acceptable test–retest reliability on an indoor multipurpose sport surface, and practitioners may compare results of run-based tests obtained on an outdoor and indoor surface.

Keywords: test–retest reliability; youth; performance; strength and conditioning; exercise

1. Introduction

Successful performance in rugby league is highly dependent on several run-based skills such as linear speed, change of direction, and aerobic capacity [1]. As a result, practitioners (i.e., coaches, sports performance, and sports science staff) seek to enhance on-field player performance by creating structured training protocols aimed at improving linear speed, change of direction, and aerobic capacity of players [2]. To ensure that the structured training protocol elicits positive training adaptations, practitioners periodically assess the effects of training on player performance of the variables they are seeking to improve [2,3]. As a result, it is common practice for rugby league practitioners to obtain several measures of linear speed (commonly assessed with 10 and 20 m sprint tests), change of direction (commonly assessed with the 505-Agility Test), and aerobic capacity (commonly assessed with the Multistage Fitness Test (MSFT)) over the duration of the season to monitor the efficacy of their training protocol [4,5].

In rugby league, particularly at the high school level, linear speed, change of direction, and aerobic capacity testing primarily occurs on outdoor turfed fields. In this regard, numerous studies have reported 10 m linear sprint speed, 20 m linear sprint speed, 505-Agility Test, and MSFT performance to be reliable on outdoor turfed fields in adolescent, male, rugby league players [6–8]. However, conducting run-based tests on outdoor turfed surfaces introduces unnecessary error into test results via extraneous variables such as weather, varied surface conditions such as turf type (e.g., various types of grass and variability in turf height), and variations in surface stiffness (e.g., moisture affecting stiffness) of the turfed surface [9,10]. Furthermore, given that the Australian adolescent rugby league season (also known as schoolboy rugby league) spans from summer through winter (i.e., the match schedule occurs from May to September), extraneous variables influencing outdoor turfed surface conditions are inevitable. Specifically, practitioners are likely to make assessments on player adaptations from outdoor test results that were collected in conditions that had substantial variations in heat [11], solar exposure [12], and moisture [13] due to rain and/or dew which effect traction, friction, and surface stiffness [14]. Each condition can affect the physiological (i.e., core body temperature and heart rate) [15] and biomechanical (i.e., ground reaction force and friction) performance of the player [9,10], which can influence test results [9,13]. Despite the limitations of conducting run-based tests on outdoor turfed surfaces, outdoor testing is the preferred mode of testing of adolescent rugby league practitioners and can be justified by the logic that rugby league is played on outdoor turfed surfaces.

Even though it is the preference of adolescent rugby league practitioners to conduct run-based tests on outdoor turfed surfaces, it is not uncommon for testing to occur on indoor multipurpose sport surfaces primarily due to weather events such as rain, snow, or lightning. As a result, it is common for adolescent rugby league practitioners to gauge player performance and progression with results of run-based tests obtained on outdoor turfed surfaces and indoor multipurpose sport surfaces. This practice raises two questions. First, are the results of run-based tests obtained on an indoor multipurpose sport surface reliable in adolescent rugby league players as no found research has been published on this topic. Second, assuming the results of run-based tests performed on an indoor multipurpose sport surface are reliable in adolescent rugby league players, can practitioners meaningfully compare results of run-based tests obtained on an outdoor turfed surface and an indoor multipurpose sport surface which is commonly occurring in practice.

2. Materials and Methods

2.1. Participants

The first aim of our study was to quantify the test–retest reliability of the 10 m sprint test, 20 m sprint test, 505-Agility test, and MSFT on an indoor multipurpose sports surface in our sample. As a result, no power analysis was required for this study aim. The second aim of our study was to determine if results from a 10 m sprint test, 20 m sprint test, 505-Agility test, and MSFT performed on an outdoor turfed field and an indoor multipurpose sports surface could be meaningfully compared by practitioners to make informed decisions about player performance and progression. As a result, we conducted an *a priori* power analysis using G*Power (3.1.9.7; Heinrich Heine University, Dusseldorf, Germany). Based on the statistical test, differences between two dependent means (matched pairs), a two-tailed test, an effect size of 0.80, an α error probability of 0.05, and a power (1-β error probability) of 0.80, the required sample size was calculated as 15. Therefore, our study was adequately powered to detect if a *large* difference occurred in the performance time of each run-based test performed on the two surface types.

Adolescent, male, rugby league players (N = 15, age: 17.1 ± 0.7 years; height: 179.96 ± 5.95 cm; mass: 83.36 ± 14.59 kg) from the same team volunteered to partake in this study. Players were recruited to participate if they were selected to compete in the first-grade schoolboy competition (e.g., equivalent to the varsity team in American high schools) and were free from injury and illness. All players had a minimum of six months of a consistent training history (i.e., rugby league skills and development training and technical/safety introductions to resistance training) and were familiarized with all tests to be completed at least once prior to the first testing session. Written informed assent was obtained from all participants and written informed consent was obtained from a legal guardian of each participant prior to the commencement of this study. The study protocol was approved by the institution's Human Research Ethics Review Committee prior to the commencement of the study (#0000023570).

2.2. Study Design

A within-participant, repeated measure, crossover design was employed for this study, which occurred at the end of the in-season training phase of the season. Players were partaking in three gym sessions (resistance training occurred on Monday, Wednesday, and Friday) and two field sessions (skills and drills training occurred on Monday and Wednesday) per week. Training occurred as follows: Monday (resistance training 15:00–15:50 followed by a field session 15:50–16:45), Wednesday (resistance training 15:00–15:50 followed by a field session 15:50–16:45), and Friday (06:00–07:00, resistance training). Data collection for this study over three weeks. During the three-week data collection period, participants trained as specified on Monday but did not train on the Wednesday (to allow for 48 h rest), and the Friday training session was replaced by testing (06:00–12:00). This modification to the training schedule allowed for a 48 h rest prior to each training session and testing sessions (Figure 1). Testing occurred in the following order: Week 1: Run-based tests performed on an outdoor turfed surface (i.e., a grass field). Weeks 2 and 3: Run-based tests performed on an indoor multipurpose sports surface. The results of run-based tests conducted during weeks 2 and 3 allowed for the examination of test–retest reliability of each run-based test on an indoor multipurpose sports surface (Aura Sports, Polyurethane Flooring; Ipswich, QLD, Australia). The results of the run-based tests conducted during weeks 1 and 2 allowed for the comparison of tests performed on an outdoor turfed surface and an indoor multipurpose sports surface. It is common practice for the reliability of run-based tests to be evaluated on different days within a timeframe of seven days to limit or prevent results of subsequent tests from being influenced by maturation in younger cohorts or a training effect in those undertaking structured training [16].

Each Friday of the testing period, players reported to the testing facility and performed a consistent 15 min warm-up protocol that was delivered prior to each testing session and was completed by all players. The warm-up comprised five minutes of light aerobic cycling, several mobility exercises which targeted major functional movements, and dynamic stretches of the lower body for four minutes. Thereafter, movement preparation exercises with body weight or resistance bands (i.e., squat, lunge, Pallof press, and single-arm row) were performed for four minutes, and a football was repeatedly passed over 10 m intervals while moving at different intensities for two minutes. Tests were always administered in the following order: 20 m linear sprint tests (from which the 10 m sprint time split was derived), 505-Agility Test, and the MSFT. The order of testing follows the recommendations of the National Strength and Conditioning Association (NSCA) [17].

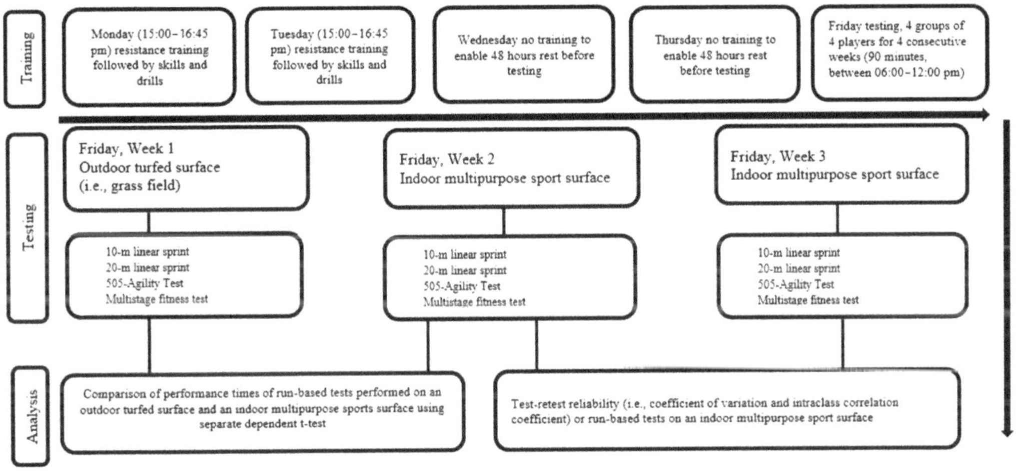

Figure 1. Schematic of the study design.

2.3. Methods

Players were instructed to consume their typical diet, refrain from vigorous activity, and continue with their normal daily schedules (i.e., nutrition, hydration, sleep, and school participation) for 48 h prior to the commencement of each testing session [6,18]. Testing sessions were conducted in three groups of four players and one group of three players. Each group of players completed testing in 90 min sessions as follows: group 1: 06:00–07:30; group 2: 07:30–09:00; group 3: 09:00–10:30; and group 4: 10:30–12:00. Each group of players was assigned to the same scheduled time for each testing session to reduce the effects of circadian rhythms [19], hormonal fluctuations [20], and feeding [21] on performance. For each testing session, participants wore regular rugby league attire (t-shirt and shorts), but footwear was altered to suit the change in surface conditions. During outdoor testing, participants wore cleats; during indoor testing, participants wore running shoes. Participants were instructed to wear the same pair of running shoes during each indoor testing session.

2.4. Linear Speed

Linear speed was assessed with 10 m and 20 m linear sprint times (s). Players were positioned with the toes of their leading foot placed 50 cm behind the first timing gate on marking tape in a split stance before initiating each sprint [22]. Each player completed three 20 m sprints with each 20 m sprint commencing upon their own volition. Single-beam electronic timing gates (SmartSpeed Pro, Fusion Sport; Brisbane, QLD, Australia) were used to record sprint times. Single-beam electric timing gates were set at 0 m, 10 m, and 20 m (at a height of 1 m) to obtain a measure of 10 m and 20 m sprint times (s). Performance times (s) were retrieved immediately after each attempt via the SmartSpeed application (version 1.0.4) for 10 m and 20 m splits to the nearest 0.001 s. Between each attempt, 60 s of passive standing rest was allocated to separate attempts, with the fastest of the three attempts for each split (10 m and 20 m) recorded for analysis [6].

2.5. Change-of-Direction

Change-of-direction was assessed with the 505-Agility test. Players began each attempt standing with the toes of their lead foot on marking tape set at the 0 m point. Players were expected to move as fast as possible on their own volition in a forward direction for 15 m before turning 180 degrees back towards the starting point, and accelerating for a further

5 m [1]. One single-beam electronic timing gate (SmartSpeed Pro, Fusion Sport; Brisbane, QLD, Australia) was positioned 10 m from 0 m starting point to record performance time to the nearest 0.001 s. Timing commenced as participants passed through the timing gate covering an additional 5 m before turning and passing the timing gate to complete the test. Performance was assessed separately for the left and right leg to initiate the COD (plant leg), requiring players to complete six total attempts in the same order on each occasion (performed first, as a right lead leg for three attempts and then left lead leg for the final three attempts, with the lead leg being the foot to make the turn). The fastest of the three attempts for each leg was recorded for analysis.

2.6. Aerobic Capacity

Aerobic capacity was assessed with the MSFT to estimate maximal oxygen uptake (VO_{2max} [$mL \cdot kg^{-1} \cdot min^{-1}$]), following an established procedure and equation [23]. The MSFT requires participants to perform repeated 20 m shuttle runs with progressive increases in speed dictated by audio cues. The MSFT concluded when players voluntarily stopped or failed to complete the necessary distance as signaled by audio cues across two successive shuttles. During testing on the outdoor turfed surface, players completed the MSFT on a regulation, grass, rugby league field with clearly marked lines to indicate the 20 m distance. During indoor testing, players completed the MSTF on an indoor multipurpose sports surface with clearly marked lines indicating the 20 m distance.

2.7. Reliability and Levels of Acceptability

Reliability of tests is often assessed by quantifying the coefficient of variation (CV) and intraclass correlation coefficient (ICC) [24]. CV represents the absolute reliability of a test and quantifies the random error between repeated measurements. CV is most relevant when assessing changes in the outcome of a test over time (i.e., the repeatability of the result in regard to average performance) [16]. In contrast, ICC represents relative reliability, which quantifies the amount of variability in the measurement that was due to differences between participants (i.e., the repeatability of the test in regard to how participants finish in the same order/hierarchy when a test is repeated over time) [16]. Using established criteria, a CV of <5.0% is considered reliable for a 10 m sprint, 20 m sprint, and 505-Agility Test, while a CV of <10.0% is considered reliable for the MSFT [25]. Given no specific thresholds of ICCs for run tests exist, ICCs were evaluated using generalized established criteria of *poor*: $\leq$0.50, *moderate*: 0.50 to 0.74, *good*: 0.75 to 0.90, or *excellent*: $\geq$0.90 and were interpreted based on the ICC value without considering the 95% confidence interval (CI) [26]. The CV and ICC of run-based tests performed on an indoor multipurpose sport surface were determined using the best attempt of each trial that occurred during each testing session (e.g., the best 10 m sprint time obtained from testing during week 2 and the best 10 m sprint time obtained from testing during week 3).

2.8. Statistical Analyses

To accomplish the first aim of our study, we quantified the CV and ICC with a 95% CI [26] for each run-based test performed on an indoor multipurpose sport surface. The CV of each run-based test was quantified using an established formula [27] with calculations being performed in Microsoft Excel (version 15, Microsoft Corp; Redmond, WA), while the ICC and 95% CI were quantified using IBM SPSS software (version 24 IBM Corp; Armo, NY, USA). To accomplish the second aim of our study, we compared the results of each run-based test performed on an outdoor turfed surface and an indoor multipurpose sport surface using separate dependent *t*-tests (i.e., outdoor turfed surface test results obtained during week 1 were compared to indoor multipurpose sport surface test results obtained during week 2). Prior to making any comparisons, each dependent variable was tested for normality with separate Shapiro–Wilk tests. Each dependent variable was normally distributed ($p > 0.05$) except for the 10 m sprint test performed on the outdoor turfed surface ($p < 0.05$). As a result, we visually inspected the distribution of data for 10 m sprint performance using Q–Q plots and determined the data to be reasonably normally distributed. As a result, all data were reported as means and standard deviations (SD). Significance testing (i.e., p-values) was utilized to determine if a repeatable difference was present for each run-based test performed on an outdoor turfed surface or indoor multipurpose sport surface with significance set *a priori* at $p < 0.05$. An effect size and 95% CI were utilized to determine if a meaningful difference was present for each run-based test performed on an outdoor turfed surface or an indoor multipurpose sport surface. Due to the sample size, Hedges' g was selected as the effect size measure [28] and was reported with a 95% CI. The effect size magnitude of Hedges' g was determined as *Trivial*: <0.20, *Small*: 0.20 to 0.49, *Medium*: 0.50 to 0.79, or *Large*: ≥0.80; however, if the 95% CI overlapped 0, the effect size magnitude was defined as *trivial*. Dependent t-tests were conducted with Jamovi (version 2.3.28; the Jamovi project) while Hedges' g and the 95% confidence intervals were quantified in Microsoft Excel (version 15, Microsoft Corp; Redmond, WA, USA) as follows:

Step 1: Quantification of Cohen's d [28]

Cohen's d = (Time Point A Mean − Time Point B Mean)/Pooled Standard Deviation

We then calculated (Outdoor testing time point − initial (week 2) indoor time point)/Pooled Standard Deviation

Step 2: Quantification of Hedges' g [28]

Hedges $g = d$*(1 − (3/(4*(Number of Pairs − 1) − 1)))

where d = Cohen's d

Step 3: Quantification of the 95% Confidence Interval for Hedges' g

95% CI for Hedges' g = g ± ($t_{\alpha/2}$*SE_g)

where g = The effect size of Hedges' g

$t_{\alpha/2}$ = The critical value from a dependent samples t-distribution table (N = 15 $t_{2.131}$ [29]

and df = N − 1)

SE_g = Standard error of Hedges' g quantified as follows:

SE_g = √((1/Number of Pairs) + (g^2/(2*Number of Pairs))))

3. Results

3.1. Test–Retest Reliability

Table 1 displays reliability statistics for each run-based test. All tests performed on an indoor multipurpose sport surface displayed an acceptable CV other than the 505-Agility test with a left leg lead (CV = 5.1%). The ICCs on an indoor multipurpose sport surface ranged from *poor* (505-Agility test, right and left leg) to *good* (10 and 20 m sprint).

Table 1. Test–retest reliability of run-based tests performed on an indoor multipurpose sports surface.

Test	n	CV (%)	Acceptable CV	ICC (95% CI)	*ICC Classification*
10 m sprint	15	1.9	Yes	0.76 (0.43 to 0.91)	*Good*
20 m sprint	15	1.4	Yes	0.86 (0.63 to 0.95)	*Good*
505-Agility Test right	15	4.6	Yes	0.19 (−0.34 to 0.63)	*Poor*
505-Agility Test left	15	5.1	No	0.21 (−0.32 to 0.64)	*Poor*
Multistage fitness test (mL·kg^{-1}·min^{-1})	15	4.1	Yes	0.63 (0.19 to 0.86)	*Moderate*

Abbreviations: n = sample; CV = coefficient of variation; ICC = intraclass correlation coefficient; CI = confidence interval. An acceptable CV of 5.0% was utilized for the 10 m sprint test, 20 m sprint test, and 505-Agility Test based on the recommendation of Currell et al. [25]. An acceptable CV of 10.0% was utilized for the multistage fitness test based on the recommendation of Currell et al. [25]. The ICC classifications were based on the ICC value independent of the 95% confidence interval [26]. The ICC classifications were defined based on the recommendations by Koo et al. [26] as follows: *poor:* ≤0.50, *moderate*: 0.50 to 0.74, *good*: 0.75 to 0.90, or *excellent*: ≥0.90.

3.2. Assessment of Significant and/or Meaningful Differences in Run-Based Tests Occurring on an Outdoor Turfed Field and an Indoor Multipurpose Sport Surface

Non-significant, *trivial* differences were revealed for each run-based test performed on an outdoor turfed surface and an indoor multipurpose sport surface (Table 2).

Table 2. Assessment of differences in run-based tests occurring on an outdoor turfed field and an indoor multipurpose sport surface.

Test	n	Outdoor Turfed Surface	Indoor Multipurpose Sport Surface		Comparison of Run-Based Tests Conducted During Week 1 and Week 2			
		Week 1 Mean ± SD	Week 2 Mean ± SD	Week 3 Mean ± SD	p-Value	Hedges' g	95% CI	Effect Size Magnitude
10 m sprint (s)	15	1.75 ± 0.05	1.77 ± 0.10	1.77 ± 0.11	0.56	0.15	−0.41 to 0.70	*Trivial*
20 m sprint (s)	15	3.05 ± 0.12	3.06 ± 0.16	3.07 ± 0.18	0.82	0.06	−0.49 to 0.61	*Trivial*
505-Agility right (s)	15	2.31 ± 0.20	2.20 ± 0.10	2.15 ± 0.17	0.05	−0.53	−1.12 to 0.06	*Trivial*
505-Agility left (s)	15	2.29 ± 0.18	2.21 ± 0.12	2.15 ± 0.19	0.13	−0.40	−0.97 to 0.17	*Trivial*
Multistage fitness test (mL·kg^{-1}·min^{-1})	15	46.09 ± 3.82	47.4 ± 3.87	46.79 ± 5.45	0.33	0.25	−0.31 to 0.81	*Trivial*

Abbreviations: n = sample; SD = standard deviation. The p-value represents significance and was set *a priori* at $p < 0.05$. Hedges' g is the effect size and represents the meaningfulness of the finding. Effect size magnitudes were determined as *trivial*: <0.20; *small*: 0.20–0.49; *medium*: 0.50–0.79; and *large*: ≥0.80 [28]. However, when the 95% overlapped 0 the effect size magnitude was determined as *trivial* [28].

4. Discussion

Commonly utilized run-based tests in adolescent rugby league include the 10 m sprint test, 20 m sprint test, 505-Agility Test with a left and right lead leg, and the MSFT [6]. Each of these run-based tests has previously been deemed reliable on an outdoor surface [6,8] but no research has examined the reliability of these tests in adolescent rugby league players on an indoor surface. Moreover, no study has examined whether practitioners can make meaningful comparisons between run-based tests performed on outdoor and indoor surfaces despite commonly occurring in practice. Findings from our study suggest that the 10 m sprint, 20 m sprint, and MSFT can be reliably performed on an indoor multipurpose sport surface, as each of these tests yielded an acceptable CV (CV <5.0%) and *moderate* to *good* ICC values (ICC range: 0.63 to 0.86). Results from our data suggest the 505-Agility Test (right and left lead leg) should be used with caution on an indoor multipurpose sport surface due to poor absolute reliability (CV right lead leg: 4.6%, CV left lead leg: 5.1%) and *poor* relative reliability (ICC right lead leg: 0.19, ICC left lead leg: 0.21). Results from the dependent t-tests suggest practitioners can make comparisons between data collected on an outdoor turfed surface and an indoor multipurpose sport surface for the 10 m sprint, 20 m sprint, 505-Agility Test, and MSFT due to the lack of significant ($p \geq 0.05$) or meaningful differences (i.e., the effect size magnitude was *trivial* for each comparison). However, we do not recommend performing the 505-Agility Tests on an indoor multipurpose sport surface due to displaying poor test–retest reliability.

Test–retest reliability of linear speed tests in adolescent, male rugby league players has previously been established on outdoor turfed surfaces [6,7]. Specifically, Carron et al. [6] assessed the test–retest reliability of the 10 m (CV = 2.1%, ICC = 0.704) and 20 m linear sprint (CV = 1.4%, ICC = 0.869) tests in adolescent, male, rugby league players (N = 50; 16.2 ± 1.3 years), while Dobbin et al. [8] assessed the test–retest reliability of 10 m (CV = 4.2%, ICC = 0.81) and 20 m linear sprint (CV = 3.6%, ICC = 0.78) tests in academy-level, male, rugby league players (N = 50, 17.1 ± 1.1 years). Moreover, Darrall-Jones et al. [7] assessed the CV of 10 m (CV = 3.1%) and 20 m linear sprint tests (CV = 1.8%) in a sample of adolescent, male rugby players (N = 28, 17.7 ± 0.6 years), but their results reflect data collected in academy rugby league (n = 14) and rugby union (n = 14) players reported together (N = 28).

Results from our study revealed the 10 m sprint (CV = 1.9%, ICC = 0.76) and 20 m sprint (CV = 1.4%, ICC = 0.86) to be reliable on an indoor multipurpose sport surface and are comparable to previously published results obtained on an outdoor surface in adolescent, male, rugby league players [6]. However, results from our study suggest the 505-Agility Test performed on an indoor surface to be unreliable, as CVs ranged from 4.6% (right foot lead) to 5.1% (left foot lead). Given that a CV of <5.0% is considered acceptable [28] and we had a small sample size (N = 15), future research conducted with a larger sample size may reveal the 505-Agility Test to have an acceptable CV on an indoor surface. However, we found the 505-Agility Test to present *poor* ICCs with a right foot lead (ICC = 0.19, 95% CI = −0.34 to 0.63) and left foot lead (ICC = 0.21, 95% CI = −0.32 to 0.64). To our surprise, our findings suggest when assessing tests of change of direction, specifically with the 505-Agility test, it may be more suitable to use an outdoor turfed surface, as previous investigations conducted in adolescent, male, high school rugby league players found the 505-Agility test to be reliable (right foot lead: CV = 1.85%, ICC = 0.787; left foot lead: CV = 2.07%, ICC = 0.860) when obtained on an outdoor surface [6]. We speculate that the degree of surface stiffness likely affects the consistency of change of direction movements when performed on an indoor multipurpose sport surface. Specifically, friction and traction are integral for cutting maneuvers [9] and the malleability (i.e., softness) of the turfed surface likely enables players to plant and stabilize their footing more efficiently by way of surface manipulation [30], particularly when wearing cleats. In this way, players may alter the surface and utilize ground reaction forces to articulate their mechanical power effectively when performing the 180-degree turn expressed in the 505-Agility test [31]. Moreover, stiffer surfaces yield less force loss via deformation of the surface resulting in improved proprioceptive feedback assisting mechanical and technical efficiency [32] when performing the sprinting component of the 505-Agility test [31]. Conversely, non-malleable surface types, such as an indoor multipurpose sport surface may introduce a slip factor negatively influencing the reliability of test results.

We found the MSFT to be reliable when performed on an indoor surface in adolescent, male, high school rugby league players (CV = 4.1%, ICC = 0.63, 95% CI = 0.19 to 0.86, *Moderate*). Our results differ from a previous study that investigated the reliability of the MSFT in male, adolescent, high school rugby league players on an outdoor turfed surface (CV = 3.04, ICC = 0.84, *Good*) [6]. The negligible differences between the reliability (CV and ICC) of the MSFT we found on an indoor multipurpose sport surface, and that which Carron et al. [6] reported on an outdoor turfed surface, suggest that practitioners can make meaningful comparisons of MSFT results obtained on these surfaces. However, due to the extraneous variables introduced by outdoor testing, best practice would suggest assessing MSFT performance on an indoor multipurpose sport surface when possible.

If accuracy is the primary concern of practitioners, the 10 m sprint, 20 m sprint, and MSFT should be performed on an indoor multipurpose sport surface in adolescent, male, rugby league players. Conducting these run-based tests on an indoor multipurpose sport surface would aid in standardizing run-based tests, resulting in greater homogeneity of testing procedures across studies and allowing for more accurate comparisons between studies. Moreover, the adoption of standardized testing procedures would enable practitioners to more accurately compare results from test outcomes obtained in practice to test outcomes presented in research. Due to the 505-Agility Test having poor reliability in our study, we cannot currently recommend performing the 505-Agility Test on an indoor multipurpose sport surface. However, future studies should attempt to replicate our findings, as we had a small sample size and we appear to be the first to report on the reliability of run-based tests on an indoor multipurpose sport surface in adolescent, male, rugby league players. Therefore, more research should be conducted before definitive conclusions about the reliability of run-based tests in adolescent, male, rugby league players and other populations can be confirmed.

Notably, we recommended that practitioners, who are using run-based tests to monitor player progression over time, perform run-based tests on an indoor multipurpose sport surface, when possible, as fewer extraneous variables are introduced to the testing protocol compared to testing on an outdoor turfed surface. In this vein, the assessment of test–retest reliability of run-based tests has previously occurred within a seven-day period [6,8]. As a result, test–retest reliability outcomes of run-based tests performed on an outdoor turfed surface are likely to occur under similar external conditions such as temperature, humidity, solar exposure, and surface conditions. However, if monitoring performance of run-based tests take place over the duration of a year, in most climates, factors such as temperature, humidity, solar exposure, and surface conditions will vary greatly from summer to winter. Our study was conducted in a subtropical climate and the average 9 a.m. conditions in February (Season: temperature: 27.2 °C, humidity: 75%, dew point: 22.1 °C, wind speed: 17.0 km/h, solar exposure: 21–24 kWh/m^2) [33,34] were notably different to the average 9 a.m. conditions in September (Season: Sprint, temperature: 21.9 °C, humidity: 69%, dew point: 15.7 °C, wind speed: 13.7 km/h, solar exposure: 21–24 kWh/m^2) [33,34].

We conducted this study as it is common for practitioners to gauge player performance and progression utilizing run-based test results obtained on outdoor turfed surfaces and indoor multipurpose sport surfaces. Therefore, we determined if there were significant or meaningful differences in performance times for the 10 m sprint test, 20 m sprint test, 505-Agility Test, and MSFT. We found there to be no significant ($p \geq 0.05$) or meaningful (a *trivial* effect size magnitude was found for each test) differences between performance outcomes of each run-based test performed on an outdoor turfed field or an indoor multipurpose sport surface. To our surprise, our results suggest that, if required, practitioners may compare results of run-based tests obtained on an outdoor turfed field and an indoor multipurpose sport surface. However, for best practice, practitioners should seek to limit as many extraneous variables as possible and, as a result, should seek to standardize their testing practice, including surface type. In this way, future research should look to monitor indoor and outdoor environmental conditions, including but not limited to temperature, humidity, solar exposure, and surface condition (i.e., grass length/type, dew, and/or water pooling). We recognize this as a limitation of our study, where conditions such as grass length/type were not recorded. Moreover, researchers should not compare the results of run-based tests obtained on an outdoor turfed surface and an indoor multipurpose sport surface due to methodological issues regarding different mechanical properties (e.g., friction or energy return) and confounding factors (e.g., altered technique or loading patterns).

5. Conclusions

The results from our study suggest that the 10 m sprint, 20 m sprint, and MSFT have acceptable absolute (CV < 5%) and relative (ICC = *moderate-good*) reliability on an indoor multipurpose sport surface. Importantly, we found the 505-Agility test to reside outside the acceptable range of absolute reliability (left leg lead: 5.1%) and to have *poor* relative reliability with a right leg and left leg lead. Researchers should not compare results of run-based tests performed on outdoor turfed surfaces and indoor multipurpose surfaces to maintain best practice. However, if necessary, practitioners may compare the results of run-based tests performed on an outdoor turfed surface and an indoor multipurpose sport surface to gauge player performance or progression. Nevertheless, best practice dictates that practitioners should standardize their testing procedures.

Author Contributions: All authors contributed equally to the current study. Conceptualization, M.A.C.; methodology, M.A.C. and V.J.D.; formal analysis, M.A.C.; investigation, M.A.C.; writing—original draft preparation, M.A.C.; writing—review and editing, M.A.C. and V.J.D.; project administration, M.A.C. All authors have read and agreed to the published version of the manuscript.

Funding: This research received no external funding.

Institutional Review Board Statement: This original investigation complies with ethical standards and practices and is approved by the Central Queensland University Human Research Ethics Review Committee (protocol code #0000023570 and approval date 19 May 2022).

Informed Consent Statement: Informed assent, and consent was obtained from both the participant and legal guardian prior to conducting this original investigation.

Data Availability Statement: The data that support the findings of this study are available from the corresponding author upon reasonable request.

Conflicts of Interest: The authors report there are no competing interests to declare.

References

1. Gabbett, T.J.; Kelly, J.N.; Sheppard, J.M. Speed, change of direction speed, and reactive agility of rugby league players. *J. Strength Cond. Res.* **2008**, *22*, 174–181. [CrossRef]
2. Carron, M.A.; Scanlan, A.T.; Doering, T.M. Quantifying the training loads and corresponding changes in physical qualities among adolescent, schoolboy rugby league players. *Sports* **2024**, *12*, 251. [CrossRef]
3. Hughes, D.C.; Ellefsen, S.; Baar, K. Adaptations to endurance and strength training. *Cold Spring Harb. Perspect. Med.* **2018**, *8*, a029769. [CrossRef] [PubMed]
4. Carron, M.A.; Scanlan, A.T.; Power, C.J.; Doering, T.M. What tests are used to assess the physical qualities of male, adolescent rugby league players? A systematic review of testing protocols and reported data across adilescent age groups. *Sports Med. Open* **2023**, *9*, 106. [CrossRef] [PubMed]
5. Verkhonshansky, Y.; Siff, M. *Supertraining*, 6th ed.; Paidotribo: Badalona, Spain, 2009.
6. Carron, M.A.; Scanlan, A.T.; Doering, T.M. The retest reliability of commo test to assess physical qualities in adolescent rugby league players. *Pediatr. Exerc. Sci.* **2024**, *37*, 212–219. [CrossRef]
7. Darrall-Jones, J.D.; Jones, B.; Roe, G.; Till, K. Reliability and usefulness of linear sprint testing in adolescent rugby union and league players. *J. Strength Cond. Res.* **2016**, *30*, 1359–1364. [CrossRef] [PubMed]
8. Dobbin, N.; Hunwicks, R.; Highton, J.; Twist, C. A reliable testing battery for assessing physical qualities of elite academy rugby league players. *J. Strength Cond. Res.* **2018**, *32*, 3232–3238. [CrossRef]
9. Choi, S.M.; Sum, K.W.R.; Leung, F.L.E. Comparison between natural turf and artificial turf on agility performance of rugby league players. *Adv. Phys. Educ.* **2015**, *5*, 273–281. [CrossRef]
10. Mathew, S.; Seetharamu, G.K.; Dileepkumar, M.; Satish, D. Grasses for sports grounds and its influence on playing quality: A review. *Sports Med.* **2021**, *36*, 19.
11. Girard, O.; Brocherie, F.; Bishop, D.J. Sprint performance under heat stress: A review. *Scand. J. Med. Sci. Sports.* **2015**, *25* (Suppl. S1), 79–89. [CrossRef]
12. Otani, H.; Kaya, M.; Tamaki, A.; Watson, P.; Maughan, R.J. Effects of solar radiation on endurance exercise capacity in a hot environment. *Eur. J. Appl. Physiol.* **2016**, *116*, 769–779. [CrossRef]
13. Gabbett, T.; Minbashian, A.; Finch, C. Influence of environmental and ground conditions on injury risk in rugby league. *J. Sci. Med. Sport.* **2007**, *10*, 211–218. [CrossRef]
14. Sanchez-Sanchez, J.; Martinez-Rodriguez, A.; Felipe, J.L.; Hernandez-Martin, A.; Ubago-Guisado, E.; Bangsbo, J.; Gallardo, L.; Garcia-Unanue, J. Effect of natural turf, artificial turf, and sand surfaces on sprint performance. A systematic review and meta-analysis. *Int. J. Environ. Res. Public Health* **2020**, *17*, 9478. [CrossRef] [PubMed]
15. Natera, A.O.; Jennings, J.; Oakley, A.J.; Jones, T.W. Influence of environmental conditions on performance and heart rate responses to the 30-15 incremental fitness test in rugby union athletes. *J. Strength Cond. Res.* **2019**, *33*, 486–491. [CrossRef]
16. de Vet, H.C.; Terwee, C.B.; Knol, D.L.; Bouter, L.M. When to use agreement versus reliability measures. *J. Clin. Epidemiol.* **2006**, *59*, 1033–1039. [CrossRef]
17. Beachle, T.; Earle, R. *Essentials Strength Training Conditioning*; National Strength and Conditioning Association (U.S.): Champaign, IL, USA; Human Kinetics: Champaign, IL, USA, 2008; Volume 3, p. 245.
18. Gabbett, T.J. Physiological characteristics of junior and senior rugby league players. *Br. J. Sports Med.* **2002**, *36*, 334–339. [CrossRef]

19. Facer-Childs, E.R.; Boiling, S.; Balanos, G.M. The effects of time of day and chronotype on cognitive and physical performance in healthy volunteers. *Sports Med. Open.* **2018**, *4*, 47. [CrossRef] [PubMed]
20. Teo, W.; Newton, M.J.; McGuigan, M.R. Circadian rhythms in exercise performance: Implications for hormonal and muscular adaptation. *J. Sports Sci. Med.* **2011**, *10940*, 600–606.
21. Hawley, J.A.; Burke, L.M. Effect of meal frequency and timing on physical performance. *Br. J. Nutr.* **1997**, *77*, S91–S103. [CrossRef]
22. Weakley, J.; McCosker, C.; Chalkley, D.; Johnston, R.; Munteanu, G.; Morrison, M. Comparison of sprint timing methods on performance, and displacement and velocity and timining initiation. *J. Strength Cond. Res.* **2023**, *37*, 234–238. [CrossRef]
23. Ramsbottom, R.; Brewer, J.; Williams, C. A progressive shuttle run test to estimate maximal oxygen uptake. *Br. J. Sports Med.* **1988**, *22*, 141–144. [CrossRef]
24. Hopkins, G. Measures of reliability in sports medicine and science. *Sports Med.* **2000**, *30*, 1–15. [CrossRef]
25. Currell, K.; Jeukendrup, A.E. Validity, reliability and sensitivity of measures of sporting performance. *Sports Med.* **2008**, *38*, 297–316. [CrossRef] [PubMed]
26. Koo, T.K.; Li, M.Y. A guideline of selecting and reporting Intraclass Correlation Coefficients for reliability research. *J. Chiropr. Med.* **2016**, *15*, 155–163. [CrossRef]
27. Sainani, K.L. Reliability Statistics. *PM R.* **2017**, *9*, 622–628. [CrossRef]
28. Cohen, J. *Statistical Power Analysis for the Behavioral Sciences*, 2nd ed.; Routledge: New York, NY, USA, 1988.
29. Beyer, W.H. *Handbook of Tables for Probability and Statistics*, 2nd ed.; CRC Press: Boca Raton, FL, USA, 2019.
30. Wannop, J.; Kowalchuk, S.; Esposito, M.; Stefanyshyn, D. Influence of Artificial Turf Surface Stiffness on Athlete Performance. *Life* **2020**, *10*, 340. [CrossRef] [PubMed]
31. Delaney, J.A.; Scott, T.J.; Ballard, D.A.; Duthie, G.M.; Hickmans, J.A.; Lockie, R.G.; Dascombe, B.J. Contributing factors to change-of-direction ability in professional rugby league players. *J. Strength Cond. Res.* **2015**, *29*, 2688–2696. [CrossRef] [PubMed]
32. Gasparetto, T.; Nesseler, C. Diverse effects of thermal conditions on performance of marathon runners. *Front. Psychol.* **2020**, *11*, 1438. [CrossRef] [PubMed]
33. Bureau of Meteorology. Average Daily Solar Exposure Maps. 2025. Available online: http://www.bom.gov.au/climate/maps/averages/solar-exposure/ (accessed on 19 February 2025).
34. Bureau of Meteorology. Climate Statistics for Australian Locations. 2025. Available online: http://www.bom.gov.au/climate/averages/tables/cw_033294.shtml (accessed on 19 February 2025).

sports

MDPI

Article

The Criterion Validity of a Newly Developed Ballroom Aerobic Test (BAT) Protocol Against Objective Methods

Tamara Despot [1,2,*] and Davor Plavec [3,4]

1 Faculty of Kinesiology, University of Zagreb, 10 000 Zagreb, Croatia
2 Dance Studio 'Dancespot', 10 000 Zagreb, Croatia
3 Facility for Medical Care 'Prima Nova', 10 000 Zagreb, Croatia; davor.plavec@primanova.hr
4 Medical Faculty Osijek, JJ Strossmayer University, 31 000 Osijek, Croatia
* Correspondence: tamdespot@gmail.com

Abstract: Although laboratory testing to assess aerobic capacity has been a 'gold standard' in sports science, its high costs and time-consuming protocols may not be feasible for monitoring and tracking progress in limited conditions. In dancesport athletes, several field-based aerobic tests have been proposed, but the majority of them have been developed for ballet or contemporary dancers at the individual level, while the data among dance couples engaging in standard dance styles is lacking. Therefore, the main purpose of this study was to validate a newly developed Ballroom Aerobic Test (BAT) protocol against objective methods. Twelve standard dancesport couples (age: 20.4 ± 3.9 years; height: 172.1 ± 8.7 cm; weight: 60.1 ± 9.4 kg) with 8.2 ± 3.4 years of training and competing experience participated in this study. Ventilatory and metabolic parameters were generated using the MetaMax® 3B portable gas analyzer (the BAT), while the KF1 (an increase in speed by 0.5 km * h^{-1} by every minute) and Bruce protocols were followed in laboratory-based settings on the running ergometer. Large to very large correlations were obtained between the BAT and KF1/Bruce protocols for the absolute maximal oxygen uptake (VO_2max; r = 0.88 and 0.87) and relative VO_2max (r = 0.88 and 0.85), respiratory exchange ratio (RER; r = 0.78 and 0.76), expiratory ventilation (VE; r = 0.86 and 0.79), tidal volume (VT; r = 0.75; 95% CI = 0.57–0.87; $p < 0.001$), ventilatory equivalent for O_2 (VE/VO_2; r = 0.81 and 0.80) and CO_2 (VE/VCO_2; r = 0.78 and 0.82), and dead space (VD/VT; r = 0.70 and 0.74). The Bland–Altman plots indicated no systematic and proportional biases between the BAT and KF1 protocols (standard error of estimate; SEE = ± 3.36 mL * kg^{-1} * min^{-1}) and the BAT and Bruce protocols (SEE = ± 3.75 mL * kg^{-1} * min^{-1}). This study shows that the BAT exhibits satisfactory agreement properties against objective methods and is a valid dance protocol to accurately estimate aerobic capacity in dancesport athletes participating in standard dance styles.

Keywords: dance; field-based test; aerobic capacity; agreement; Bruce protocol; KF1 protocol; MetaMax® 3B portable gas analyzer

1. Introduction

Dance has often been defined as a combination of art and sport, with some intermittent intensity elements which are performed at higher levels [1]. Regardless of the style of dance, the ability to withstand the training and competition schedules is a prerequisite, and these physiologic capabilities are essential. Evidence suggests that aerobic capacity plays a significant role for success in dance [2]. Prioritizing the efficiency of the uptake, transport, and oxygen use efficiently is crucial for dance performance [3]. However, it has been noted that both semi-professional and professional dancers tend to have lower levels of maximal oxygen uptake (VO_2max) in comparison to other athletes [4]. The VO_2max in dancesport athletes is approximately 30% lower, in comparison to mono-structural and team sport athletes [1]. A further explanation for the VO_2max hypothesis in dance might relate to the limited capacity of dance to stimulate positive training adaptations. Research has shown that improvements in aerobic capacity are not linked to rehearsal activities but rather to the intensity and duration of physical performances [5]. During specific dance movements or training protocols, the level of VO_2max should ideally be maintained at a level between 70% and 80% of an individual's VO_2max, and the duration should exceed 20 min in order to effectively boost the aerobic capacity [1]. From a practical view, complex dance movements do not necessarily mean intensity but rather complexity. The shortcoming of dance is that there is no methodology for developing aerobic capacity and defined dance structures through which both intensity and duration are achieved. Thus, aerobic endurance is maintained or even increased through multiple repetitions of dance routines and choreography.

In the field of dance, assessing aerobic capacity using objective measures such as heart rate monitors and ergometers is crucial for tailoring training programs at an individual level [4]. Determining an individual's cardiovascular and respiratory capabilities is important for effectively managing the training load and focusing on achieving positive aerobic outcomes during the preparatory period. However, evaluating 'maximal' aerobic levels in dance presents challenges due to its non-competitive nature and the predetermined intensity by a choreographer [6]. Traditional objective methods for assessing aerobic performance, such as running- or cycling-based ergometers, are not well-suited for dance as they are costly, difficult to administer, and do not replicate the intricate movements involved in dance. Furthermore, dancers may experience biomechanical constraints during running or walking, stemming from limited dorsiflexion movements in the ankle and the highly developed turn out of the feet, leading to potential stress on the knee and hip joints [7]. When running, dancers often experience discomfort and pain in the shin area and uneven force distribution between tendons, ligaments, and muscles (especially in the calf area), leading to a higher risk of injuries or strain-related musculoskeletal problems [8]. To address these limitations, previous studies have endeavored to develop on-field aerobic tests specifically tailored for dance. A systematic review by Tiemens et al. [4] identified several common cardiorespiratory fitness test protocols in dance, including the Aerobic Power Index (API) [9], the Ballet-Specific Aerobic Fitness Test (B-DAFT) [10], the Dance Aerobic Fitness Test (DAFT) [11], the High-Intensity Dance Performance Fitness Test (HIDT) [12], and the Seifert Assessment of Functional Capacity for Dancers (SAFD) [13].

Although an effort has been made to adequately predict aerobic outcomes derived from objective methods from dance-specific testing protocols [9–13], most previous studies have correlated the VO_2max and maximal heart rate (HRmax) from a single device [10,11]. Also, the agreement between correlation coefficients for the VO_2max and associated factors ranged from −0.12 [13] to 0.91 [11], limiting the 'true' validity in dancesport athletes. Finally, the available tests have been primarily developed for ballet or contemporary dancers [10–13] at the individual level, while the validity properties in ballroom dance couples engaging in standard dance styles have yet to be investigated. Ballet and contemporary dancers have different training routines and movement patterns compared to the standard dance practitioners [14]. Also, ballet dancers have been shown to have an even lower accumulated fat mass %, which often goes below 10%, while ballroom style dancers tend to maintain their fat mass % between 10 and 20%, respectively [15]. Standard male and female ballroom dancers tend to have higher average VO_2max values [15], compared to ballet or contemporary dancers [10,11]. This would imply that higher levels of the VO_2max

and peak heart rate (HRpeak) are generally needed to maintain performance at a high level and to cope with training and competition demands [15]. From a sport-specific point of view, ballroom dancesport athletes who come from modern dance typically develop aerobic capacity and maximal performance at different rates, while athletes from other endurance activities tend to increase their aerobic capacities linearly throughout their career [15]. On the other hand, by comparing the maximal aerobic capacity of dancers to other endurance sport athletes, the average VO_2max is 48.0 mL * kg^{-1} * min^{-1}, while it ranges between 55.0 and 77.0 mL * kg^{-1} * min^{-1} in swimmers, middle- and long-distance runners, rowers, and triathlon athletes [1]. Interestingly, the VO_2max in dancers is similar to sedentary behaviors (≈44.0 mL * kg^{-1} * min^{-1}), highlighting that the endurance in dancesport athletes is only developed throughout dance routines, while the development-oriented endurance training has yet to be investigated [1]. Thus, aerobic capacities and field-based tests in these athletes cannot be generalized to other dance styles, due to different physiological profiles and training/performance regimes during the preparatory and competition periods [1,4]. By examining the regular training and performance by using a specific test to assess aerobic capacity, coaches and choreographers would be able to monitor and track both cardiovascular and respiratory demands of different standard dance styles and could adjust the training volume to tackle physiological enhancements.

Because of the shortcomings from previously developed and validated dance protocols, the primary purpose of this study was to develop and validate a newly established Ballroom Aerobic Test (BAT) protocol specifically designed for dance couples performing in various standard dance styles. A secondary purpose was to establish the typical error of measurement and Bland–Altman agreement between the protocols. Based on the available evidence, we hypothesized that the BAT protocol would yield large to very large criterion validity properties against treadmill-based methods (KF1 and Bruce protocols) for measuring aerobic capacity.

2. Materials and Methods

2.1. Experimental Approach

In this study, a within subject test–retest sub-study was utilized to examine the validity properties of the BAT in standard dancesport athletes. This study was part of a project entitled 'Construction and validation of a test protocol to assess aerobic capacity in dancesport athletes from standard dance styles.' The project was divided into four segments to examine (i) reliability and usefulness; (ii) validity; (iii) sensitivity; and (iv) pragmatic validity of the BAT. For the purpose of this study, two standard progressive treadmill tests (the KF1 and Bruce protocols) were assessed to determine aerobic capacity, followed by the BAT protocol one week later. The testing procedure was initiated during the preparatory period of dancesport athletes. Measurements were conducted by the same experienced researcher to avoid possible measurement errors. During testing, the participants wore their standard dance equipment (light T-shirt, tights, dance shoes). The air temperature conditions of indoor facility and laboratory were controlled to be between 22 °C and 24 °C with a humidity of ≈55%.

2.2. Study Participants

Through a public call between April 2025 and June 2025, a convenience sample of twenty-four standard dancesport athletes (12 dance couples; age: 20.4 ± 3.9 years; height: 172.1 ± 8.7 cm; weight: 60.1 ± 9.4 kg) with 8.2 ± 3.4 years of training and competing experience participated in the study. All participants were members of certified dance clubs who competed at national and internation levels. The inclusion criteria to enter the study were as follows: (i) being free from any kind of injury, acute or chronic illness, and disease, confirmed by a certified dance association doctor; (ii) age range between 16 and 35 years; and (iii) complete both measurements for validity properties of the BAT protocol. The exclusion criteria included having dance experience < 5 years, suffering from musculoskeletal or any other injury that precluded them from entering and completing the testing procedures, being without a training partner, which could not mimic conditions from competition, and not being able to complete the field- and laboratory-based protocols. The a priori power analysis calculated by the G*Power software ver. 3.1.9.7 [16] showed that by setting the input parameters of a two-tailed $\alpha < 0.05$, a minimum required correlation between the two methods at $r > 0.69$, and statistical power of $1 - \beta = 0.95$, the required total sample size was n = 16. Because of a possible drop-out rate, we enlarged the sample size by 50% to $n = 24$. Before the study began, all participants had signed a written informed consent form to participate in the study and to use data solely for scientific purposes. All procedures in this study were anonymous and in accordance with the Declaration of Helsinki [17]. The Ethical Committee of the Faculty of Kinesiology approved this study on 29 April 2020 (ethical code number: 77/2020).

2.3. The BAT Protocol

To assess the level of aerobic capacity of dancesport athletes, we constructed a field-based BAT protocol. The protocol was standardized by 5 standard dance styles with the following order: (i) English waltz; (ii) slow fox; (iii) tango; (iv) Viennese waltz; and (v) quick step. Every dance style had multiple levels of dancing that were progressively linked, where the speed of dancing (tempo) was defined by individual beats per minute (bpm). The English waltz consisted of 6 levels, danced in 3/4 time in the range of or 75–110 bpm. The slow fox included 5 levels, danced in 4/4 time in the range of 117–145 bpm. The tango had 5 levels, danced in 4/4 time in the range of 152–180 bpm. The Viennese waltz was carried out through 3 levels, danced in 3/4 time in the range of 187–201 bpm. Finally, the quick step consisted of 6 levels, danced in 4/4 time in the range of 208–243 bpm. At each level, dance couples had to perform standard dance figures for 30 s at a defined speed without the melody (Table 1), while the time was cumulatively summed from the beginning of the BAT protocol. The speed expressed in beats progressively increased throughout the protocol by 7 bpm. The initial speed of the dance protocol was set at 75 bpm. Participants danced to a pre-defined dance tempo and rhythm by following the metronome. The elements for each dance style were basic and easy to perform, with the freedom of dance couples to create their own choreography. The duration of the BAT protocol was cumulatively added up and each pair danced until exhaustion.

2.4. The MetaMax® 3B Outcomes

To examine the reliability properties of the BAT protocol, we used the MetaMax® 3B (CORTEX Biophysik GmbH, Leipzig, Germany), a reliable and valid portable breath-by-breath ventilatory and metabolic measurement system specifically designed for field- and laboratory-based testing [18]. The device was composed of two parts designed to be worn on the chest. By using an electrochemical cell and an infrared analyzer, the MetaMax® 3B was able to calculate O_2 and CO_2 concentrations based on standard metabolic equations [19]. Based on manufacturer's recommendations and previous studies [17], the system was turned on for at least 20 min and calibrated prior to the testing. The calibration process included adjusting the gas analyzers by using reference gas values of O_2 (14.97%), CO_2 (4.96%), and N_2 (±0.02%) and volume with a standardized 3 L syringe (5530 series, Hans Rudolph, Inc., Kansas City, MO, USA). The MetaMax® 3B software generated data regarding absolute (L * min^{-1}) and relative VO_2max (mL * kg^{-1} * min^{-1}) and associated variables including respiratory exchange ratio of CO_2 produced to O_2 consumed during metabolism (RER), expiratory ventilation as the total volume of air inhaled or exhaled per min (VE; L * min^{-1}), tidal volume as the volume inhaled or exhaled during a normal breath (VT; L), ventilatory equivalent for O_2 (VE/VO_2) and CO_2 (VE/VCO_2) as determinants of breathing efficiency, and dead space to tidal volume ratio (VD/VT), which indicated the air that failed to participate in O_2 and CO_2 exchange process during breathing.

Table 1. The BAT dance protocol for every dance style.

Dance Styles	Stage 1	Stage 2	Stage 3	Stage 4	Stage 5	Stage 6
English waltz						
Beats	75	82	89	96	103	110
Time	30 s	60 s	1.5 min	2 min	2.5 min	3 min
Slow fox						
Beats	117	124	131	138	145	
Time	3.5 min	4.0 min	4.5 min	5.0 min	5.5 min	
Tango						
Beats	152	159	166	173	180	
Time	6.0 min	6.5 min	7.0 min	7.5 min	8.0 min	
Viennese waltz						
Beats	187	194	201			
Time	8.5 min	9.0 min	9.5 min			
Quick step						
Beats	208	215	222	229	236	243
Time	10.0 min	10.5 min	11.0 min	11.5 min	12.0 min	12.5 min

Time = cumulative time from BAT start.

The testing procedure indicated that both male and female dancers (one dance couple) were simultaneously measured with the MetaMax® 3B in order to simulate conditions from competitions in real-life settings. Although the order of trial was fixed, where dance couples first had to be tested for the BAT protocol and 48h after with the KF1 and 72 h after the KF1 protocol with the Bruce protocol in laboratory conditions, the possibility of a learning effect was vastly diminished. Each dance couple was tested individually to other dance couples for both field-and laboratory-based protocols. Also, they were told to keep the dance protocols and procedures to themselves and not to unveil them to the next dance couple. The BAT protocol was performed in an environment specific to dance, regarding the floor and dance attire that needed to be worn, while the KF1 and Bruce protocols were examined in laboratory conditions.

2.5. The KF1 and Bruce Testing Protocols

VO_2max and associated ventilatory and metabolic parameters were assessed by a breath-by-breath pulmonary gas exchange system (Quark b^2, COSMED, Roma, Italy) during an incremental treadmill test (KF1 and Bruce). KF1 is a standard test for the assessment of aerobic and anaerobic energy capacity [20]. The starting speed of the KF1 was 3 km * h^{-1} at a slope of 1% (continuous) for a duration of 2 min, after which the speed increased by 0.5 km * h^{-1} at the end of the third min and after that every 30 s until volitional exhaustion. During recovery after each test protocol, the subjects walked at 5 km * h^{-1} for 3 min.

In the Bruce protocol, the participants started exercising at a treadmill speed of 2.7 km * h^{-1} and an incline of 10% gradient for 3 min. Workloads (speed and inclination) were subsequently increased each 3 min period in a simultaneous way until volitional exhaustion was reached [21]. Both protocols generated equal cardiorespiratory data as the MetaMax® 3B, which were filtered and averaged on a 5 s basis.

2.6. Data Analysis

Shapiro–Wilk's (S-W) test was used to assess data normality. Data were checked for the critical W values, Q-Q plot inspection and the homogeneity of the variance was confirmed using the Leven test. If a calculated W value was larger than tabulated W value, this denoted that we did not reject the null hypothesis. All variables included in further analysis came from a hypothetical normal distribution, so data were presented as means and standard deviations (SDs) with 95% confidence interval limits (95% CI). To examine whether there was a couple dependence present during the BAT protocol, we utilized a linear-mixed effects model (LMM) with random intercept for couples and showed that there was no dependence effect within each couple for VO_2max, as our primary outcome of the study ($F = 1.533$, $p = 0.244$). Differences between each protocol were examined with repeated measures analysis of variance (RM ANOVA). The magnitude of the change between the two measurements (the BAT protocol vs. KF1 and Bruce protocols) was examined with a standardized mean difference and the following effect sizes (ESs) proposed by Hopkins et al. [22]: trivial (ES < 0.2), small (0.2 < ES < 0.5), moderate (0.5 < ES < 0.8), large (0.8 < ES < 1.6), and very large (ES > 1.6). Degree of coherence between ventilatory and metabolic parameters of the BAT protocol vs. KF1 and Bruce protocols was assessed using Pearson's product–moment correlation (r). Correlation values denoted association between variables and tests as small ($r = 0.1$–0.3), moderate ($r = 0.3$–0.5), large ($r = 0.5$–0.7), very large ($r = 0.7$–0.9), and almost perfect ($r = 0.9$–1.0) [23]. Since VO_2max is considered as one of the most important determinants of performance in dancesport athletes [1,4,5], a Bland–Altman plot was created to present a graphical visualization of the agreement between the BAT and KF1/Bruce protocols for relative VO_2max. In brief, the difference between the BAT and KF1 (BAT and Bruce) protocol was calculated on the y-axis, while the average of the two measurements was presented on the x-axis. To be able to determine the mean difference ideally close to (0) and the upper and lower limits of agreement ($\pm$1.96 SD), we created three horizontal lines. Based on data representation, we were able to (i) determine visual agreement between the two methods; (ii) identify possible bias where the mean difference was significantly different from 0; (iii) assess the presence of magnitude of random error; and (iv) establish the limits of agreement to confirm whether the differences between the two methods were clinically meaningful [24]. Finally, we calculated Lin's concordance coefficient of correlation (ρc), an analysis which tests both precision and accuracy of bivariate pairs of observations relative to a 'gold standard' or another set of data. According to Altman [25], the cut-off points for 'poor' vs. 'excellent' agreement were <0.20 and >0.80. In addition, a Passing–Bablok regression analysis was considered as a non-parametric technique for comparing the BAT with the KF1 and Bruce protocols to observe a potential error in both measurements [26]. All statistical analyses were performed in SPSS v27.0 software (IBM, Armonk, NY, USA), with an alpha level set a priori at $p < 0.05$ to denote statistical significance.

3. Results

3.1. Primary Outcomes

According to the objective termination criteria of an RER $\geq$ 1.10, of the 24 participants, the proportion of the participants who reached this cut-off was 20.8% for the BAT protocol and 45.8% and 37.5% for the KF1 and Bruce protocols. Basic descriptive statistics of the study participants are presented in Table 2. No significant differences between the KF1 and BAT nor between the Bruce and BAT protocols were observed for the absolute VO_2max ($F_{1,3} = 0.206$; $p = 0.816$; $\eta^2_p = 0.02$) and relative VO_2max ($F_{1,3} = 1.502$; $p = 0.245$; $\eta^2_p = 0.12$), RER ($F_{1,3} = 2.272$; $p = 0.094$; $\eta^2_p = 0.24$), VE ($F_{1,3} = 1.956$; $p = 0.165$; $\eta^2_p = 0.15$), VT ($F_{1,3} = 2.833$; $p = 0.065$; $\eta^2_p = 0.31$), VE/VO_2 ($F_{1,3} = 2.514$; $p = 0.104$; $\eta^2_p = 0.19$) and VE/VCO_2 ($F_{1,3} = 2.737$; $p = 0.087$; $\eta^2_p = 0.20$), and VD/VT ($F_{1,3} = 2.878$; $p = 0.078$; $\eta^2_p = 0.21$). ESs showed trivial to small changes. Large to very large correlations were calculated between the KF1 and BAT protocols for absolute VO_2max ($r = 0.88$; 95% CI = 0.75–0.95; $p < 0.001$) and relative VO_2max ($r = 0.88$; 95% CI = 0.76–0.95; $p < 0.001$), RER ($r = 0.78$; 95% CI = 0.59–0.90; $p < 0.001$), VE ($r = 0.86$; 95% CI = 0.62–0.96; $p < 0.001$), VT ($r = 0.75$; 95% CI = 0.57–0.87; $p < 0.001$), VE/VO_2 ($r = 0.81$; 95% CI = 0.55–0.91; $p < 0.001$) and VE/VCO_2 ($r = 0.78$; 95% CI = 0.65–0.94; $p < 0.001$), and VD/VT ($r = 0.70$; 95% CI = 0.40–0.87; $p < 0.001$). Large to very large correlations were obtained between the Bruce and BAT protocols for absolute VO_2max ($r = 0.87$; 95% CI = 0.72–0.95; $p < 0.001$) and relative VO_2max ($r = 0.85$; 95% CI = 0.71–0.93; $p < 0.001$), RER ($r = 0.76$; 95% CI = 0.50–0.91; $p < 0.001$), VE ($r = 0.79$; 95% CI = 0.50–0.94; $p < 0.001$), VT ($r = 0.83$; 95% CI = 0.71–0.91; $p < 0.001$), VE/VO_2 ($r = 0.80$; 95% CI = 0.64–0.92; $p < 0.001$) and VE/VCO_2 ($r = 0.82$; 95% CI = 0.75–0.94; $p < 0.001$), and VD/VT ($r = 0.74$; 95% CI = 0.44–0.89; $p < 0.001$).

Table 2. Basic descriptive statistics, mean difference (diff.), and ES between the BAT protocol against the KF1 and Bruce protocols.

Study Variables	KF1	Bruce	BAT	Absolute Diff. (95% CI)		Relative Diff. (%)		ES	
	Mean ± SD	Mean ± SD	Mean ± SD	KF1-BAT	Bruce-BAT	KF1–BAT	Bruce–BAT	KF1–BAT	Bruce–BAT
Absolute VO_2 ($L * min^{-1}$)	3.05 ± 0.74	3.05 ± 0.75	3.00 ± 0.65	−0.05 (−0.19–0.10)	−0.05 (−0.20–0.11)	1.64%	1.64%	0.07 (trivial)	0.07 (trivial)
Relative VO_2 ($mL * kg^{-1} * min^{-1}$)	50.92 ± 7.47	49.98 ± 7.55	50.21 ± 5.96	−0.71 (−2.24–0.83)	0.23 (−1.47–1.93)	1.39%	0.46%	0.11 (trivial)	0.03 (trivial)
RER	1.09 ± 0.05	1.08 ± 0.04	1.07 ± 0.06	−0.02 (−0.03–0.02)	−0.01 (−0.02–0.02)	1.83%	0.93%	0.36 (small)	0.20 (small)
VE ($L * min^{-1}$)	110.21 ± 28.43	110.43 ± 28.75	104.20 ± 26.37	−6.01 (−12.22–0.20)	−6.23 (−13.83–1.37)	5.45%	5.64%	0.22 (small)	0.23 (small)
VT (L)	1.93 ± 0.42	1.98 ± 0.54	1.77 ± 0.36	−0.16 (−0.28–−0.04)	−0.22 (−0.54–−0.28)	8.29%	11.11%	0.41 (small)	0.46 (small)
VE/VO_2	33.65 ± 3.82	33.85 ± 3.46	32.93 ± 2.93	−0.71 (−1.67–0.24)	−0.91 (−1.78–0.04)	2.11%	2.69%	0.21 (small)	0.29 (small)
VE/VCO_2	30.90 ± 3.83	30.16 ± 2.67	31.04 ± 3.51	0.14 (−0.89–1.17)	0.88 (−0.03–1.73)	0.45%	2.92%	0.04 (trivial)	0.28 (small)
VD/VT	0.15 ± 0.03	0.14 ± 0.03	0.15 ± 0.02	0.003 (−0.005–0.01)	0.009 (−0.001–0.02)	2.00%	6.43%	0.01 (trivial)	0.39 (small)

Lin's analysis indicated an excellent concordance between the KF1 and BAT protocols for the absolute VO_2max ($\rho c = 0.93$; 95% CI = 0.84–0.97) and relative VO_2max ($\rho c = 0.92$; 95% CI = 0.82–0.97), RER ($\rho c = 0.86$; 95% CI = 0.68–0.94), VE ($\rho c = 0.92$; 95% CI = 0.82–0.97), VT ($\rho c = 0.85$; 95% CI = 0.66–0.94), VE/VO_2 ($\rho c = 0.88$; 95% CI = 0.71–0.95) and VE/VCO_2 ($\rho c = 0.88$; 95% CI = 0.71–0.95), and VD/VT ($\rho c = 0.81$; 95% CI = 0.57–0.92). Similarly, the data showed an excellent concordance between the Bruce and BAT protocols for the absolute VO_2max ($\rho c = 0.93$; 95% CI = 0.83–0.97) and relative VO_2max ($\rho c = 0.90$; 95% CI = 0.78–0.96), RER ($\rho c = 0.83$; 95% CI = 0.62–0.93), VE ($\rho c = 0.88$; 95% CI = 0.73–0.95), VT ($\rho c = 0.87$; 95% CI = 0.70–0.94), VE/VO_2 ($\rho c = 0.89$; 95% CI = 0.73–0.95) and VE/VCO_2 ($\rho c = 0.88$; 95% CI = 0.73–0.95), and VD/VT ($\rho c = 0.84$; 95% CI = 0.63–0.93).

3.2. Secondary Outcomes

Figure 1 shows the Bland–Altman scatterplot of the VO_2max agreement between the BAT and KF1 protocols. The mean difference between the two methods yielded a value of −0.71, indicating no measurement bias ($p > 0.05$). Although a negative linear trend was observed, a linear regression analysis showed no potential proportional bias ($\beta = -0.24$; 95% CI -0.46–0.02; $p = 0.066$), with a standard error for the estimate (SEE) of 3.36 mL * kg^{-1} * min^{-1}. The linear regression equation to predict the relative VO_2max from the KF1 protocol was as follows: VO_2max_{KF1} (mL * kg^{-1} * min^{-1}) = $-4.305 + (1.100 * VO_2max_{BAT})$ ($R^2 = 0.77$; $p < 0.001$). The slope coefficient between the BAT and KF1 protocols was b = 1.625 with a 95% CI (0.90, 2.25), while the intercept coefficient was $a = -18.43$ with a 95% confidence interval (-64.65, 42.13). According to Passing and Bablok [26], if one was included in the CI for the slope and zero was included for the intercept, the BAT procedure yielded similar measurements to the KF1 procedure.

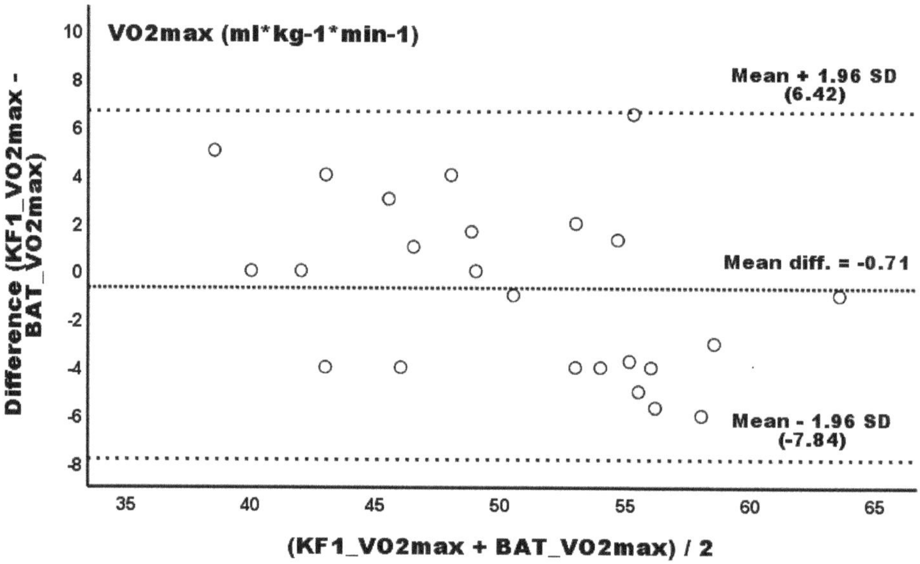

Figure 1. Bland–Altman plot of differences between the BAT and KF1 protocols (y-axis) and the average of the two measurements (x-axis) for relative VO_2max.

The Bland–Altman scatterplot of the VO_2max agreement between the BAT and Bruce protocols is presented in Figure 2. The mean difference between the two methods yielded a value of 0.23, indicating no measurement bias ($p > 0.05$). Similarly to the BAT-KF1, a negative linear trend between the BAT and Bruce protocols was observed; however, no potential proportional bias was shown ($\beta = -0.26$; 95% CI -0.51–0.15; $p = 0.087$). The generated SEE of the VO_2max was 3.75 mL * kg^{-1} * min^{-1}. Similarly to the KF1 protocol, the linear regression equation to predict the relative VO_2max from the Bruce protocol was as follows: VO_2max_{BRUCE} (mL * kg^{-1} * min^{-1}) = $-3.996 + (1.075 * VO_2max_{BAT})$ ($R^2 = 0.72$; $p < 0.001$). The slope coefficient between the BAT and KF1 protocols was $b = 1.10$ with a 95% CI (0.80, 1.30), while the intercept coefficient was $a = -1.05$ with a 95% confidence interval (-10.17, 9.90), indicating that the BAT protocol yielded similar measurements to the Bruce protocol.

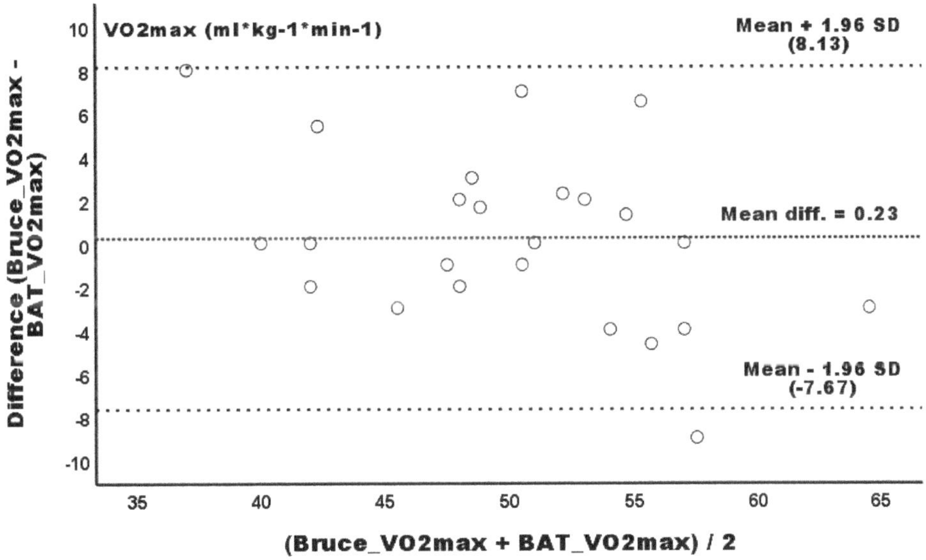

Figure 2. Bland–Altman plot of differences between the BAT and Bruce protocols (y-axis) and the average of the two measurements (x-axis) for relative VO_2max.

4. Discussion

The main purpose of this study was to develop and examine the criterion validity and Bland–Altman agreement of the BAT protocol against the KF1 and Bruce laboratory protocols in dancesport athletes performing in standard dance styles. Findings suggest that the ventilatory and metabolic parameters derived from the MetaMax® 3B portable gas analyzer during the BAT protocol correlate as large to very large with the KF1 and Bruce aerobic outcomes. The level of agreement calculated from the Bland–Altman plots for the relative VO_2max shows no systematic nor proportional biases between the two methods with the SEE of 3.36 mL * kg^{-1} * min^{-1} (KF1) and 3.75 mL * kg^{-1} * min^{-1} (Bruce).

To the best of the authors' knowledge, this is the first study examining the development and validity of a progressive test to assess aerobic capacity in standard dancesport athletes. Our results should be interpreted in light of previous studies. To date, several progressive field-based tests to assess the level of aerobic capacity in dance have been proposed and validated against more objective methods. For example, a study by Wallmann et al. [9] showed that the API submaximal exercise fitness test correlated well with the VO_2max (r = 0.89 and 0.90), with a technical error of measurement (TEM) of a power output = 0.07 W * kg^{-1} and VO_2max = 0.71 mL * $kg^{-1}min^{-1}$. Another dance protocol designed for ballet dancers indicated that the mean squared root (s_w^2) for the test was 5.01, with a SEE of 6.20 mL * $kg^{-1}min^{-1}$ [10]. One of the most common fitness protocols to examine aerobic capacity is the DAFT, a five-stage 4 min progressive test [10]. In a study by Wyon et al. [11], data generated from the portable telemetric gas analyzer (Cosmed K4 b2, Italy) indicated that the HRmax and VO_2max correlated very strongly for the test (r = 0.91; SEE = 5.60 b * min^{-1}). Similar observations were noted for the HIDT dance protocol, where five participants (n = 5) undertook both the treadmill and dance tests to estimate the VO_2max [12]. During the treadmill protocol, the mean VO_2max was 46.40 ± 3.60 mL * $kg^{-1}min^{-1}$, and during the HIDT, the VO_2max value was 51.00 ± 6.60 mL * $kg^{-1}min^{-1}$. A pairwise comparison between the treadmill and dance protocols showed no significant differences in VO_2max (p = 0.100) [12]. The same study also showed that the mean % of the

HRmax was significantly lower in the HIDT compared to the treadmill test (97.50 vs. 101.00%, $p = 0.020$), while the validity of blood lactate values were high (HIDT = 6.10 ± 1.90 mmol*L^{-1} vs. treadmill = 6.30 ± 1.70 mmol * L^{-1}, $p = 0.860$) [12]. The most recent SAFD test to evaluate the functional capacity of collegiate dancers revealed large to very large correlations with the peak treadmill test for the relative VO_2max ($r = 0.78$), HRmax ($r = 0.85$), blood lactate ($r = 0.72$), and rate of perceived exertion (RPE; $r = 0.84$), while trivial to moderate correlations were found for time ($r = 0.60$) and the RER ($r = -0.12$) [13].

Although the existing progressive dance protocols to assess aerobic capacity exhibited satisfactory validity properties against objective measures [9–13], our newly developed BAT protocol yielded high agreements with the treadmill test following two protocols (KF1 and Bruce). The incremental difference and the novelty between our and other dance protocols lies in the fact that it is specifically designed for dance couples who engage in standard dance styles. This is very important, because both individuals need to cope with each other during the rehearsal/training or competition. This would suggest that their aerobic capacity needs to be at equal level in order to keep up with the partner. Despite the fact that the VO_2max tends to be low in dancesport athletes, compared to other athletes [4–6], the intention of the BAT protocol is to enhance the aerobic system and to physiologically prepare for stress during training and/or performance. Dance movements in standard dance styles are often characterized by sway components and the interplay between rises and falls, which are considered key elements for preserving or increasing functional performance in competitive dancesport athletes [27]. Moreover, the complexity of figures and faster pace during training and competition in standard dance styles is not comparable to ballet or contemporary dance styles, where the movements are often performed in static conditions, emphasizing esthetic rather than functional components of dance. Therefore, the BAT protocol can serve as an avenue for screening and tracking aerobic capacity within the narrow niche of standard style dance athletes.

The practical application of the BAT protocol is reflected in the development of a completely new model for measuring aerobic capacity and an algorithm for estimating the VO_2max in standard dances under the conditions of the sport-specific activity. This enables a realistic assessment of physical and energy loads specific to the activity, in comparison with the existing tests for assessing aerobic capacity. Since standard dance styles have been often categorized as high-intensity physical activities that need aerobic and anaerobic energy systems to perform [28], the newly established dance protocol would be able to increase aerobic capacity and to optimize dance training. Indeed, correct and timely diagnostic procedures for measuring and/or assessing energy capacities in dance are needed to achieve primary goals and positive trends towards sports success [1,4].

This study is not without limitations. First, a cross-sectional design prevents us from confirming a causal relationship between field- and laboratory-based testing protocols for assessing aerobic capacity. Second, we did not include the HRmax nor blood lactate parameters as indicators of aerobic and anaerobic capacities, limiting our findings to data generated from the MetaMax® 3B and treadmill devices. Previous studies have shown a strong relationship between HRmax and VO_2max [10,11] and adequate sensitivity in HRmax and blood lactate changes following the dance protocol [13]. Third, a relatively small sample size might have underpowered the validity properties of the BAT protocol. Although we performed a sample size calculation (for more information, please see the 'Study Participants' section), we cannot exclude the lack of statistical power. Fourth, we failed to examine the rate of perceived exertion (RPE) and collect blood samples for lactate concentrations following the BAT, KF1, and Bruce protocols. These physiological measures have been constantly used as potential markers for determining fatigue and should be considered in further research in dancesport athletes. Fifth, the BAT protocol was measured with the MetaMax® 3B, while the treadmill tests used COSMED Quark b^2. The difference in devices could introduce systematic errors independent of the protocol. Finally, the BAT protocol was not cross-validated in other athletes from different dance styles (ballet, contemporary, or Latin American), limiting its applicability. Nevertheless, the authors suggest that the BAT protocol is a valid training and performance tool for measuring aerobic capacity and associated factors in dancesport athletes from standard dance styles.

5. Conclusions

In summary, this study shows that the BAT protocol has a strong to excellent criterion validity against the KF1 and Bruce protocols. Also, the Bland–Altman analysis indicated that the SEE for the KF1 and Bruce protocols against the BAT protocol was 3.36 mL * kg^{-1} * min^{-1} and 3.75 mL * kg^{-1} * min^{-1}. The advantage of the BAT protocol is that it simulates classical movements from five dance styles and mimics competition conditions. The current findings have provided evidence of its validity properties and potential guidelines for monitoring and tracking ventilatory and metabolic parameter changes under different training conditions. The authors suggest that this test can be implemented within the dance training program in preparatory and competitive periods, as it gives important and valid information about the agreement between field and laboratory aerobic performance variables among standard dancesport athletes.

Author Contributions: T.D. and D.P. designed the study and collected and analyzed the data. All authors contributed to interpretation of the data, drafting, and revising the manuscript and approved the final version of the manuscript. All authors have read and agreed to the published version of the manuscript.

Funding: This research received no external funding.

Institutional Review Board Statement: This study was conducted in accordance with the Declaration of Helsinki, and the Ethical Committee of the Faculty of Kinesiology approved this study on 29 April 2020 (ethical code number: 77/2020).

Informed Consent Statement: Written informed consent was obtained from all subjects involved in this study.

Data Availability Statement: The data that support the findings of this study are available upon reasonable request from the corresponding author. The data are not publicly available due to privacy or ethical restrictions.

Acknowledgments: We are particularly grateful to all the dancesport athletes who voluntarily participated in this study.

Conflicts of Interest: Author Tamara Despot is professionally engaged through her own company, Dancespot d.o.o. The company served solely as the legal entity through which the author conducts her professional activities and has no financial, commercial, or other interests that could be considered a potential conflict of interest in relation to the present study. Author Davor Plavec is employed at Polyclinic Prima Nova. The institution had no financial, commercial, or other involvement that could be construed as a potential conflict of interest in relation to the present study.

References

1. Koutedakis, Y.; Jamurtas, A. The dancer as a performing athlete: Physiological considerations. *Sports Med.* **2004**, *34*, 651–661. [CrossRef] [PubMed]
2. Sánchez-Alcalá, M.; Carcelén-Fraile, M.D.C.; Vico-Rodríguez, P.; Cano-Orihuela, M.; Carcelén-Fraile, M.D.M. Effects of dance-based aerobic training on functional capacity and risk of falls in older adults with mild cognitive impairment. *J. Clin. Med.* **2025**, *14*, 5900. [CrossRef] [PubMed]
3. Yang, Y.; Deng, N.; Yang, X. A meta-analysis of the effects of strength training on physical fitness in dancers. *Front. Physiol.* **2025**, *16*, 1511833. [CrossRef] [PubMed]

4. Tiemens, A.; van Rijn, R.M.; Koes, B.W.; Stubbe, J.H. A systematic review of cardiorespiratory fitness tests used in dance. *J. Danc. Med. Sci. Off. Publ. Int. Assoc. Danc. Med. Sci.* **2023**, *27*, 27–40. [CrossRef]
5. Wyon, M.A.; Abt, G.; Redding, E.; Head, A.; Sharp, N.C. Oxygen uptake during modern dance class, rehearsal, and performance. *J. Strength Cond. Res.* **2004**, *18*, 646–649.
6. Zaferiou, A.M. Dance-themed National Biomechanics Day community engagement to inspire our future STEAM leaders. *J. Biomech.* **2023**, *150*, 111511. [CrossRef]
7. Russell, J.A. Preventing dance injuries: Current perspectives. *Open Access J. Sports Med.* **2013**, *4*, 199–210. [CrossRef]
8. Giustino, V.; Patti, A. Biomechanics and sports performances. *Sports* **2025**, *13*, 73. [CrossRef]
9. Wallman, K.; Goodman, C.; Morton, A.; Grove, R.; Dawson, B. Test-retest reliability of the aerobic power index component of the tri-level fitness profile in a sedentary population. *J. Sci. Med. Sport* **2003**, *6*, 443–454. [CrossRef]
10. Twitchett, E.; Nevill, A.; Angioi, M.; Koutedakis, Y.; Wyon, M. Development, validity, and reliability of a ballet-specific aerobic fitness test. *J. Danc. Med. Sci. Off. Publ. Int. Assoc. Danc. Med. Sci.* **2011**, *15*, 123–127. [CrossRef]
11. Wyon, M.; Redding, E.; Abt, G.; Head, A.; Sharp, N.C. Development, reliability, and validity of a multistage Dance Specific Aerobic Fitness Test (DAFT). *J. Danc. Med. Sci.* **2003**, *7*, 80–84. [CrossRef]
12. Redding, E.; Weller, P.; Ehrenberg, S.; Irvine, S.; Quin, E.; Rafferty, S.; Wyon, M.; Cox, C. The development of a high intensity dance performance fitness test. *J. Danc. Med. Sci. Off. Publ. Int. Assoc. Danc. Med. Sci.* **2009**, *13*, 3–9. [CrossRef]
13. Seifert, A.M.; Mullin, E.M.; Zehnder, S.; Paolone, V.J. Development and Validation of a Functional Capacity Test for Collegiate Dancers. *J. Danc. Med. Sci. Off. Publ. Int. Assoc. Danc. Med. Sci.* **2021**, *25*, 131–138. [CrossRef] [PubMed]
14. Ngo, J.K.; Lu, J.; Cloak, R.; Wong, D.P.; Devonport, T.; Wyon, M.A. Strength and conditioning in dance: A systematic review and meta-analysis. *Eur. J. Sport Sci.* **2024**, *24*, 637–652. [CrossRef]
15. Liiv, H.; Jürimäe, T.; Mäestu, J.; Purge, P.; Hannus, A.; Jürimäe, J. Physiological characteristics of elite dancers of different dance styles. *Eur. J. Sport Sci.* **2014**, *14*, 429–436. [CrossRef]
16. Kang, H. Sample size determination and power analysis using the G*Power software. *J. Educ. Eval. Health Prof.* **2021**, *18*, 17. [CrossRef]
17. World Medical Association. World Medical Association Declaration of Helsinki: Ethical principles for medical research involving human subjects. *JAMA* **2013**, *310*, 2191–2194. [CrossRef]
18. Van Hooren, B.; Souren, T.; Bongers, B.C. Accuracy of respiratory gas variables, substrate, and energy use from 15 CPET systems during simulated and human exercise. *Scand. J. Med. Sci. Sports* **2024**, *34*, e14490. [CrossRef]
19. Wasserman, K.; Hansen, J.; Sue, D.; Casaburi, R.; Whipp, B. *Principles of Exercise Testing and Interpretation: Including Pathophysiology and Clinical Applications*, 3rd ed.; Lippincott Williams & Wilkins: Philadelphia, PA, USA, 1999; Appendix C; pp. 531–540.
20. Kjertakov, M.; Dalip, M.; Hristovski, R.; Epstein, Y. Prediction of lactate threshold using the modified Conconi test in distance runners. *Physiol. Int.* **2016**, *103*, 262–270. [CrossRef]
21. Bruce, R.A. Exercise testing of patients with coronary heart disease. Principles and normal standards for evaluation. *Ann. Clin. Res.* **1971**, *3*, 323–332.
22. Hopkins, W.G.; Schabort, E.J.; Hawley, J.A. Reliability of power in physical performance tests. *Sports Med.* **2001**, *31*, 211–234. [CrossRef]
23. Hopkins, W.G. How to interpret changes in an athletic performance test. *Sportscience* **2004**, *8*, 1–7.
24. Mansournia, M.A.; Waters, R.; Nazemipour, M.; Bland, M.; Altman, D.G. Bland-Altman methods for comparing methods of measurement and response to criticisms. *Glob. Epidemiol.* **2020**, *3*, 100045. [CrossRef]
25. Altman, D.G. *Practical Statistics for Medical Research*; Chapman and Hall: London, UK, 1991.
26. Passing, H.; Bablok, W. Comparison of several regression procedures for method comparison studies and determination of sample sizes. Application of linear regression procedures for method comparison studies in Clinical Chemistry, Part II. *J. Clin. Chem. Clin. Biochem. Z. Klin. Chem. Klin. Biochem.* **1984**, *22*, 431–445. [CrossRef]
27. Fotaki, A.; Triantafyllou, A.; Papagiannis, G.; Stasi, S.; Georgios, P.; Olga, S.; Tsolakis, C.K.; Koulouvaris, P. The science of biomechanics can promote dancers' injury prevention strategies. *Phys. Ther. Rev.* **2020**, *26*, 94–101. [CrossRef]
28. Pilch, W.; Tota, Ł.; Pokora, I.; Głowa, M.; Piotrowska, A.; Chlipalska, O.; Zuziak, R.; Czerwińska, O. Energy expenditure and lactate concentration in sports dancers in a simulated final round of the standard style competition. *Hum. Mov.* **2017**, *18*, 62–67. [CrossRef]

sports

MDPI

Brief Report

Power–Load Relationship of Bench Press, Ballistic Bench Press, and Prone Bench Pull in International Medal-Winning Canoeists and Kayakers

Oscar Crisafulli [1,2,†], Matteo Fortunati [1,3,†], Tiziano Gemelli [1], Massimiliano Febbi [3,4], Patrik Drid [2], Stefano Ramat [5] and Giuseppe D'Antona [1,6,*]

1 Centro di Ricerca Interdipartimentale Attività Motorie e Sportive (CRIAMS)-Sport Medicine Centre Voghera, University of Pavia, 27058 Voghera, Italy; oscar.crisafulli@unipv.it (O.C.); matteo.fortunati01@gmail.com (M.F.); tiziano.gemelli@unipv.it (T.G.)
2 Faculty of Sport and Physical Education, University of Novi Sad, 21000 Novi Sad, Serbia; patrikdrid@gmail.com
3 Department of Industrial Engineering, University of Roma "Tor Vergata", 00133 Roma, Italy; massimilianofebbi@gmail.com
4 Laboratory for Rehabilitation, Medicine and Sport (LARM), 00133 Roma, Italy
5 Department of Electrical, Computer and Biomedical Engineering, University of Pavia, 27100 Pavia, Italy; stefano.ramat@unipv.it
6 Department of Public Health, Experimental and Forensic Medicine, University of Pavia, 27100 Pavia, Italy
* Correspondence: giuseppe.dantona@unipv.it
† These authors contributed equally to this work.

Abstract: Paddler athletes use resistance training (RT) to optimize power output (PO) during competitions. Understanding the power–load relationship (P–Lr) is essential for effective RT prescription. Moreover, the push-to-pull ratio (PU/PR)—the one-repetition maximum (1RM) of a pulling exercise divided by the one of a pushing exercise—has been suggested as a metric associated with sprint kayak performance. This study aimed to describe P–Lr in three guided exercises (bench press (BP), ballistic bench press (BBP), and prone bench pull (PBP)), along with PU/PR in international-level canoeing and kayaking athletes. Nine male athletes (21.0 ± 1.5 years) were monitored during two sessions of an incremental testing protocol. Load ranged from 30 to 100 kg in BP, 30 to 95 kg in PBP, and 20 to 60 kg in BBP. Instantaneous displacement was measured using a linear position transducer, and PO was computed for each repetition and exercise. PU/PR was calculated upon PBP and BP. A two-way repeated-measures ANOVA was used to explore differences among exercises and relative load from 20% to 90% 1RM. PBP displayed a higher PO between 40% and 90% 1RM compared to BP and BBP), while no statistical difference was found between BP and BBP at any relative load. Additionally, mean PU/PR resulted 0.96. This study provides preliminary values regarding P–Lr and PU/PR in elite paddlers, which may assist in designing training programs for those targeting major competitions.

Keywords: resistance training; velocity-based training; paddle sport; linear encoder

1. Introduction

Canoe and kayak flat water competitions can vary between an effort of approximately thirty seconds (200 m sprint races) and 1 h 45 min (20 km marathon races). Even if athletes specialize either in short or long races, they must have, at the same time, a high level of maximal strength, power output (PO) and muscular endurance [1–4]. The PO is necessary for a successful outcome; in fact, a recent investigation found that international medal-winning canoe sprinters have a slightly higher PO than their non-trophy counterparts in resistance training (RT) exercises [3].

Power–load relationship (P–Lr) is a curve that, for a given subject, associates a value of PO (W) to any load (Kg) of a lifting exercise, showing a unimodal, bell-shaped trend [5]. It differs between the type of exercise (i.e., upper or lower-body) [6–9], gender [10], and age [11]. Measuring P–Lr is essential for trainers to prescribe PO-oriented training to improve a specific part of the competition. For example, knowing that kayak paddlers during a 2 min kayak ergometer test show a maximum PO during an all-out start of 747 ± 151 W and an average 2 min PO of 348 ± 47 W [12], coaches can prescribe a load of a specific resistance training exercise that mimics these PO to further improve them.

The RT sessions of canoeists and kayakers' athletes frequently involve bench press (BP), prone bench pull (PBP), and ballistic bench press (BBP). Even if such exercises have been previously used to study P–Lr in other populations of athletes [13,14], to the best of our knowledge, no studies have utilized this paradigm to investigate P–Lr in elite canoeists and kayakers.

Moreover, in paddle sports, the push-to-pull ratio (PU/PR) obtained by dividing the 1RM of bench pull or weighted chin-up (PU) against the 1RM of bench press (PR) or similar exercises is a valuable information. Indeed, previous studies in sub-elite male kayakers have reported that, during a three-year longitudinal monitoring, improvements in all-out sprint kayak performance over 200 m and 500 m distances were observed alongside the approach and stabilization of the PU/PR at around 1.3 [4,15]. Therefore, the authors proposed it as a reference value for ameliorating paddling sprint performance (i.e., achieving a shorter time to complete the race) [4,15]. However, despite this valuable information, data regarding PU/PR in international-level medalist kayakers has not been previously analyzed.

The main goal of this work is to describe the P–Lr between 20% and 90% one-repetition maximum (1RM) in the guided BP, guided BBP, and guided PBP in international kayakers and canoeists. The secondary aim is to compare these relationships between exercise types, and the tertiary objective is to investigate the PU/PR ratio. We hypothesize that PO on PBP is superior to pushing exercises, that there is no difference in P–Lr between BBP and BP, and that PU/PR on canoeists and kayakers is around 1.3. To achieve these goals, we applied an incremental protocol, over two complementary testing sessions, investigating PO from an absolute load of 30 kg to 100 kg in BP, from 30 kg to 95 kg in PBP, and from 20 kg to 60 kg in BBP, in a group of international medal-winning athletes.

2. Materials and Methods

2.1. Study Design

The research is an observational pilot study design.

2.2. Participants

A total of 9 athletes (all males, mean ± SD; age: 21.0 ± 1.5 years; weight: 80.3 ± 4.8 kg; height: 183.3 ± 4.6 cm; kayak/canoe training experience: 8.8 ± 2.6 years; resistance training experience: 5.7 ± 1.9 years) completed the experimental sessions. All subjects were international medal-winning kayakers and canoeists specializing in sprint–endurance competitions (200 m–5000 m) who participated in the 2020 European Championship (October 2020, Poznan). The sample of kayakers consisted of national team members who secured 4 gold, 5 silver, 4 bronze medals, and multiple Final A placements (the final heat determining podium positions) at U23 World or European Championships over their careers. Their weekly training volume consisted of 2 to 3 resistance training sessions and 4 to 5 kayak training sessions conducted both on (kayak) and off-water (paddle ergometer).

Each training session typically lasted between 60 and 120 min. Additionally, the values of maximum oxygen consumption, lactatemia response, and power output of eight athletes of this cohort, evaluated during a specific, off-water incremental test until exhaustion, can be appreciated elsewhere [16]. Participants were free from physical limitations, health problems, or musculoskeletal injuries that could negatively impact performance and the full range of motion in BP, BBP, and PBP. Participants were required to abstain from alcohol and exercise for 48 h before all experimental trials. After an exhaustive explanation of the aim of the research, risks, and benefits, all the volunteers have read and signed an informed consent form. The research protocol was approved by the Sport and Physical Education Ethics Committee of the University of Novi Sad, Serbia (n°47-06-02/2021-3). Data and sensible information were protected by the General Data Protecting Regulation (GDPR).

2.3. Procedure

2.3.1. Warm-Up Protocol

Each session began with a 5 min warm-up on the kayak ergometer at an intensity between 68% and 72% of the heart rate maximum, which was previously measured during an all-out water test. Then, athletes performed 3 sets of 10 repetitions on dumbbell chest press and the exact same amount on bodyweight push-up, and 5 min of self-selected upper mobility exercises. Overall, the warm-up procedure lasted 20 min, and the incremental protocol followed in the order BP, BBP, PBP.

2.3.2. Incremental Protocol

Due to the high number of repetitions required, the study was conducted in two days, 48 hours apart, at the same time of the day. The incremental protocol comprised two complementary testing sessions, termed Test 1 (T1) and Test 2 (T2), that, when combined, allowed to obtain P–Lr. On T1, the starting absolute load was set at 30 kg for PBP and BP, while at 20 kg for BBP. On T2, it was set at 35 kg for PBP and BP and at 25 kg for BBP. Subsequently, on each testing day, the load was increased by 10 kg at every set until reaching, on T1, an absolute ending load of 90 kg for PBP, 100 kg for BP, and 60 kg for BBP, or until subjects reached their 1RM if it was below this arbitrary weight. On T2, the end of the incremental test was set at 95 kg for PBP, 95 kg for BP, and 55 kg for BBP, or again, if 1RM was reached directly. Regarding sets and repetitions, in the PBP and BP testing: five repetitions with lighter loads ($\leq$55 kg), three repetitions with medium loads (60 kg and 65 kg), and a set consisting of a single repetition for heavier loads ($\geq$70 kg) were used. In contrast, a single effort was monitored in the BBP due to the high repeatability of the exercise [17]. For the subsequent analysis, we considered the highest mean value for each load of T1 and T2 when more than one repetition was performed (e.g., loads $\leq$ 65 kg in BP and PBP). Conversely, when only a single repetition was performed (i.e., loads $\geq$ 70 kg for BP and PBP, and $\geq$20 kg for BBP), we considered the single value at each load for both T1 and T2. Regarding recovery, in BP, BBP, and PBP the inter-sets rest period was fixed at five minutes [18]. Passive rest between exercises was established at 15 min to allow a complete recovery.

2.3.3. One Repetition Maximum

The direct achievement of 1RM was possible in 2 athletes regarding BP, and 4 on PBP; for the others, it was indirectly estimated through the load–velocity relationship (L–Vr) [19]. Specifically, a linear regression was fitted to the velocity $V\text{–}Lr_{BP}$ experimentally recorded values considering a minimum velocity (V_{1RM}) of 0.15 m/s to estimate 1RM in BP. In contrast, the same function, including $V\text{–}Lr_{PBP}$ and a V_{1RM} of 0.45 m/s, was used for PBP. The 1RM for BBP press was set at 80% of the maximum weight lifted in BP [20].

2.3.4. Calculation of the Standardized Relative Load

Once the 1RM had been directly or indirectly achieved, standardized absolute load [kg] from 20% to 90% 1RM at each 10% interval was extrapolated.

2.3.5. Calculation of the Power Output at a Standardized Relative Load

Once the absolute load [kg] was extrapolated at the standardized percentage of 1RM, PO was indirectly calculated based on the work (*W*) performed during each movement and its execution time as PO = W/Δt where W = m × g × Δh, m represents mass in Kg, g is gravitational acceleration constant 9.8 m/s^2, Δt is the execution time and Δh is the vertical displacement. The overall P–Lr curve was then found using the individual data and the P–Lr polynomial equation for data interpolation:

$$PO(m) = a^*m^2 + b^*m + c$$

where PO indicates power in Watts. The values for the a, b, and c parameters were estimated by interpolation of the experimental data through the appropriate Microsoft Excel function. An example of such analysis for one representative subject is shown in Figure 1.

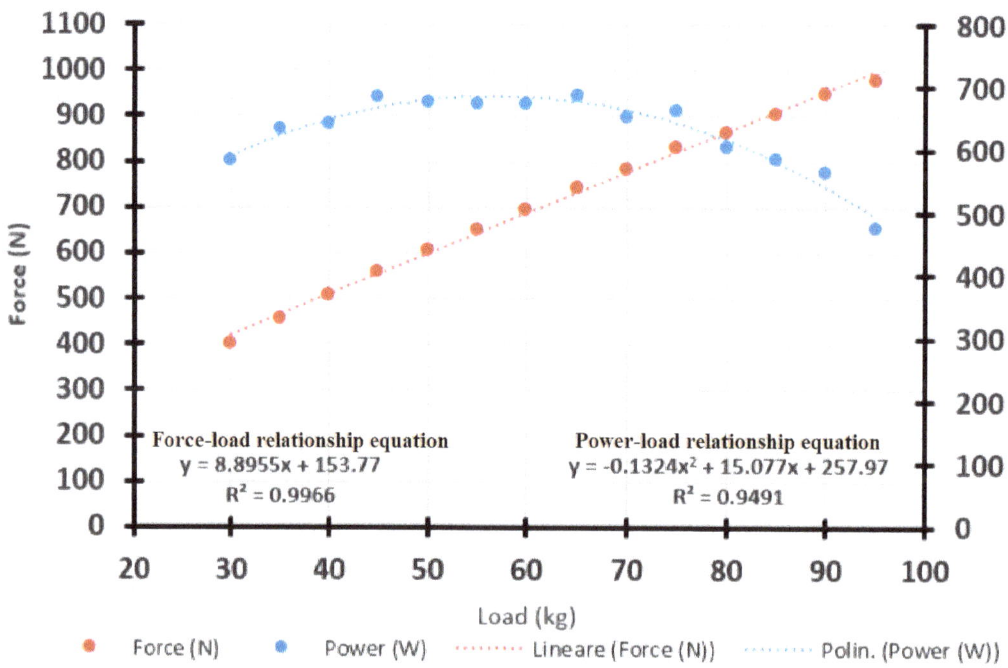

Figure 1. Example of data analysis and computation of the Power–Load relationship by interpolation of the experimental data.

2.4. Exercises

Guided eccentric–concentric bench press and ballistic bench press. BP and BBP were performed on a Smith Machine (Multipower®, Technogym®, Cesena, Italy). Repetitions began with a rapid but controlled eccentric movement, immediately followed by a straight explosive vertical push. In BP, all the repetitions of the sets were performed continuously without intra-set rest. In BBP, the athlete had to let go of the barbell after each repetition.

Guided concentric-only prone bench pull. On the same Smith Machine (Multipower®, Technogym®, Cesena, Italy), PBP was built using two commercial wooden plyometric boxes of 76.2 cm (30 inch) (Lacertosus®, Parma, Italy) as bases, and a bench (thickness of 8 cm) was then placed on them. The bench was raised by another 20 cm to let each subject start with the arms extended during the pulling movement. Even at the lowest load, the sets were performed as a sum of single repetitions inserting a self-paced pause of approximately 2 s to eliminate the contribution of the rebound effect.

2.5. Instrumentation

A linear position transducer (LPT) (MuscleLab™, Model 4000e, Ergotest Technology, Bjønnveien, Norway) with a sampling frequency of 200 Hz was used for data collection, as previously carried out in similar research [3,21], to determine instantaneous displacement during the concentric phase of the lift. Mean velocity (m/s) and mean PO (W) were computed from these data.

2.6. Statistical Analysis

Data were summarized by the mean and standard deviation (sd). We applied a two-way repeated-measures ANOVA to explore differences among different exercises and relative load from 20% to 90% 1RM. For ANOVAs, Mauchly's sphericity test was performed, and where this assumption was violated, Greenhouse Geisser adjustments were used. Bonferroni correction for multiple comparisons was applied. Effect sizes (Cohen's d) were calculated to quantify the magnitude of differences in mean PO between exercises at various %1RM. Statistical significance level was set at $p < 0.05$, analysis was performed using STATA16 (StataCorp LLC, College Station, TX, USA). Of note, due to the small sample size, the results of the statistical analyses should be considered solely for descriptive and not inferential purposes.

3. Results

3.1. Performance Characteristics of the Sample

The subjects' average 1RM in BP, PBP and BBP was, respectively: 99.2 ± 11.1 kg, 95.1 ± 10.1 kg, and 79.3 ± 8.8 kg. Related to their average body weight (BW), 1RM was, respectively: 1.2 ± 0.1 kg^{-1}, 1.2 ± 0.2 kg^{-1}, and 1.0 ± 0.1 kg^{-1}. Overall, PU/PR was 0.96.

3.2. Power–Load Relationship

3.2.1. Between Exercises

Overall, PBP shows the greatest values of PO compared to BP and BBP from the relative load of 40% to 90% 1RM. In contrast, amongst BP and BBP, no significant difference at any relative load was found. Post hoc analysis shows that the relative load that maximizes PO differs between exercises; 60% 1RM for PBP, 50% 1RM for BBP and 40% for BP; while the minimum PO's relative load is 20% 1RM for PBP and 90% 1RM for BBP and PB (Figure 2, Table 1). The magnitude of differences in mean PO between exercises at various %1RM is reported in Table 2.

Table 1. Values of average power output across different loads (from 20% to 90% 1RM) and exercises.

Different Loads	20% a	30% b	40% c	50% d	60% e	70% f	80% g	90% h
Prone bench pull-1, ($n = 9$)								
mean ± sd	424.64 ± 74.93	531.41 ± 77.24	607.83 ± 93.53	653.92 ± 102.56	669.66 ± 98.2	655.05 ± 79.73	610.11 ± 51.20	534.82 ± 47.72
Loads comparison	a vs. all	b vs. a,d,e,f	c vs. a	d vs. a,b,h	e vs. a,b,h	f vs. a,b,h	g vs. a,h	h vs. a,d,e,f,g
Bench press-2, ($n = 9$)								
mean ± sd	452.10 ± 76.81	487.64 ± 90.36	503.11 ± 98.80	498.51 ± 100.99	473.84 ± 96.49	429.10 ± 85.14	364.29 ± 66.99	279.41 ± 42.72
Loads comparison	a vs. g,h	b vs. f,g,h	c vs. f,g,h	d vs. f,g,h	e vs. g,h	f vs. b,c,d,g,h	g vs. f,h	h vs. all
Ballistic bench press-3, ($n = 9$)								
mean ± sd	363.48 ± 34.79	448.08 ± 50.74	498.35 ± 63.89	514.29 ± 71.18	495.91 ± 75.23	443.19 ± 82.40	356.14 ± 100.90	234.76 ± 135.48
Loads comparison	a vs. b,c,d,e,f,h	b vs. a,d,g,h	c vs. g,h	d vs. a,f,g,h	e vs. a,g,h	f vs. a,d,g,h	g vs. b,c,d,e,f,h	h vs. all
Exercises comparison	1 vs. 3	1 vs. 3	1 vs. 2, 3	1 vs. 2, 3	1 vs. 2, 3	1 vs. 2, 3	1 vs. 2, 3	1 vs. 2, 3

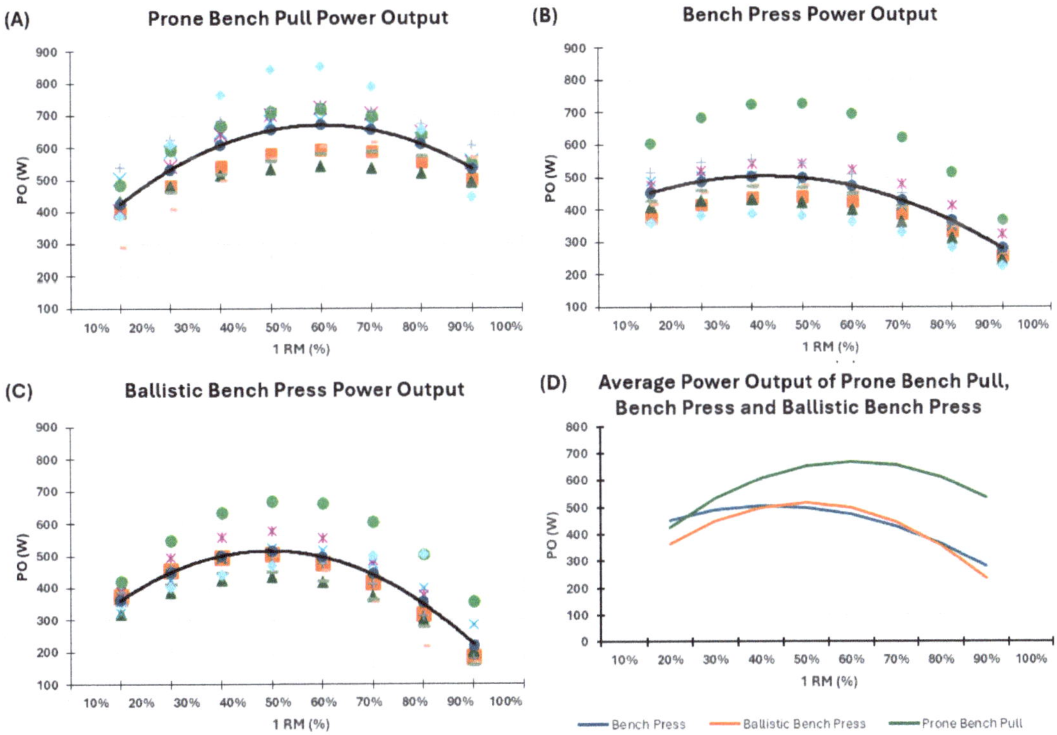

Figure 2. Individual values of power output for each of the three exercises, along with the average power output across the different exercises.

Table 2. Cohen's d Effect Sizes for mean power output across different %1RM in prone bench pull, bench press, and ballistic bench press.

Exercise	Percentage of One Repetition Maximum							
	20%	30%	40%	50%	60%	70%	80%	90%
PBP vs. BP	−0.36	0.52	1.08	1.52	2.01	2.73	4.12	5.64
PBP vs. BBP	1.05	1.27	1.36	1.57	1.98	2.62	3.22	5.56
BP vs. BBP	1.50	0.53	0.05	−0.17	−0.25	−0.16	0.09	1.09

PBP—prone bench pull; BP—bench press; BBP—ballistic bench press.

Figure 2 reports the individual and mean power output for the following exercises: Panel A, Prone Bench Pull; Panel B, Bench Press; Panel C, Ballistic Bench Press. Different individuals are represented with distinct symbols within the same Panel, but are constant between Panels; the black marked line of Panels A, B, and C represents the average power output. Finally, in Panel D, a graphical comparison of the mean power output across the three exercises is available. 1RM—One repetition maximum; %—Percentage; PO—power output; W—Watts.

3.2.2. Within Exercises

Within each exercise, the PO was not statistically different from 40% to 80% 1RM in PBP, from 40% to 60% 1RM in BBP, and from 20% to 60% in BP (Table 1).

4. Discussion

To our knowledge, this study is the first to describe P–Lr from 20% to 90% 1RM in BP, BBP, and PBP in international medal-winning canoeists and kayakers. The main finding is that P–Lr differs between PBP, BP and BBP, with the highest PO in PBP compared to BP and BBP.

4.1. Pull-to-Push Ratio

Our sample shows an overall PU/PR of 0.96, which, if compared with the investigation of McKean and Burkett in sub-elite kayakers (2010, 2014) could be considered low. Indeed, the cited studies found that improvements in all-out sprint kayak performance were correlated with the PU/PR ratio approaching 1.3 during three-year longitudinal monitoring. However, compared to the present study, some methodological differences about the modality of PU/PR investigation emerge. In fact, in these investigations [4,15], it was obtained by dividing the maximum weight lifted during a chin-up (plus body mass) versus 1RM in BP, while our study divided the 1RM in PBP versus 1RM in BP. Such a discrepancy may explain the different results, since, although the chin-up is a pulling exercise, the primary muscles involved act at different joint positions compared to the PBP. This hypothesis would be confirmed by observing results obtained in studies which utilized our same exercises, reporting similar PU/PR values: equal to 1.0 [22,23] or 0.92 [2].

Another difference could be attributed to the composition of our sample, which included kayakers specialized in sprint and endurance disciplines (i.e., kayak marathon), whereas the cited studies focused exclusively on sprint specialists. Therefore, it seems that a high PU/PR could be appropriate for sprint events, where explosive upper-body strength is critical, while in longer distances, other factors such as endurance, may play a more significant role in performance, thus reducing the overall PU/PR. However, further research is needed to determine the most effective method for calculating the PU/PR ratio through exercise and to identify discipline-specific reference values.

4.2. Power–Load Relationship

4.2.1. Power–Load Relationship Between Exercises

The greatest values of PO in the PBP than those observed for BP and BBP, from 40% to 90% 1RM are in line with previous investigations [13,24]. This finding may reflect the sport-specific demands placed on this type of athlete. Indeed, kayakers and canoeists rely heavily on pulling motions to generate propulsion, as outlined as one of the most important characteristics of paddlers by coaches of this discipline [25]. This could contribute to greater PO development in pulling exercises like the PBP as opposed to pushing tasks such as the BP. Similarities with other studies could be explained by the fact that Sánchez-Medina et al. (2014) recruited strength-trained athletes mainly from combat sports (judo and wrestling) [13], and Pearson et al. (2009) a group of sailors [24], both activities that require a strong pull, the first to immobilize the opponent, while the second to pulling ropes to control the sails. Moreover, the difference in the PO between pushing and pulling exercises might also derive from different mechanical advantages during execution; indeed, we know that BP, unlike PBP, has a sticking point that could be up to half of the concentric effort [13]. Finally, no statistically relevant difference was found between BP and BBP in the P–Lr as assumed.

4.2.2. Power–Load Relationship Within Exercises

In PBP, the maximum PO was found at 60% 1RM, with non-significantly different values between 40 and 80% 1RM. This result slightly differs from previous research that observed the maximum at 78.6 ± 5.7% 1RM without distinction between 60 and 100%

1RM [24] or at 70 ± 4% without difference in the range 50–90% 1RM [13]. This difference may be attributed to the fact that, the strength-trained athletes in Sánchez-Medina et al. (2014) may have been able to optimize their annual training specifically to enhance PO and strength in pulling exercises [13]. In contrast, international-level kayakers typically engage in twice as many on- and off-water sessions compared to resistance training sessions, potentially limiting the extent of PO adaptations due to reduced RT volume. In contrast, the entire P–Lr is consistent with that measured in elite rowers [21]. Maximum PO is comparable to those of a Spanish Olympic rowing championship team [21]; however, from the overall P–Lr, we assume that the Spanish team trains more with a heavy relative load than our sample because their maximum PO was attained near 75% 1RM. Indeed, training with a high percentage of 1RM shifts the bell-shape P–Lr to the right [26]. This difference could be partially explained by the relatively lower competitive level of our sample. Although all participants were international-level medalists, none had competed in the Olympic Games. Consequently, they lacked access to the training volume, recovery strategies, and support systems typically available to Olympic-level athletes, who may have modestly limited their overall physical conditioning and adaptations.

In BP, the highest PO occurred at 40% 1RM and was not significantly different from the values reported between 20% and 60% of 1RM. This result slightly differs from previously published data in a cohort of strength-trained athletes, primarily from combat sports such as judo and wrestling, that found the maximum PO at 56 ± 2%, without differences from 40% to 70% 1RM [13]. We hypothesize that the athletes in our research use lighter loads on the bench press than the cited sample because the pushing exercise is not the primary goal in paddle sports. Indeed, training with a lighter relative load shifts the P–Lr to the left with the expected highest PO to move toward the lower %s of the curve [26]. Moreover, it can be speculated that the specific loads encountered during sport participation influence PO adaptation. Indeed, combat athletes require higher pushing forces to quickly overcome an opponent's resistance and avoid being controlled or taken down, demanding powerful pushing actions and as suggested before, they may have been able to optimize their annual training specifically to enhance PO and strength in this movement [13]. Of note, the pushing action in paddling does not have the same fundamental importance for specific on-water performance. In our investigation, the maximum PO in BBP peaked at 50% 1RM, without a significant difference from 20% to 60% 1RM. Our result is similar to the one performed on professional rugby players that have found a non-statistical difference in PO from 20% to 60% 1RM, even if it was shown that their maximum PO was at 30% 1RM [14]. The difference in maximum PO could be due to the different sports as well as training regimes. In this context, when comparing two cohorts from different sports that prioritize sport-specific (on-pitch and on-water) training over RT in terms of volume, our results are consistent—and in this case superior—in terms of the percentage in which maximum PO is achieved. This further reflects the high performance level of our participants.

Possible Elements for Power-Based Resistance Training Prescription

Considering that during the paddling stroke the paddle blade is submerged in water and acts as a fixed point of resistance, the muscle action involved in pulling closely resembles a contraction against a high resistance. Therefore, contextualizing the result in our sample of kayakers, it would be ideal to obtain maximum PO at higher relative loads (such as the one reported in a rowing championship team [21]), because this indicates the ability to generate greater PO under conditions that closely mimic the high-resistance demands encountered during actual paddling. This ability reflects a superior capacity to apply strength and power effectively during the phases of the stroke, which are critical for maximizing propulsion and overall performance. To achieve this, training should focus on loads that shift the maximum PO of the PBP toward higher intensities [26]. Therefore, from a strength training perspective, this would likely be accomplished by training within the higher portion of the P–Lr (i.e., 60–80% 1RM) and even near-maximal loads (≥85% 1RM). Additionally, we suggest focusing on the higher end of the P–Lr, as training at these loads is more likely to enhance strength and neuromuscular adaptations [27].

Moreover, since we have observed that PO is maximized at 60% 1RM (669.66 ± 98.2 W) in PBP, and that paddlers generate 747 ± 151 W during an all-out start of 10 s [12], prescribing training loads around 50–70% of 1RM in PBP may be effective for improving this part of the race. Specifically, coaches must count the number of strokes performed at maximal intensity during the initial start, which could be approximately 20. With that information in mind, coaches could prescribe to athletes several long sets performing the exact number of pulling movements (i.e., 3 sets per 20 repetitions, with 5 min of rest in between) or could opt to break down these long sets into smaller groups of reps with short rest periods in between (10 to 30 s) [28] and, again, complete rest between sets. For example, a set of 20 repetitions can be broken into a set of four blocks of five repetitions with 20 s of rest between blocks (i.e., 3 sets × (4 blocks × 5 reps, 20 s rec)/5 min). This approach would maintain PO mainly constant throughout all the repetitions of a set to increase muscle adaptations and minimize neuromuscular fatigue [28].

Moreover, considering that a PO of 424.64 ± 74.93 W was observed at 20% 1RM in PBP, and that paddlers generate 374 ± 63 W in the first half and 323 ± 36 W in the second half of a 2 min all-out kayaking performance [12], a training prescription aimed at simulating the full race effort could be developed based on these values. For example, during the competitive phase, coaches might prescribe a full, 2 min set on the PBP using lighter loads (i.e., 20–30% 1RM) to target in-water power–endurance. However, during the preparatory phase, this could be structured as repeated sets of 30 s of pulling movements followed by 30 s of rest, continued until a total of 2 min of RT is completed.

Another approach to closely simulate race demands involves starting with a load corresponding to the all-out start PO (60% 1RM), and then progressively reducing the load as PO declines, allowing the athlete to complete the 2 min set. In this scenario, teammates assist by deloading the barbell for the athlete performing the exercise, minimizing dead time between repetitions.

Regarding exercise selection, considering that paddling is a predominantly pulling activity, from our perspective, PBP must have priority in all the RT sessions. However, BP and BBP must be implemented to avoid upper-body's agonist and antagonist muscle imbalances.

Limitations and Future Directions

The major limitations of this study are the number of athletes recruited (n = 9) and the measurement of a guided exercise. The restricted cohort of international-level medal-winning athletes has been analyzed for descriptive purposes only and does not allow for drawing broader inferences to a cohort of matched kayakers, nor comparisons with paddlers of different levels (sub-elite, Olympic paddlers). Moreover, no gender stratification was possible. For these aims, future studies on larger cohorts, better representing both sexes, and involving groups of paddlers of different levels would be necessary. For the measurement of a guided exercise, we chose this modality because the BBP is usually performed on a guided machine due to the potential danger associated with its execution with a free barbell.

Moreover, future investigations on PU/PR should consider standardizing the methodology (i.e., exercises from which this ratio is calculated), along with the identification of discipline-specific (i.e., kayak sprint versus kayak endurance competitions) reference values. Additionally, the exercise order was not randomized because all athletes were tested simultaneously (i.e., in the same training session) due to time constraints imposed by a rigid calendar of structured training. Additionally, the exercise order was chosen because, for the PBP, we needed to completely change the starting position of the barbell and set up the bench using two wooden plyometric boxes, as described in the method. Therefore, it would have been impossible to quickly and repeatedly change this setup after a bench press set by another athlete. Therefore, a future study that will randomize the exercise order would add scientific rigor.

Finally, a dedicated study that answers how a training prescription at peak PO might impact sprint kayak performance in international-level elite kayakers is warranted, along with one aiming to correlate gym-based P–Lr profiles with on-water paddling stroke characteristics (force, velocity, and power). Such investigations would enhance understanding of how RT adaptations transfer to paddling performance, thereby refining training specificity for sprint kayak athletes.

5. Conclusions

This study is the first to describe the P–Lr from 20% to 90% 1RM in BP, BBP, and PBP in international-level, medalist-winning canoeists and kayakers. The main findings are that pulling in PBP showed an overall higher PO than the pushing movement (BP and BBP), and that the maximum PO was found at 60% 1RM in PBP, 40% 1RM in BP, and 50% 1RM BBP. Moreover, our elite cohort of paddlers has a PU/PR < 1. Although necessitating confirmation in a wider sample, these data may provide preliminary reference values useful to prescribe athlete-specific power-based oriented training in paddle-sports.

Author Contributions: Conceptualization, O.C., M.F. (Matteo Fortunati), and G.D.; methodology, O.C., M.F. (Matteo Fortunati), T.G., P.D. and G.D.; investigation, O.C., M.F. (Matteo Fortunati), T.G., M.F. (Massimiliano Febbi), P.D., S.R. and G.D.; data curation, O.C., M.F. (Matteo Fortunati), and P.D. writing—original draft preparation, O.C., M.F. (Matteo Fortunati), and G.D.; writing—review and editing, O.C., M.F. (Matteo Fortunati), T.G., M.F. (Massimiliano Febbi), P.D., S.R. and G.D.; supervision, O.C., P.D. and G.D. All authors have read and agreed to the published version of the manuscript.

Funding: This research received no external funding.

Institutional Review Board Statement: The research protocol was approved by the Sport and Physical Education Ethics Committee of the University of Novi Sad, Serbia (n°47-06-02/2021-3) is compliance with ethics standards committee.

Informed Consent Statement: Informed consent was obtained from all subjects involved in the study.

Data Availability Statement: The data associated with the paper are not publicly available but are available from the corresponding author on reasonable request.

Conflicts of Interest: The authors declare no conflicts of interest.

References

1. Gäbler, M.; Prieske, O.; Elferink-Gemser, M.T.; Hortobágyi, T.; Warnke, T.; Granacher, U. Measures of Physical Fitness Improve Prediction of Kayak and Canoe Sprint Performance in Young Kayakers and Canoeists. *J. Strength Cond. Res.* **2023**, *37*, 1264–1270. [CrossRef] [PubMed]
2. Kristiansen, M.; Pedersen, A.S.K.; Sandvej, G.; Jørgensen, P.; Jakobsen, J.V.; de Zee, M.; Hansen, E.A.; Klitgaard, K.K. Enhanced Maximal Upper-Body Strength Increases Performance in Sprint Kayaking. *J. Strength Cond. Res.* **2023**, *37*, e305–e312. [CrossRef] [PubMed]
3. Bielik, V.; Lendvorský, L.; Vajda, M.; Lopata, P.; Ružbarský, P.; Masselli Dos Reis, I.G.; Messias, L.H.D. Comparison of Aerobic and Muscular Power Between Junior/U23 Slalom and Sprint Paddlers: An Analysis of International Medalists and Non-medalists. *Front. Physiol.* **2020**, *11*, 617041. [CrossRef] [PubMed]

4. McKean, M.R.; Burkett, B. The relationship between joint range of motion, muscular strength, and race time for sub-elite flat water kayakers. *J. Sci. Med. Sport* **2010**, *13*, 537–542. [CrossRef]
5. Kawamori, N.; Haff, G.G. The optimal training load for the development of muscular power. *J. Strength Cond. Res.* **2004**, *18*, 675–684.
6. Cormie, P.; McCaulley, G.O.; Triplett, N.T.; McBride, J.M. Optimal loading for maximal power output during lower-body resistance exercises. *Med. Sci. Sports Exerc.* **2007**, *39*, 340–349. [CrossRef]
7. Comfort, P.; Haff, G.G.; Suchomel, T.J.; Soriano, M.A.; Pierce, K.C.; Hornsby, W.G.; Haff, E.E.; Sommerfield, L.M.; Chavda, S.; Morris, S.J.; et al. National Strength and Conditioning Association Position Statement on Weightlifting for Sports Performance. *J. Strength Cond. Res.* **2023**, *37*, 1163–1190. [CrossRef]
8. Siegel, J.A.; Gilders, R.M.; Staron, R.S.; Hagerman, F.C. Human muscle power output during upper- and lower-body exercises. *J. Strength Cond. Res.* **2002**, *16*, 173–178. [PubMed]
9. Soriano, M.A.; Suchomel, T.J.; Marín, P.J. The Optimal Load for Maximal Power Production During Upper-Body Resistance Exercises: A Meta-Analysis. *Sports Med.* **2017**, *47*, 757–768. [CrossRef]
10. Miller, R.M.; Freitas, E.D.; Heishman, A.D.; Kaur, J.; Koziol, K.J.; Galletti, B.A.; Bemben, M.G. Maximal power production as a function of sex and training status. *Biol. Sport.* **2019**, *36*, 31–37. [CrossRef]
11. Thomas, G.A.; Kraemer, W.J.; Spiering, B.A.; Volek, J.S.; Anderson, J.M.; Maresh, C.M. Maximal power at different percentages of one repetition maximum: Influence of resistance and gender. *J. Strength Cond. Res.* **2007**, *21*, 336–342. [CrossRef] [PubMed]
12. Bishop, D.; Bonetti, D.; Dawson, B. The influence of pacing strategy on VO_2 and supramaximal kayak performance. *Med. Sci. Sports Exerc.* **2002**, *34*, 1041–1047. [CrossRef] [PubMed]
13. Sánchez-Medina, L.; González-Badillo, J.J.; Pérez, C.E.; Pallarés, J.G. Velocity- and power-load relationships of the bench pull vs. bench press exercises. *Int. J. Sports Med.* **2014**, *35*, 209–216. [CrossRef] [PubMed]
14. Bevan, H.R.; Bunce, P.J.; Owen, N.J.; Bennett, M.A.; Cook, C.J.; Cunningham, D.J.; Newton, R.U.; Kilduff, L.P. Optimal loading for the development of peak power output in professional rugby players. *J. Strength Cond. Res.* **2010**, *24*, 43–47. [CrossRef] [PubMed]
15. McKean, M.R.; Burkett, B.J. The influence of upper-body strength on flat-water sprint kayak performance in elite athletes. *Int. J. Sports Physiol. Perform.* **2014**, *9*, 707–714. [CrossRef]
16. Crisafulli, O.; Fortunati, M.; Gemelli, T.; Grattarola, L.; Quintiero, V.; Febbi, M.; Drid, P.; Ramat, S.; D'antona, G. Power Output, Lactatemia, and Maximum Oxygen Consumption During a Specific Off-Water Incremental Test in International-Level Podium-Winner Kayak and Rowing Athletes. *J. Funct. Morphol. Kinesiol.* **2025**, *10*, 203. [CrossRef]
17. García-Ramos, A.; Padial, P.; García-Ramos, M.; Conde-Pipó, J.; Argüelles-Cienfuegos, J.; Štirn, I.; Feriche, B. Reliability Analysis of Traditional and Ballistic Bench Press Exercises at Different Loads. *J. Hum. Kinet.* **2015**, *47*, 51–59. [CrossRef]
18. Hultman, E.; Bergström, J.; Anderson, N.M. Breakdown and resynthesis of phosphorylcreatine and adenosine triphosphate in connection with muscular work in man. *Scand. J. Clin. Lab. Investig.* **1967**, *19*, 56–66. [CrossRef]
19. Jidovtseff, B.; Harris, N.K.; Crielaard, J.M.; Cronin, J.B. Using the load-velocity relationship for 1RM prediction. *J. Strength Cond. Res.* **2011**, *25*, 267–270. [CrossRef]
20. Loturco, I.; McGuigan, M.R.; Suchomel, T.; Freitas, T.T.; Rodríguez-Rosell, D.; Pereira, L.A.; Pareja-Blanco, F. Determining the One Repetition Maximum in the Ballistic Bench Press Exercise. *J. Strength Cond. Res.* **2020**, *34*, 3321–3325. [CrossRef]
21. Izquierdo-Gabarren, M.; Expósito, R.G.; de Villarreal, E.S.; Izquierdo, M. Physiological factors to predict on traditional rowing performance. *Eur. J. Appl. Physiol.* **2010**, *108*, 83–92. [CrossRef] [PubMed]
22. Pickett, C.W.; Nosaka, K.; Zois, J.; Hopkins, W.G.; Blazevich, A.J. Maximal Upper-Body Strength and Oxygen Uptake Are Associated With Performance in High-Level 200-m Sprint Kayakers. *J. Strength Cond. Res.* **2018**, *32*, 3186–3192. [CrossRef] [PubMed]
23. Akra, F.; Muniroglu, S. Anthropometric-Somatotype and Strength Profiles and On-Water Performance in Turkish Elite Kayakers. *Int. J. Appl. Sports Sci.* **2008**, *20*, 22–34.
24. Pearson, S.N.; Cronin, J.B.; Hume, P.A.; Slyfield, D. Kinematics and kinetics of the bench-press and bench-pull exercises in a strength-trained sporting population. *Sports Biomech.* **2009**, *8*, 245–254. [CrossRef] [PubMed]
25. Teunissen, J.W.A.; Ter Welle, S.S.; Platvoet, S.S.; Faber, I.; Pion, J.; Lenoir, M. Similarities and differences between sports subserving systematic talent transfer and development: The case of paddle sports. *J. Sci. Med. Sport* **2021**, *24*, 200–205. [CrossRef]
26. Haff, G.G.; Nimphius, S. Training Principles for Power. *Strength Cond. J.* **2012**, *34*, 2–12. [CrossRef]
27. Lopez, P.; Radaelli, R.; Taaffe, D.R.; Newton, R.U.; Galvão, D.A.; Trajano, G.S.; Teodoro, J.L.; Kraemer, W.J.; Häkkinen, K.; Pinto, R.S. Resistance Training Load Effects on Muscle Hypertrophy and Strength Gain: Systematic Review and Network Meta-analysis. *Med. Sci. Sports Exerc.* **2021**, *53*, 1206–1216. [CrossRef]
28. Davies, T.B.; Tran, D.L.; Hogan, C.M.; Haff, G.G.; Latella, C. Chronic Effects of Altering Resistance Training Set Configurations Using Cluster Sets: A Systematic Review and Meta-Analysis. *Sports Med.* **2021**, *51*, 707–736. [CrossRef]

sports

MDPI

Article

Physiological Correspondence Between Different Indexes of High-Intensity Endurance Exercise in Young Male Runners

Danilo A. Massini [1,2], Renato A. C. Caritá [3], Tiago A. F. Almeida [1,2,4], Anderson G. Macedo [1,2,5], Víctor Hernández-Beltrán [6], José M. Gamonales [6,7], Mário C. Espada [8,9,10,11,12,*] and Dalton M. Pessôa Filho [1,2]

1 Department of Physical Education, School of Sciences, São Paulo State University (UNESP), Bauru 17033-360, Brazil; dmassini@hotmail.com (D.A.M.); tiagofalmeida.w@gmail.com (T.A.F.A.), andersongmacedo@yahoo.com.br (A.G.M.); dalton.pessoa-filho@unesp.br (D.M.P.F.)
2 Postgraduate Program in Human Development and Technology, São Paulo State University (UNESP), Rio Claro 13506-900, Brazil
3 Faculty of Americana-(FAM), Americana 13477-360, Brazil; renatocarita@fam.edu.br
4 Centre for Research in Economics and Comparative Development (CIEDEC), Lusíada University of Lisbon, 1349-001 Lisbon, Portugal
5 Postgraduate Program in Rehabilitation Sciences, Institute of Motor Sciences, Federal University of Alfenas, Alfenas 37133-840, Brazil
6 Training Optimization and Sports Performance Research Group (GOERD), Faculty of Sport Science, University of Extremadura, 10005 Cáceres, Spain; vhernandpw@alumnos.unex.es (V.H.-B.); martingamonales@unex.es (J.M.G.)
7 Faculty of Education and Psychology, University of Extremadura, 06006 Badajoz, Spain
8 Instituto Politécnico de Setúbal, Escola Superior de Educação, 2914-504 Setúbal, Portugal
9 Life Quality Research Centre (CIEQV-Leiria), Complexo Andaluz, Apartado, 2040-413 Rio Maior, Portugal
10 Centre for the Study of Human Performance (CIPER), Faculdade de Motricidade Humana, Universidade de Lisboa, Cruz Quebrada-Dafundo, 1499-002 Lisboa, Portugal
11 Comprehensive Health Research Centre (CHRC), Universidade de Évora, 7004-516 Évora, Portugal
12 SPRINT Sport Physical Activity and Health Research & Innovation Center, Centro de Investigação e Inovação em Desporto Atividade Física e Saúde, 2001-904 Santarém, Portugal
* Correspondence: mario.espada@ese.ips.pt

Abstract: Critical speed (CS), the respiratory compensation point (RCP), and the midpoint between gas exchange threshold and maxial oxygen uptake (VO_{2max}) (i.e., 50%Δ) have been considered indexes able to demarcate the boundary between the heavy and severe exercise domains. However, the agreement between these indexes—and therefore the validity of using them reciprocally—remains to be reported in running. The current study analyzed the agreement between RCP, 50%Δ, and CS. Twelve young runners performed an incremental test to assess VO_{2max}, RCP, and 50%Δ, with CS estimated by the linear model of time-limited trials at 90, 95, and 110% of the speed corresponding to VO_2max. One-way ANOVA showed no differences when comparing VO_2 and running speed at CS vs. 50%Δ vs. RCP (47.5 ± 4.4 vs. 46.6 ± 4.4 vs. 47.8 ± 4.5 $mLO_2 \cdot kg^{-1} \cdot min^{-1}$; and 13.9 ± 1.3 vs. 13.7 ± 1.3 vs. 14.0 ± 1.4 $km \cdot h^{-1}$; $p > 0.05$ for all comparisons). The bias for 50%Δ vs. CS was −0.82 ± 1.55 $mLO_2 \cdot kg^{-1} \cdot min^{-1}$ and −0.23 ± 0.55 $km \cdot h^{-1}$, and for RCP vs. CS, it was 0.36 ± 1.21 $mLO_2 \cdot kg^{-1} \cdot min^{-1}$ and 0.05 ± 0.46 $km \cdot h^{-1}$. Therefore, the agreement between RCP, 50%Δ, and CS in estimating VO_2 responses and running speed did not preclude their reciprocal similarity in exercise intensity, although the observed individual variability in physiological variables is a constraint on considering these indexes interchangeable.

Keywords: critical speed; respiratory compensation point; running; youth

1. Introduction

To define the zones for exercise training, the profiles of physiological variables like oxygen uptake (VO_2) and blood lactate concentration ($[La^-]$) during running or cycling have been used to account for the interplay of energy systems (aerobic vs. anaerobic activation) and acid–base balance control (metabolites (H+, Pi) clearance ability) [1,2]. Basically, the transition from an evenly steady state to an uncontrolled rise toward maximal values of VO_2 and $[La^-]$, passing through an intermediary state of uneven but still controlled responses, characterizes the range of exercise intensities across the moderate (i.e., highly tolerable), heavy (fairly tolerable), and severe (poorly tolerable) domains [1–3]. To demarcate these domains, the responses of VO_2, $[La^-]$, pulmonary ventilation (V_E), and gas exchange variables (like carbon dioxide production (VCO_2), ventilatory equivalents for O_2 and CO_2, and pulmonary end-tidal O_2 and CO_2) have been analyzed during incremental or constant-load exercises and applied to parametrize the transitions between physiological profiles in each exercise domain [4,5].

In this context, the onset of additional VCO_2 release through the buffering process of H+ (due to the increased demand on the glycolytic pathway) drives $[La^-]$, V_E, and VCO_2 to rise more sharply, marking the transition from the moderate to heavy domain. This transition has been indexed by the lactate threshold (LT), the gas exchange threshold (GET), and the first ventilatory threshold (VT_1) [4,5]. The heavy domain marks the upper limit of exercise at which blood lactate concentration ($[La^-]$) and oxygen uptake (VO_2) responses [2–4] remain high but stable, i.e., an isocapnic buffering region [5]. In this region, an exercise intensity can also be observed eliciting the maximal balance between the rate of metabolite efflux from the muscle and the rate of metabolite clearance from the blood (known as the maximal lactate steady state, MLSS) [2]. Above the heavy domain, the responses of $[La^-]$ and VO_2 are projected to their respective maximal values [6,7]; thus, the transition from the heavy to severe domain is characterized by respiratory compensation for metabolic acidosis (i.e., V_E rises exponentially (hyperventilation) to reduce the excess of CO_2 in the blood), which has been indexed by the lactate turn point (LTP), respiratory compensation point (RCP), and second ventilatory threshold (VT_2) [4,5].

In running, critical speed (CS) has been recognized and well supported as the exercise intensity demarcating the upper limit of the heavy domain [2,6–8]. Thus, below CS, there is a range of exercise intensities eliciting physiological [1,2,8] and metabolic [2,3,9] responses without inducing sufficient accumulation of metabolites to disturb the acid–base balance [9,10]. However, the determination of CS yields values subjected to protocol influence (i.e., time limit (t_{Lim}) between 2 and 15 min) [1–3] and mathematical adjustments (linear and non-linear equations) [2,11] and is often expensive and physically demanding for athletes [12].

In addition, other indexes able to parametrize the zone of heavy but still sustainable exercise, mainly those assessed during incremental exercise tests, have been compared to CS regarding their observed similarities [6,13]. For example, it has been proposed that the exercise intensity at half the difference (i.e., Δ 50%) between maximal oxygen consumption (VO_{2max}) and GET would also delimit the upper boundary of exercise intensities with physiological responses still characterizing the heavy domain [14]. Despite all normalization efforts, information from incremental exercise tests is dependent on the specificity of training status and movement pattern [15–18]. Lansley et al. [19] reported more consistent physiological responses during exercise when the level of intensity was prescribed at a given %Δ rather than at $\%VO_{2max}$. Moreover, another study reported that the transition from the heavy to severe domain in running can be observed in a wide range between 40 and 60%Δ [20]. However, typical physiological responses of the heavy domain were reported during cycling at 50%Δ [14], whereas responses at 60, 70, and 80%Δ were typical of the physiological profile in the severe domain [21]. Therefore, there is enough theoretical support for the assumption that 50%Δ might be a reliable index of the transition between sustainable and exhaustive exercises [14].

As already mentioned, another index from the incremental exercise test able to characterize the heavy sustainable exercise intensity is RCP [22,23], which has shown similarity to CS [3,11]. The physiological significance of RCP corresponds to an exercise intensity beyond which the mechanisms for controlling the acid–base balance lose the capacity to buffer hydrogen anion production due to the increased demand for ATP resynthesis from anaerobic glycolytic metabolism [4,5,10,11,13]. Thus, the concept of RCP is best aligned with the assumption that it represents an exercise intensity around which the physiological response can transition from the heavy to severe domain [24,25]. Therefore, if CS is an index from a time-limited model able to evidence agreement with threshold indexes of incremental exercise, then CS can be a reliable and feasible index to support high-intensity training planning for young runners. It is notable that the insufficient number of investigations to support the agreement or disagreement between CS and indexes from incremental exercise, particularly RCP and 50%Δ, contrasts with the substantial evidence supporting their roles in demarcating exercise zones characterized by submaximal and sustainable physiological responses. In addition, previous studies did not refute that both RCP and CS are indexes eliciting comparable load/speed intensities or physiological responses [11,26], although the interchangeability in physiological responses is still being questioned [5,18].

Thus, the present study aimed to analyze metabolic (VO_2) and speed ($km \cdot h^{-1}$) agreement at 50%Δ and RCP with CS during treadmill running in trained young runners. The hypothesis was that these indexes would show statistical similarities in terms of oxidative demand. However, when comparing running speeds, differences were expected to reduce compatibility due to the influence of individual anthropometric characteristics on stride length and frequency and their association with running economy [17].

2. Materials and Methods

2.1. Participants

Twelve young male runners (15.7 ± 1.8 years; 1.7 ± 0.1 m; and 57.1 ± 11.7 kg), regularly involved in a running training program for at least two years, participated in this study. Assessments were conducted during the third microcycle of the base training period. The participants were selected after an initial screening of 20 young athletes to exclude those who were recently injured or sick, those experiencing pain or discomfort during the training, and those who were not endurance-trained runners. All participants obtained permission from their guardians and signed an informed consent form acknowledging the procedures. All research procedures were conducted following the Declaration of Helsinki and the ethical standards in sport and exercise science research [27], and were previously approved by the local University Ethics Committee (CAEE: 36936714.6.0000.5398).

2.2. Experimental Design

Figure 1 illustrates the experimental design. Participants underwent four testing sessions: (1) a progressive ramp test to determine GET, RCP, 50%Δ, and VO_2max, along with their respective intensities (vGET, vRCP, v50%Δ, and vVO_2max, respectively), and (2) three constant-velocity exercise bouts to voluntary exhaustion at 90%, 95%, and 110% of vVO_2max, which were performed for CS prediction. A 24 h interval was maintained between each exercise bout [8]. All tests were conducted on a motorized treadmill (HP/Cosmos Pulsar, Nussdorf-Traunstein, Germany) with a fixed 1.0% incline [26] in an indoor environment with controlled temperature (21–23 °C) and air humidity (50–60%). Participants were instructed to avoid exhaustive training, refrain from drinking alcoholic and caffeinated beverages the day before the assessment, and arrive in a fed and hydrated state [7,8].

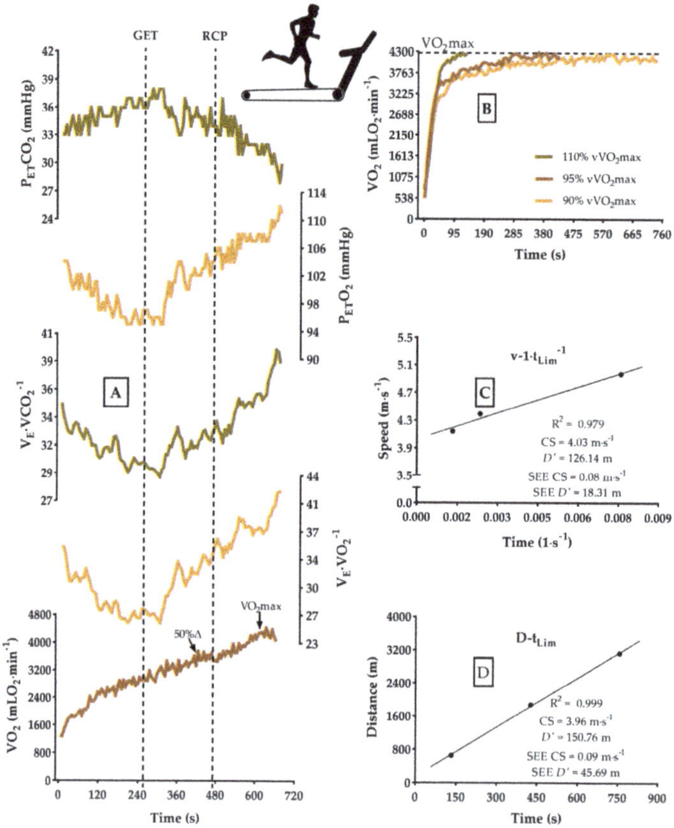

Figure 1. An example of estimating a participant's physiological and speed variables in the study. Panel (**A**) depicts the maximal incremental test for determining GET, RCP, 50%Δ, and VO_{2max}. Panel (**B**) illustrates the VO_2 response during the predictive trials for CS. Panels (**C**,**D**) show the determination of CS using the v-tLim^{-1} and d-t$_{Lim}$ models, respectively.

2.3. *Maximal Incremental Test*

During the maximal incremental test (Figure 1, Panel A), the speed progressed by 1.0 km·h^{-1}·min^{-1}, starting from 7.0 km·h^{-1} [28] until voluntary exhaustion. VO_2 was breath-by-breath sampled throughout the test (QuarkPFTergo, Cosmed, Rome, Italy). The O_2 and CO_2 concentration analysis system was calibrated before each test using ambient air and a gas with known O_2 and CO_2 concentrations, and the turbine analysis was calibrated using a three-liter syringe, according to the manufacturer's recommendations. VO_2 values were smoothed by a three-second filter and averaged every six seconds. [La$^-$] was analyzed at rest and in the first minute after test completion, and its analysis was performed using the enzymatic method (YSL 2500STAT, Yellow Spring, CO, USA) from 25 μL of arterial blood diluted in 50 μL of 1% NaF solution [11].

VO_2max was considered the highest value smoothed by a 30 s moving average. VO_2max was determined as the lowest speed in the incremental test that elicited the maximum VO_2 elevation [17]. GET was determined following Whipp's [4] recommendations based on the responses of $V_E \cdot VCO_2^{-1}$, $V_E \cdot VO_2^{-1}$, $P_{ET}CO_2$, and $P_{ET}O_2$. It involved observing an increase in the responses of $VE{\cdot}VO_2^{-1}$ and $P_{ET}O_2$ without a change in the response of $V_E{\cdot}VCO_2^{-1}$ and $P_{ET}CO_2$. Identification of the metabolic fatigue threshold at 50%Δ was performed using VO_2 at GET and VO_{2max} (50%Δ = GET + [(VO_{2max} − GET) × 0.5]) [14,16]. The corresponding speed was determined by trend fitting between running speed ($km{\cdot}h^{-1}$) and its VO_2 during the incremental test. GET, RCP, 50%Δ, and VO_{2max} determinations were conducted independently by three experienced researchers [29].

2.4. Critical Speed (CS) Determination

The predictive trials for CS (90%, 95%, and 110% of vVO_{2max}) (Figure 1, Panel B) were randomly performed with a minimum interval of 24 h [8]. The value of t_{Lim} was recorded in seconds and associated with the prediction speed using the speed vs. time-limited ($v\text{-}t_{Lim}^{-1}$) model (Figure 1, Panel C) and the distance vs. time-limited ($d\text{-}t_{Lim}$) model (Figure 1, Panel D) (Equations (1) and (2)) [12]. The selection of the CS value for each participant was based on the smallest standard error of the estimate (SEE) as the criterion [30].

(a) Speed vs. inverse of time to exhaustion ($v\text{-}1{\cdot}t_{Lim}^{-1}$)

$$v = D' \times \frac{1}{(t)} + CS \quad (1)$$

(b) Total distance vs. time ($D\text{-}t_{Lim}$)

$$d = D' \times t + CS \quad (2)$$

where v = running speed; D' = amount of work from bioenergetic reserves; t = the time limit (t_{Lim}) of predictive trials; and CS = critical speed. The VO_2 corresponding to CS was determined using the trend relationship between VO_2 and running speed during the incremental test [7,30].

2.5. Statistical Analysis

The sample size was previously estimated using G*Power, considering a security level of 95% ($Z_1\text{-}\alpha/2$ = 1.960) and power of 85% ($Z_1\text{-}\beta$ = 1.036), as well as a high correlation level of 0.80 [31]. The estimated size was 10 participants, which was increased by 20% (N = 12) to avoid statistical underpower with participants withdrawing.

Data were expressed as mean ± SD with a 95% confidence interval ($CI_{95\%}$). Outliers and normality were checked using a 1.5·IQR range (interquartile range = Q3–Q1) and the Shapiro–Wilk test. Homogeneity, variance, and differences between 50%Δ, RCP, and CS (VO_2 and $km{\cdot}h^{-1}$) analysis were examined using the Levene test and one-way ANOVA, supplemented by Fisher's LSD test.

The normality, independence, and homoscedasticity of the residuals for the regression analyses between 50%Δ, RCP, and CS were assessed using the Shapiro–Wilk, Durbin–Watson, and Breusch–Pagan tests, respectively. Influential residuals or leverage points were identified through Cook's distance. For agreement analysis, the difference between the means of variables was checked using the two-tailed Student's *t*-test for a single sample, and the proportional bias of differences was assessed through linear regression analysis between the mean (independent variable) and the difference (dependent variable) of the measurement. An analysis of dispersion was performed using the sample-adjusted coefficient of determination (R^2adj.) and SEE, whilst agreement was analyzed with Bland–Altman plots [32] and the standard error of the mean (SEM = SD ÷ $\sqrt{n}$).

The effect size for ANOVA and R^2adj. was calculated using eta squared (η^2) considering threshold values as follows: <0.04 [trivial], 0.04–0.24 [weak], 0.25–0.63 [medium], and ≥0.64 [strong] [33]. The correlations between the variables were assessed using the coefficient of correlation (r) derived from the coefficient of determination (R^2), with which the sample power was determined (Equation (3)) [31].

$$Z_{1-\beta} = \sqrt{n-3}\,\frac{1}{2}Ln\left(\frac{1+r}{1-r}\right) - Z_{1-\frac{\alpha}{2}} \quad (3)$$

where $Z_{1-\beta}$ provides the coefficient for determining the sample power by the bicaudal normal distribution of the value r [31]. The IBM SPSS Statistics software (version 27, 2021, IBM Co., Ltd., Armonk, NY, USA) was used to conduct statistical analyses. Statistical significance was determined at $\alpha < 0.05$.

3. Results

The value of VO_{2max} reached 53.0 ± 5.1 ($CI_{95\%}$ = 49.8–56.2) $mLO_2{\cdot}kg^{-1}{\cdot}min^{-1}$, and the corresponding speed reached 16.1 ± 1.7 ($CI_{95\%}$ = 15.0–17.2) $km{\cdot}h^{-1}$. The lower limit of the heavy domain was indexed by GET, corresponding to 76.2 ± 4.2% VO_2max (70.1 ± 6.2% vVO_2max), and CS marked the upper limit at 89.6 ± 3.1% VO_2max (86.5 ± 3.6% vVO_2max). The VO_2 responses during predictive trials for CS reached 53.0 ± 4.9 (110% vVO_2max), 53.9 ± 4.4 (95% vVO_2max), and 56.2 ± 7.2 $mLO_2{\cdot}kg^{-1}{\cdot}min^{-1}$ (90% vVO_{2max}), providing greater prediction rigor for the $v^{-1}{\cdot}t_{Lim}{}^{-1}$ fit with R^2 = 0.98 ± 0.03 (SEE = 2.89 ± 1.69% and $CI_{95\%}$ = 0.25–0.55 $km{\cdot}h^{-1}$). Figure 2 presents the metabolic and speed values of the indexes used in the upper limit of the heavy domain. Another variable for sustainable exercise was RCP, which was situated at 90.2 ± 2.8% VO_2max (86.8 ± 3.7% vVO_2max). Both 50%Δ (88.0 ± 3.7% VO_{2max} and 85.1 ± 3.1% vVO_{2max}) and RCP showed no significant differences when compared to CS, respectively, regarding VO_2 ($F_{[2,35]}$ = 0.227, η^2 = 0.014 [trivial], p = 0.65 and p = 0.84, respectively) and running speed ($F_{[2,35]}$ = 0.151, η^2 = 0.009 [trivial], p = 0.68 and p = 0.92, respectively). Similarly, there was no difference in RCP compared to 50%Δ for VO_2 (p = 0.51) and $km{\cdot}h^{-1}$ (p = 0.61), confirming the hypothesis regarding the statistical similarity between them.

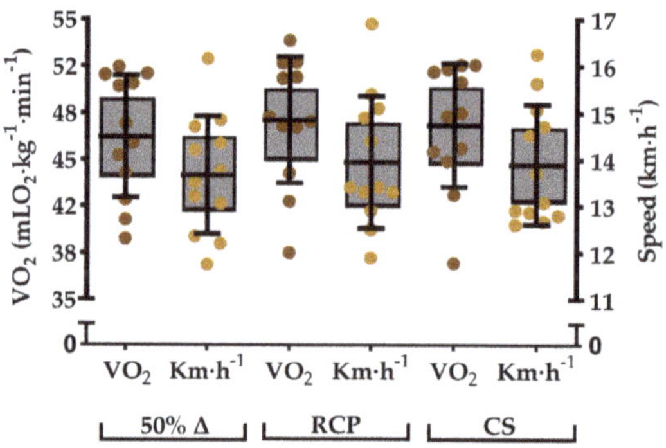

Figure 2. Individual values (circles), mean ± SD (line and whiskers), and 95% confidence interval (gray box) of $VO_2{}^-$ (brown) and running speed (light brown) associated with 50%Δ, RCP, and CS.

The regression and agreement analyses between 50%Δ, RCP, and CS regarding VO_2 and running speed are shown in Figures 3 and 4, respectively. The agreement analyses in relative values of VO_2 and $km{\cdot}h^{-1}$ are shown in Figure 5. Both 50%Δ ($F_{[1,10]}$ = 72.13, p < 0.01) and RCP ($F_{[1,10]}$ = 128.6, p < 0.01) were able to account for the variance in VO_2 at CS with a potential of 86.6% [strong] and 92.1% [strong], respectively (Figure 3A,C), and a bias ($t_{[11]}$ = −1.830, p = 0.94 and $F_{[1,11]}$ = 0.003, p = 0.96; $t_{[11]}$ = 1.046, p = 0.32 and $F_{[1,11]}$ = 0.065, p = 0.80) of −0.82 ± 1.55 and 0.36 ± 1.21 $mLO_2{\cdot}kg^{-1}{\cdot}min^{-1}$ (SEM = 3.0 and 2.4 $mLO_2{\cdot}kg^{-1}{\cdot}min^{-1}$ or 6.9 and 4.9%, respectively, Figure 3B,D) or −1.74 ± 3.54

and 0.76 ± 2.52%, respectively ($t_{[11]}$ = −1.701, p = 0.12 and $F_{[1,11]}$ = 0.004, p = 0.94; $t_{[11]}$ = 1.041, p = 0.32 and $F_{[1,11]}$ = 0.016, p = 0.90, Figure 5A,C).

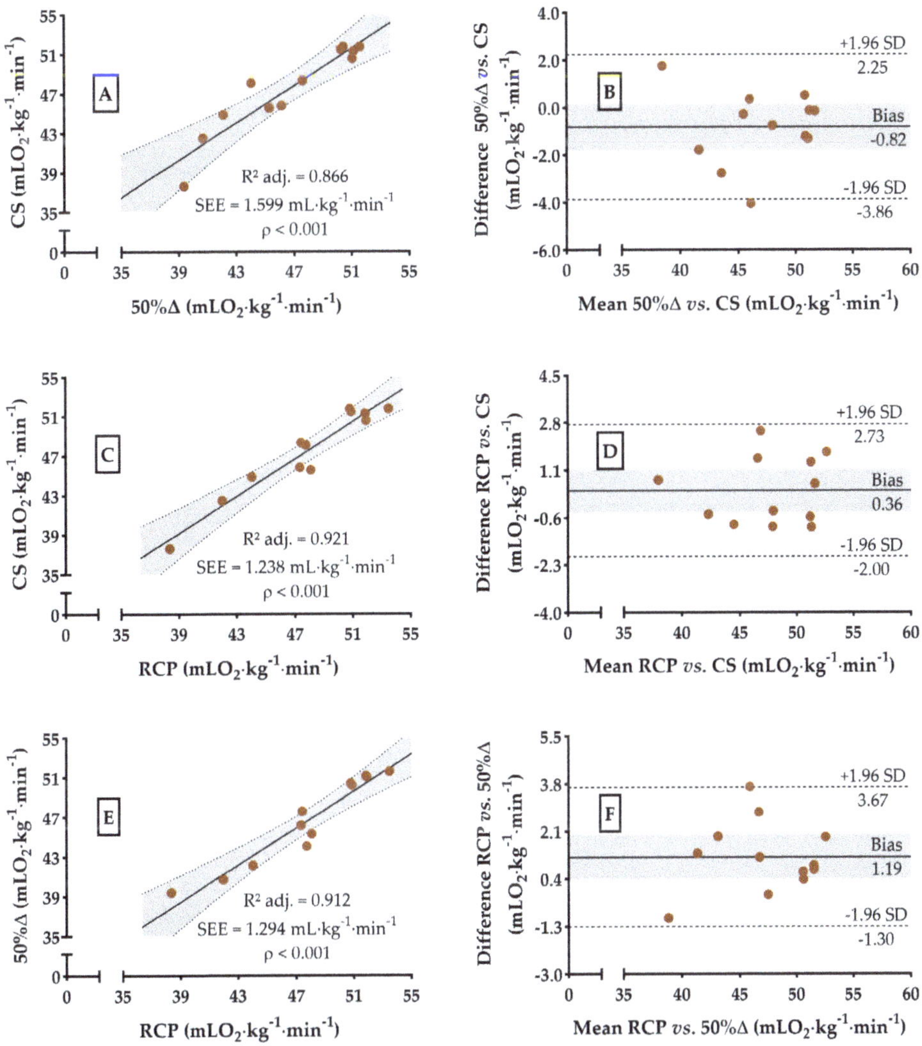

Figure 3. Dispersion and Bland–Altman plots for VO_2 values at CS, RCP, and 50%Δ. Dispersion between VO_2 at 50%Δ vs. CS (99.9% power, Panel (**A**)), VO_2 at RCP vs. CS (99.9% power, Panel (**C**)), and VO_2 at RCP vs. 50%Δ (99.9% power, Panel (**E**)). Agreements analysis between VO_2 at 50%Δ vs. CS (Panel (**B**)), RCP vs. CS (Panel (**D**)), and RCP vs. 50%Δ (Panel (**F**)). The gray area in all the panels represents the 95% confidence interval.

On the other hand, RCP ($F_{[1,10]}$ = 115. 3, p < 0.01) has the potential to predict VO_2 at 50%Δ, explaining 92.1% of the variance [strong] (Figure 3E), but lacks statistical agreement ($t_{[11]}$ = 3.234, p < 0.01 and $F_{[1,11]}$ = 0.096, p = 0.76), with a bias of 1.19 ± 1.27 $mLO_2{\cdot}kg^{-1}{\cdot}min^{-1}$ (SEM = 2.5 $mLO_2{\cdot}kg^{-1}{\cdot}min^{-1}$ or 5.5%, Figure 3F) or 2.50 ± 2.84% ($t_{[11]}$ = 3.049, p = 0.01 and $F_{[1,11]}$ = 0.037, p = 0.85, Figure 5E). For running speed, a lack of statistical compatibilities was also observed, confirming our second hypothesis. Both 50%Δ ($F_{[1,10]}$ = 47.16, p < 0.01) and RCP ($F_{[1,10]}$ = 87.84, p < 0.01) were able to account for the variance in km·h^{-1} at CS with a potential of 80.4% [strong] and 88.8% [strong], respectively (Figure 4A,C), and a bias ($t_{[11]} = -1.431$, $p = 0.18$ and $F_{[1,11]} = 0.014$, $p = 0.91$; $t_{[11]} = 0.392$, $p = 0.70$ and $F_{[1,11]} = 0.957$, $p = 0.35$) of -0.23 ± 0.55 and 0.05 ± 0.46 km·h^{-1} (SEM = 1.0 and 0.9 km·h^{-1} or 8.0 and 4.9%, respectively, Figure 4B,D) or -1.66 ± 4.13 and 0.29 ± 3.26%, respectively ($t_{[11]} = -1.391$, $p = 0.19$ and $F_{[1,11]} = 0.006$, $p = 0.94$; $t_{[11]} = 0.310$, $p = 0.76$ and $F_{[1,11]} = 0.835$, $p = 0.38$, Figure 5B,D).

Finally, RCP ($F_{[1,10]} = 73.51$, $p < 0.01$) explained 86.8% of the variance in running speed (km·h^{-1}) at 50%Δ [strong] (Figure 5E), with a bias ($t_{[11]} = 1.955$, $p = 0.08$ and $F_{[1,11]} = 1.095$, $p = 0.32$) of 0.28 ± 0.49 km·h^{-1} (SEM = 1.0 km·h^{-1} or 7.0%, Figure 4F) or 1.95 ± 3.54% ($t_{[11]} = 1880$, $p = 0.09$ and $F_{[1,11]} = 0.541$, $p = 0.48$, Figure 5F).

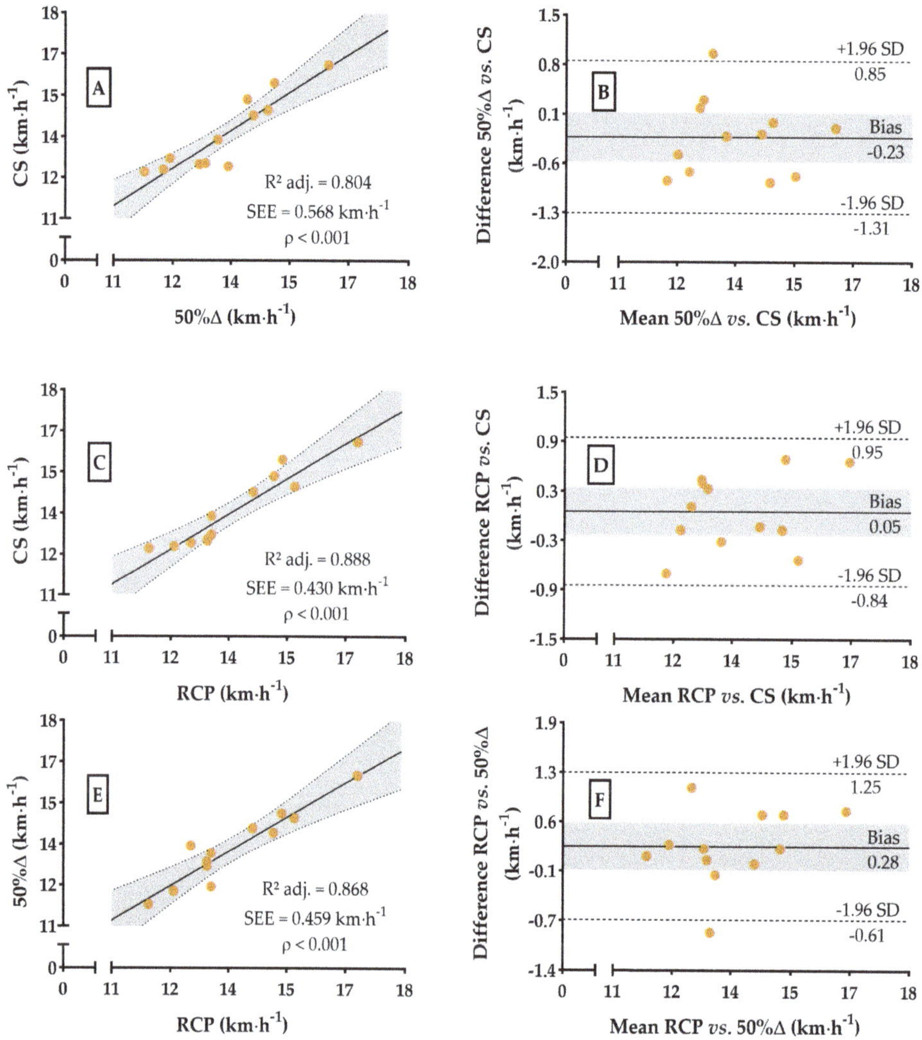

Figure 4. Dispersion and Bland–Altman plots for speed (km·h^{-1}) values at CS, RCP, and 50%Δ. Dispersion for 50%Δ vs. CS (99.4% power, Panel (**A**)), RCP vs. CS (99.9% power, Panel (**C**)), and RCP vs. 50%Δ (99.9% power, Panel (**E**)). Agreements analysis between velocities at 50%Δ vs. CS (Panel (**B**)), RCP vs. CS (Panel (**D**)), and RCP vs. 50%Δ (Panel (**F**)). The gray area in all the panels represents the 95% confidence interval.

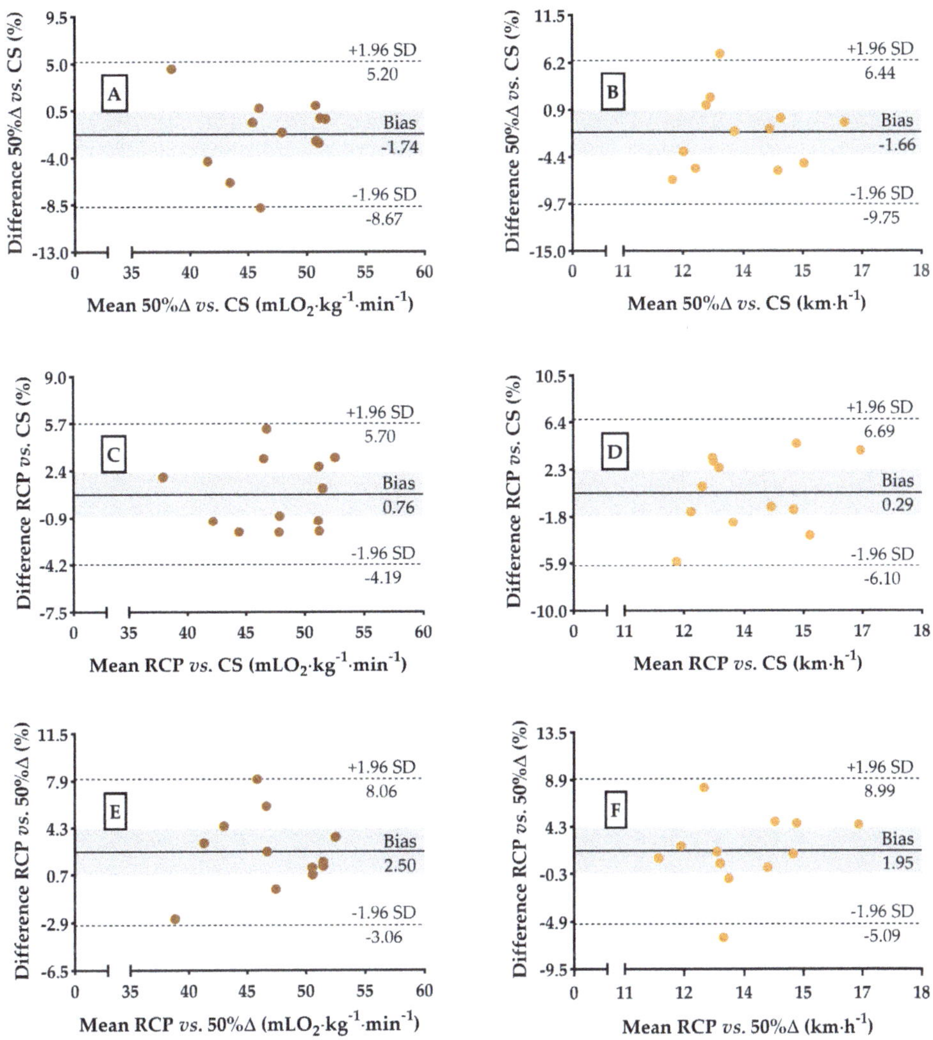

Figure 5. Bland–Altman plots showing the percentage difference between VO_2 values and running speed (respectively) for 50%Δ vs. CS (Panel (**A**,**B**)), RCP vs. 50%Δ (Panel (**C**,**D**)), and RCP vs. 50%Δ (Panel (**E**,**F**)). The gray area in all the panels represents the 95% confidence interval.

4. Discussion

This study analyzes the agreement between physiological indexes in running speed at different fatigue thresholds in young runners. By assessing 50%Δ and RCP during an incremental ramp test, no differences were significant when comparing these indexes in terms of metabolic rate and running speed, nor when comparing these responses from both indexes with those estimated for CS. In light of these findings, this study demonstrates that all three indexes might be applied to determine the transition between the heavy and severe exercise intensity domains for young runners, showing similarities with the age group and training status of the participants. However, the Bland–Altman analysis [32] showed wide and biased confidence intervals, indicating error in metabolic rate and speed between 50%Δ and CS, which is a finding consistent with previously reported variability in cycling [12]. Also, the speeds corresponding to 50%Δ and RCP were not in agreement (i.e., comparisons differed from zero significantly) and showed a considerably high estimation error (7.0%). Since the errors exceed 5%, the planning of training (e.g., targeting an athlete's periodization) and/or the design of experimental protocols (e.g., targeting analysis of exercise intensity) may not provide a reliable estimate of exercise conditions [12,13]. Indeed, previous research has suggested that exercising at 5% above CP reduces tolerance and elicits muscular and blood metabolic imbalance [34]. Taking this into account, only the comparisons of VO_2 and speed between RCP and CS might be considered closely reciprocal and likely to provide high confidence in determining different exercise domains around these thresholds.

Thus, the lack of statistical differences between the indexes (RCP vs. 50%Δ vs. CS) regarding the VO_2 response should be interpreted with caution since the individual variability of the responses observed might preclude the assumption of similar metabolic responses for the entire sample of participants in each index, in line with previous studies reporting a lack of similarity in cycling [13,26,35] and running [6]. Individual variability in physiological thresholds across exercise domains has been reported to be influenced by slight differences in training experience, conditioning level, and running economy [10,35,36]. For example, altering the slope of the relationship between VO_2 and speed to the right allows a previously required metabolic demand to be maintained at a higher running speed or enables a given running speed to be sustained for a longer duration [10]. Although this tendency is well reported for training in the moderate exercise domain, there is a large variance among individuals regarding the changes, as was observed by Philp et al. [36] after four weeks of training with moderately trained runners (VO_{2max} = 45 $mLO_2 \cdot min^{-1} \cdot kg^{-1}$), in which the increases in the lactate threshold (LT) (7–9%), maximal lactate steady state (5–8%), and VO_{2max} (6–10%) showed variability. Consequently, the relative allocation (%VO_{2max} and/or %vVO_{2max}) of the physiological thresholds changes, and the boundaries of the heavy domain (lower and upper, e.g., LT, CS) move up accordingly [16]. In addition, further considering that the relative location of these indexes depends on individual adaptation to training [19,37], as well as on the sensitivity of each index to adjustments based on the specialized plan of training [16], the interchangeability between RCP, 50%Δ, and CS remains a critical concern, due to the particular contribution of energetics (aerobic vs. anaerobic) and tolerance to exercise [25,38], even when differences in exercise intensity among these indexes are slight [13,18]. However, the current study observed very close values at a given %VO_{2max} and %vVO_{2max} between RCP and CS, suggesting that exercise 1% below and/or above these indexes tends to fall in different domains, which indicates a closer overlap of boundaries.

Therefore, an aspect to consider is individual variability, which is intrinsic to the relative allocation of RCP, 50%Δ, and CS in terms of %VO_{2max} and/or %vVO_{2max}. The current study observed a very small underestimation of CS by 50%Δ (~1.6%). When observing the current results in terms of Δ, two participants had CS located above 60%Δ, which would imply an underestimation of the upper limit of the heavy domain by 50%Δ. However, considering the study of Lansley et al. [19] recommending a safety margin (±10%Δ) to define the boundary between heavy and severe domains based on 50%Δ, the current mean difference between CS and 50%Δ is well aligned with this suggestion, supporting the use of 50%Δ to parametrize exercise domains. However, it is important to note the probability of observing different physiological responses (VO_2 and heart rate), metabolic responses ([La^-]), and exercise tolerance between individuals when predicting exercise intensity in a given domain [1,34]. An attempt to account for this variability was proposed by Souza et al. [12], whose study suggested an even larger "safe zone" of ±20%Δ (i.e., heavy domain <30%Δ and severe >70%Δ) to accommodate major sources of interindividual variability in physiological responses, such as (i) training status [35];

(ii) central and peripheral limitations to oxygen uptake during exercise, muscle fiber contractile properties, and metabolic profile [18]; and (iii) age and sex [35]. In spite of the possible large variability in physiological responses reported in these previous studies when exercising at different paces near the boundary between the heavy and severe domains, the current study emphasizes that the proportional similarity between CS and 50%Δ is strong (i.e., showing a rate above 80%) for speed or VO_2 comparisons.

In addition, the comparison between RCP and CS showed the strongest similarities (~90%) when comparing the speed and estimated VO_2 for these indexes. Nevertheless, the SEM can attain ~5%, which might result in allocating RCP within the severe intensity domain in different sport modalities, such as running, cycling [1,2,4,24], and swimming [23]. There are many studies comparing RCP with CS (or CO, which is the equivalent for power measurements) that have observed statistical equivalence, as shown in cycling (286 ± 28 W or 85.3 ± 5.6% VO_2max vs. 278 ± 22 W or 85.4 ± 4.8% VO_2max, respectively) [22], in running (RCP vs. CS: 11.5 ± 2.3 vs. 11.7 ± 2.3 km·h^{-1}, respectively) [6], and in oxidative demand while running (2.88 ± 0.80 vs. 2.83 ± 0.72 L·min^{-1}, respectively) [6]. Therefore, the current results reinforce the lack of difference between RCP and CS, in line with previous findings [22,23] for either absolute (VO_2 and speed) or relative (%VO_{2max} and/or %vVO_{2max}) measures. In practical terms, the closest similarities between RCP and CS suggest a reciprocal confidence for planning high-intensity exercise in the heavy and severe domains, with each index being suitable for control running intensity during training and conditioning adjustments over a planning period, despite the availability of a metabolic chart being mandatory for RCP assessment.

The current study showed some limitations regarding the measurements, experimental conditions, and population. The first concern is related to the assessment of CS, since the variability of the values is associated with the number of predictive trials [2] and mathematical adjustments (linear and non-linear) [2,30]. However, the current study ensured that the t_{Lim} of the predictive trials lay around the recommended range (2 to 15 min), and that VO_2max was reached during the trials at 90%, 95%, and 110% VO_{2max} [2,6,9]. The fact that VO_2 responses were not analyzed during exercise (e.g., VO_2 on-kinetics) around each index (RCP, 50%Δ, and CS) limits the ability to assert metabolic equivalence between these indexes and prevents a definitive recommendation regarding their interchangeability for demarcating the transition from the heavy to severe exercise domain. In addition, the findings of the current study are restricted to the analyzed group regarding the age and training level of the runners; therefore, extrapolation of the results to a larger sample of young runners should be interpreted with caution. Moreover, we recommend future studies investigating the similarity between different training conditions and age groups of runners.

5. Conclusions

The results indicated that during maximal progressive exercise, certain indexes of speed and VO_2 demand were highly correlated with CS, suggesting their ability to represent the transition from high-intensity, yet sustainable, exercise to poorly tolerated zones. Therefore, the indexes 50%Δ and RCP can be considered useful references for identifying the transition between heavy and severe exercise domains, due to their physiological (VO_2) and speed (km·h^{-1}) similarities with CS. However, interindividual variabilities should be considered a source of estimation errors of these variables, and, thus, the interchangeability between these indexes must be interpreted with caution. This consideration is essential for planning training and experimental designs demanding a high level of specificity regarding the physiological responses in young runners, since large variability might allocate different subjects in distinct exercise zones. In addition, the current analysis also evidenced that CS might be an excellent index for characterizing the heavy domain in athletes of comparable age and training levels (or experience) to the present participants, considering that RCP and 50%Δ both showed a tendency to overestimate CS. Therefore, although the reliability of RCP, 50%Δ, and CS for planning training in the heavy and severe domains for young runners remains a questionable issue due to the lack of detailed physiological comparisons among these indexes, the current findings support a high degree of similarity in exercise intensity, at least from running speed comparisons, between RCP and CS.

Author Contributions: Conceptualization, D.A.M., R.A.C.C. and D.M.P.F.; methodology, D.A.M., R.A.C.C., A.G.M. and D.M.P.F.; formal analysis, D.A.M., A.G.M., T.A.F.A. and D.M.P.F.; investigation, D.A.M., A.G.M., T.A.F.A. and D.M.P.F.; supervision, T.A.F.A. and D.M.P.F.; data curation, D.A.M. and D.M.P.F.; writing—original draft preparation, D.A.M., R.A.C.C., A.G.M., T.A.F.A., M.C.E. and D.M.P.F.; writing—review and editing, D.A.M., A.G.M., T.A.F.A., V.H.-B., J.M.G., M.C.E. and D.M.P.F.; visualization, D.A.M., A.G.M., T.A.F.A., V.H.-B., J.M.G., M.C.E. and D.M.P.F.; funding acquisition, A.G.M., T.A.F.A., V.H.-B., M.C.E. and D.M.P.F. All authors have read and agreed to the published version of the manuscript.

Funding: T.A.F.A. acknowledges the scholarships granted by CAPES, in the scope of the Program CAPES-PrInt, process number 88887.310/2018-00, mobility number 88887.580265/2020-00, and A.G.M acknowledges the fellowship from Coordenação de Aperfeiçoamento de Pessoal de Nível Superior-Brazil (CAPES—Finance Code 001). All the authors would like to thank the São Paulo Research Foundation (FAPESP—processes 2017/23717-9 and 2016/04544-3) for the financial support. D.A.M. would like to thank the National Council for Scientific and Technological Development (CNPq) for the fellowship (number: 150328/2024-9). This study was supported by the Portuguese Foundation for Science and Technology, I.P. under Grant UID04045/2020, and Instituto Politécnico de Setúbal. Also, the research was partially funded by the Optimisation of Training and Sports Performance Research Group (GOERD) of the Faculty of Sports Sciences of the University of Extremadura and the Aid for Research Groups (GR24133) from the Regional Government of Extremadura (Department of Education, Science and Professional Training), with a contribution from the European Union from the European Funds for Regional Development.

Institutional Review Board Statement: The study was conducted following the ethical standards laid down in the 1964 Declaration of Helsinki and approved by the local University Ethical Committee (CAAE), approval date (05/03/2015) (study protocol: 36936714.6.0000.5398).

Informed Consent Statement: Informed consent was obtained from all subjects involved in the study.

Data Availability Statement: The data that support the findings of this study are available from the corresponding and last author (dalton.pessoa-filho@unesp.br) upon reasonable request.

Conflicts of Interest: The authors declare no conflict of interest.

Abbreviations

The following abbreviations are used in this manuscript:

VO_2	Oxygen uptake
VO_{2max}	Maximal oxygen uptake
vVO_{2max}	Speed corresponding to the VO_{2max} in the incremental test
VCO_2	Carbon dioxide
H+	Hydrogen ion
Pi	Inorganic phosphate
[La-]	Blood lactate concentration
GET	Gas exchange threshold
vGET	Speed corresponding to the GET in incremental test
50%Δ	Middle point of the difference GET and VO_{2max}
v50%Δ	Speed corresponding to 50%Δ in the incremental test
LT	Lactate threshold

VT_1	First ventilatory threshold
MLSS	Maximal lactate steady state
V_E	Pulmonary ventilation
RCP	Respiratory compensation point
vRCP	Speed corresponding to the RCP in the incremental test
VT_2	Second ventilatory threshold
LTP	Lactate turn point
CS	Critical speed
t_{Lim}	Time limit
v-t_{Lim}	Time-limited model for the assessment of CS using trials with different velocities
d-t_{Lim}	Distance-limited model for the assessment of CS using trials with different distances

References

1. Burnley, M.; Jones, A.M. Power–duration relationship: Physiology, fatigue, and the limits of human performance. *Eur. J. Sport Sci.* **2018**, *18*, 1–12. [CrossRef] [PubMed]
2. Jones, A.M.; Burnley, M.; Black, M.I.; Poole, D.C.; Vanhatalo, A. The maximal metabolic steady state: Redefining the 'gold standard'. *Physiol. Rep.* **2019**, *7*, e14098. [CrossRef] [PubMed]
3. Jones, A.M.; Wilkerson, D.P.; DiMenna, F.; Fulford, J.; Poole, D.C. Muscle metabolic responses to exercise above and below the "critical power" assessed using ^{31}P-MRS. *Am. J. Physiol. Regul. Integr. Comp. Physiol.* **2008**, *294*, 585–593. [CrossRef] [PubMed]
4. Sietsema, K.E.; Rossiter, H.B. Exercise physiology and cardiopulmonary exercise testing. *Semin. Respir. Crit. Care Med.* **2023**, *44*, 661–680. [CrossRef]
5. Whipp, B.J. Physiological mechanisms dissociating pulmonary CO_2 and O_2 exchange dynamics during exercise in humans. *Exp. Physiol.* **2007**, *92*, 347–355. [CrossRef]
6. Broxterman, R.M.; Ade, C.J.; Craig, J.C.; Wilcox, S.L.; Schlup, S.J.; Barstow, T.J. The relationship between critical speed and the respiratory compensation point: Coincidence or equivalence. *Eur. J. Sport Sci.* **2015**, *15*, 631–639. [CrossRef]
7. Jones, A.M.; Kirby, B.S.; Clark, I.E.; Rice, H.M.; Fulkerson, E.; Wylie, L.J.; Wilkerson, D.P.; Vanhatalo, A.; Wilkins, B.W. Physiological demands of running at 2-hour marathon race pace. *J. Appl. Physiol.* **2021**, *130*, 369–379. [CrossRef]
8. Poole, D.C.; Burnley, M.; Vanhatalo, A.; Rossiter, H.B.; Jones, A.M. Critical power: An important fatigue threshold in exercise physiology. *Med. Sci. Sports Exerc.* **2016**, *48*, 2320–2334. [CrossRef]
9. Vanhatalo, A.; Fulford, J.; DiMenna, F.J.; Jones, A.M. Influence of hyperoxia on muscle metabolic responses and the power-duration relationship during severe-intensity exercise in humans: A ^{31}P magnetic resonance spectroscopy study. *Exp. Physiol.* **2010**, *95*, 528–540. [CrossRef]
10. Zoladz, J.A.; Majerczak, J.; Grassi, B.; Szkutnik, Z.; Korostyński, M.; Gołda, S.; Grandys, M.; Jarmuszkiewicz, W.; Kilarski, W.; Karasinski, J.; et al. Mechanisms of attenuation of pulmonary VO_2 slow component in humans after prolonged endurance training. *PLoS ONE* **2016**, *11*, e0154135. [CrossRef]
11. Massini, D.A.; Pessôa Filho, D.M.; Caritá, R.A.C.; Denadai, B.S. Physiological and perceptual response at critical speed and respiratory compensation point. *Braz. J. Sports Med.* **2016**, *22*, 439–444. [CrossRef]
12. Souza, K.M.; Lucas, R.D.; Salvador, P.C.N.; Helal, L.C.A.S.; Guglielmo, L.G.A.; Greco, C.C.; Denadai, B.S. Agreement analysis between critical power and intensity corresponding to 50% in cycling exercise. *Braz. J. Kinanthropom Hum. Perform.* **2016**, *18*, 197–206. [CrossRef]
13. Sitko, S.; Ciper-Sastre, R.; Corbi, F.; López-Laval, I. Relationship between functional threshold power, ventilatory threshold and respiratory compensation point in road cycling. *J. Sports Med. Phys. Fit.* **2022**, *62*, 626–632. [CrossRef]
14. Pringle, J.S.M.; Doust, J.H.; Carter, H.; Tolfrey, K.; Campbell, I.T.; Jones, A.M. Oxygen uptake kinetics during moderate, heavy and severe intensity "submaximal" exercise in humans: The influence of muscle fibre type and capillarisation. *Eur. J. Appl. Physiol.* **2003**, *89*, 289–300. [CrossRef]
15. Caputo, F.; Denadai, B.S. Does 75% of the difference between VO_2 at lactate threshold and VO_2max lie at the severe-intensity domain in well-trained cyclists? *Sci. Sports* **2009**, *24*, 257–261. [CrossRef]
16. Caritá, R.A.C.; Caputo, F.; Greco, C.C.; Denadai, B.S. Aerobic fitness and amplitude of the exercise intensity domains during cycling. *Braz. J. Sports Med.* **2013**, *19*, 271–274. [CrossRef]
17. Denadai, B.S.; Greco, C.C. Can the critical power model explain the increased peak speed/power during incremental test after concurrent strength and endurance training? *J. Strength Cond. Res.* **2017**, *31*, 2319–2323. [CrossRef]
18. Rossiter, H.B. Exercise: Kinetic considerations for gas exchange. *Compr. Physiol.* **2011**, *1*, 203–244. [CrossRef]
19. Lansley, K.E.; DiMenna, F.J.; Bailey, S.J.; Jones, A.M. A 'new' method to normalise exercise intensity. *Int. J. Sports Med.* **2011**, *32*, 535–541. [CrossRef]

20. Carter, H.; Pringle, J.S.; Jones, A.M.; Doust, J.H. Oxygen uptake kinetics during treadmill running across exercise intensity domains. *Eur. J. Appl. Physiol.* **2002**, *86*, 347–354. [CrossRef]
21. Burnley, M.; Davison, G.; Baker, J.R. Effects of Priming exercise on VO_2 Kinetics and the power-duration relationship. *Med. Sci. Sports Exerc.* **2011**, *43*, 2171–2179. [CrossRef]
22. Dekerle, J.; Baron, B.; Dupont, L.; Vanvelcenaher, J.; Pelayo, P. Maximal lactate steady state, respiratory compensation threshold and critical power. *Eur. J. Appl. Physiol.* **2003**, *89*, 281–288. [CrossRef]
23. Pessôa Filho, D.M.; Alves, F.; Reis, J.; Greco, C.; Denadai, B.S. VO_2 kinetics during heavy and severe exercise in swimming. *Int. J. Sports Med.* **2012**, *33*, 744–748. [CrossRef]
24. Almeida, T.A.F.; Espada, M.C.; Massini, D.A.; Macedo, A.G.; Castro, E.A.; Ferreira, C.C.; Reis, J.F.; Pessôa Filho, D.M. Stroke and physiological relationships during the incremental front crawl test: Outcomes for planning and pacing aerobic training. *Front. Physiol.* **2023**, *14*, 1241948. [CrossRef]
25. Massini, D.A.; Espada, M.C.; Macedo, A.G.; Santos, F.J.; Castro, E.A.; Ferreira, C.C.; Robalo, R.A.M.; Dias, A.A.P.; Almeida, T.A.F.; Pessôa Filho, D.M. Oxygen uptake kinetics and time limit at maximal aerobic workload in tethered swimming. *Metabolites* **2023**, *13*, 773. [CrossRef]
26. Broxterman, R.M.; Ade, C.J.; Barker, T.; Barstow, T.J. Influence of pedal cadence on the respiratory compensation point and its relation to critical power. *Respir. Physiol. Neurobiol.* **2015**, *208*, 1–7. [CrossRef]
27. Harriss, D.J.; Jones, C.; MacSween, A. Ethical standards in sport and exercise science research: 2022 update. *Int. J. Sports Med.* **2022**, *43*, 1065–1070. [CrossRef]
28. Vucetić, V.; Sentija, D.; Sporis, G.; Trajković, N.; Milanović, Z. Comparison of ventilation threshold and heart rate deflection point in fast and standard treadmill test protocols. *Acta Clin. Croat* **2014**, *52*, 190–203.
29. Scheuermann, B.W.; Kowalchuk, J.M. Attenuated respiratory compensation during rapidly incremented ramp exercise. *Respir. Physiol.* **1998**, *114*, 227–238. [CrossRef]
30. Massini, D.A.; Caritá, R.A.C.; Siqueira, L.O.; Simionato, A.R.; Denadai, B.S.; Pessôa Filho, D.M. Assessment of critical speed in track and treadmill: Physiological profiles and relationship with 3000-meter performance. *Braz. J. Kinanthropom Hum. Perform.* **2018**, *20*, 432–444. [CrossRef]
31. Díaz, S.P.; Fernández, S.P. Determinación del tamaño muestral para calcular la significación del coeficiente de correlación lineal. *Cad. Aten. Primaria* **2002**, *9*, 209–211.
32. Bland, J.M.; Altman, D.G. Statistical methods for assessing agreement between two methods of clinical measurement. *Lancet* **1986**, *327*, 307–310. [CrossRef]
33. Ferguson, C.J. An effect size primer: A guide for clinicians and researchers. *Prof. Psychol. Res.* **2009**, *40*, 532–538. [CrossRef]
34. Vanhatalo, A.; Black, M.I.; DiMenna, F.J.; Blackwell, J.R.; Schmidt, J.F.; Thompson, C.; Wylie, L.J.; Mohr, M.; Bangsbo, J.; Krustrup, P.; et al. The mechanistic bases of the power-time relationship: Muscle metabolic responses and relationships to muscle fibre type. *J. Physiol.* **2016**, *594*, 4407–4423. [CrossRef]
35. Murgatroyd, S.R.; Wylde, L.A.; Cannon, D.T.; Ward, S.A.; Rossiter, H.B. A 'ramp-sprint' protocol to characterise indices of aerobic function and exercise intensity domains in a single laboratory test. *Eur. J. Appl. Physiol.* **2014**, *114*, 1863–1874. [CrossRef]
36. Philp, A.; Macdonald, A.; Carter, H.; Watt, P.; Pringle, J. Maximal lactate steady state as a training stimulus. *Int. J. Sports Med.* **2008**, *29*, 475–479. [CrossRef]
37. Neder, J.A.; Jones, P.W.; Nery, L.E.; Whipp, B.J. The effect of age on the power/duration relationship and the intensity-domain limits in sedentary men. *Eur. J. Appl. Physiol.* **2000**, *82*, 326–332. [CrossRef]
38. Busso, T.; Chatagnon, M. Modelling of aerobic and anaerobic energy production in middle-distance running. *Eur. J. Appl. Physiol.* **2006**, *97*, 745–754. [CrossRef]

sports MDPI

Article

Does Birth Month Matter? Effects of Birth Subgroupings on Motor Performance and Ball-Involving Tests in a Youth Soccer Academy

Lorenzo Marcelli [1], Fioretta Silvestri [1], Gianluca Di Pinto [1,2,3,*], Andrea Colombo [1], Federica Marzoli [1], Maria Chiara Gallotta [4], Laura Guidetti [1], Fabrizio Perroni [5,†] and Davide Curzi [1,†]

1 Department of Economic, Psychological, Communication, Education and Movement Science, University Niccolò Cusano, 00166 Rome, Italy
2 BIND-Behavioral Imaging and Neural Dynamics Center, University "G. d'Annunzio" Chieti-Pescara, 66100 Chieti, Italy
3 Department of Medicine and Aging Sciences, University "G. d'Annunzio" Chieti-Pescara, 66100 Chieti, Italy
4 Department of Physiology and Pharmacology "Vittorio Erspamer", Sapienza University of Rome, 00185 Rome, Italy
5 Department of Biomolecular Sciences, Section of Exercise and Health Sciences, Carlo Bo University of Urbino, 61029 Urbino, Italy
* Correspondence: gianluca.dipinto@phd.unich.it
† These authors contributed equally to this work.

Abstract: Youth motor performance changes are not strictly linear during their sports career, and within-year birth timing may introduce relative age differences, known as the relative-age effect. In a cross-sectional study of 170 male young soccer players (8–12 years old), field tests were compared between adjacent age groups and within each of them: countermovement jump (with and without arm swing); 15 m linear sprint and agility test with and without the ball. Non-parametric tests with post hoc comparisons revealed significant differences between consecutive birth years in physical skills, particularly between the youngest and oldest groups. Specifically, differences were noted in the jumping test between U12 and U11, and between U10 and U9. Additionally, linear sprint and agility tests showed significance in U13 versus U12 and U10 versus U9. Finally, dribbling skills mature later (in both tests, U13 v U12, U12 v U11; with the ball, U10 v U9). Differences were found within the groups based on the semester, but not the trimester of birth, confirming a progressive yet non-linear pattern and semester-level within-year differences. These findings suggest the key role of motor skills development trajectories in creating individualized training programs tailored to the needs of individual young soccer players.

Keywords: football; relative age effect; young players; chronological age; talent identification; agility; CMJ; dribbling; technical skills; player development

1. Introduction

Soccer is an open-skill team sport involving a combination of motor (e.g., strength, endurance and flexibility) and technical skills as key indicators of performance, particularly in young players [1,2]. Some physical characteristics, such as cardiovascular fitness, follow a direct improvement with age, while others follow a non-linear trend (e.g., vertical countermovement jump, slalom agility) [3].

Fundamental motor skills, being the foundation of movement in children, play a crucial role in overall motor competence [4,5]. The object control skills, a subcategory of fundamental motor skills, involve the manipulation of objects with hands, feet, or tools, requiring high levels of coordination [4]. Its development at an early age is considered essential to facilitate skills transfer [4]. Indeed, studies have shown that the most successful players possess advanced motor abilities from an early stage and maintain their advantage over future non-elite players throughout their development [6]. Furthermore, object control skills are positively related to age [7], and specific physical exercise interventions have significantly improved object control skills in children [5]. The evidence regarding soccer-specific skills is unclear, with some authors [2] claiming a strong relationship between physical and technical skills, while others have not reported any direct correlation [8]. Indeed, Duncan and colleagues [8] suggest that the main predictors of performance development should be identified in the fundamental motor skills and perceived competence, regardless of the player's chronological age. Research findings confirm that physical maturity is a determining factor in physical performance, particularly in strength and muscular power. Biologically more mature athletes often outperform their less mature peers, although this relationship may vary according to chronological age, sex and the specific fitness component analyzed [1,9,10].

Although differences in physical performance across age groups are more closely related to differences in physical maturity, within the same birth years, selection processes often show a bias toward athletes born in the first months of the year, a phenomenon known as the Relative Age Effect (RAE) [11–13]. The advantage of being born in the first months of the year has been attributed to biological maturation, but it is also present when the differences in performance were corrected by somatic maturation [14]. RAE is more evident in younger age groups and tends to decrease with growth [15]. It appears to be present across all aspects of life (school, sport, lifestyle, etc.). Despite that, youth competitions are traditionally organized into age groups based on a fixed cut-off date (i.e., 1 January), but there is a growing interest in grouping players based on biological rather than chronological age, to address developmental differences [16,17]. Even by aligning the cut-off date to the academic year (September to August), RAE remains present as it should be addressed as an intrinsic factor of athletes, being non-eliminable [13]. In addition to physical performance, RAE also influences cognitive development and reflects broader maturation processes [18]. Studies have shown that growth goes hand in hand with improvements in both physical and academic performance [1,2,8,9,16,19].

Although the scientific literature has investigated the different levels of motor skills among young soccer players born in adjacent years, through field-based motor tests [2,9], few studies have examined differences in subjects born in the same year. Therefore, the aims of this study were to compare motor and dribbling skills in young soccer players through field-based tests (1) across consecutive age groups and (2) within the same birth year through birth-based subgrouping strategies. In our hypothesis, relatively older players (born earlier in the selection year) would demonstrate superior motor (sprint, CMJ, agility, flexibility) and technical (speed dribbling) performance compared to later-born peers.

2. Materials and Methods

2.1. Participants

One hundred and seventy young male soccer players were included in this study and were firstly divided into the following groups, based on their age range: Under 9 (n = 23, age = 8.2 ± 0.3 years), Under 10 (n = 31, age = 9.4 ± 0.3 years), Under 11 (n = 39, age = 10.4 ± 0.3 years), Under 12 (n = 42, age = 11.3 ± 0.3 years) and Under 13 (n = 35, age = 12.3 ± 0.3 years). The division into traditional age groups (U9–U13) reflects the official categories used in Italian and European youth competitions (FIGC/UEFA). To investigate the relative age effect (RAE) within the same age category, each group was further divided into two subgroups based on the period of birth: the oldest athletes (O), born in the first half of the year (January–June, subgroup O) and the youngest athletes (Y), born in the second half of the year (July–December, subgroup Y). Despite the limited sample size, an explorative analysis was performed to check magnitudes and potential differences within a shorter birth timeframe. The trimestral subdivision was organized as follows: Q1: January–March; Q2: April–June; Q3: July–September; and Q4: October–December [20,21].

Participants were selected from an Italian amateur soccer club (Soccer Club Frascati, Rome, Italy), based on their regular participation in both training and official matches. The club is located in a suburban Rome area with a relatively homogeneous socioeconomic population. Position-specific analysis was not conducted as young players at these ages often rotate between positions and do not have fixed tactical roles. To be included in the study, athletes had to have been active for the entire competitive season and be free from chronic or acute injuries in the three months preceding the study and during the whole season. Additionally, all participants had to have played soccer for at least two years prior to the start of the study.

All tests were conducted in October, at the beginning of the competitive season, after one month of training from the start of the activity in September, ensuring that players had adapted to the initial training phase before the test. The participants were homogeneous regarding their training status (e.g., average training hours per week: 4.5, divided into three training sessions; total training weeks per season: 40), as none of the participants underwent any strenuous activity or training outside of their normal training schedule.

Athletes and their parents were informed about the project through a written document, and informed consent was obtained from the athletes' parents or legal guardians, as all participants were minors. Ethical approval was granted by the Institutional Review Board of the University Niccolò Cusano, study protocol number MO 8/22, in accordance with the 1964 Helsinki Declaration and its later amendments or comparable ethical standards.

2.2. Testing Procedures

During the two weeks prior to the data collection, all participants attended four familiarization sessions in which each test was explained, demonstrated, and practiced. To assess the physical and technical abilities (i.e., dribbling skills) of the players, the following tests were conducted on a synthetic grass field under stable weather conditions (temperature 18–22 °C, minimal wind). All participants wore standard soccer boots and uniform sports clothing. The selected tests represent fundamental components of youth soccer performance and were chosen based on their relevance to soccer-specific skills and established validity in youth populations. Tests were administered in a fixed order (warm-up; flexibility; CMJ; sprint; agility) with 3 min of recovery between different test types to minimize fatigue effects. On test day, participants were allowed an additional warm-up attempt before official recording.

Test:

- Counter Movement Jump (CMJ) and Counter Movement Jump with Arm Swing (CMJA). The players performed three consecutive vertical jumps from a standing position, which were measured using the Optojump System (96 LEDs, 1.0416 cm resolution, Microgate, Bolzano, Italy). The system allowed precise measurement of the jump height by analyzing the flight time of each jump [22]. The highest jump among the three attempts was recorded for analysis. Arm movements were standardized: in CMJ, arms remained positioned on the hips throughout the movement, while in CMJA, free arm swing was permitted to assess coordination improvements. These tests were selected as they evaluate lower limb power and coordination, fundamental components for soccer performance, particularly in jumping for headers and explosive movements [23]. Slinde and colleagues [24] showed a high test–retest stability coefficient (range 0.80–0.98) for CMJ performances.

- 15-Meter Linear Sprint (LS) and 15-Meter Sprint with Ball Control (LSB). For the sprint test, the players completed a 15 m linear sprint in the shortest possible time. These tests measure fundamental speed capabilities and technical-coordinative abilities essential for soccer performance, with the ball control variant specifically assessing the integration of technical skills under speed demands [25]. The time spent in the sprint test was detected by a photocell system (Witty, Microgate, Bolzano, Italy). The fastest time among multiple trials was recorded for analysis. Altmann and colleagues [26] showed a high test–retest stability for these tests.
- 15-Meter Agility Test (AT) and 15-Meter Agility Test with Ball Control (ATB). Agility was assessed using a 15 m slalom sprint. These tests evaluate the ability to change direction rapidly, a crucial skill in soccer for evading opponents and creating space, with the ball variant assessing technical execution under coordinative demands [25]. The time spent in the sprint test was detected by a photocell system (Witty, Microgate, Bolzano, Italy). The fastest time among multiple trials was recorded for analysis. Altmann and colleagues [26] showed a high test–retest stability for these tests.
- Sit and Reach Test (SeR). Lower limb and spine flexibility were evaluated using the Sit and Reach test. Players sat with their legs extended and their feet resting on a graduated panel, and their best maximum forward reach distance among multiple attempts was measured [27]. This test was included as flexibility is important for injury prevention and overall movement quality in young athletes.

2.3. Statistical Analysis

Variables were not normally distributed, even after natural log transformation. Thus, a non-parametric Kruskal–Wallis test for independent samples was used to detect differences among age groups. Considering the total number of five groups and the smallest group sample size, a post hoc power analysis conducted with G*Power (v 3.1.9.7) indicated a statistical power of 0.93 for detecting a large effect size (f = 0.40), with an alpha error probability of 0.05.

Since significant differences between younger and older athletes could be expected due to athletes' growth, the post hoc analysis by the non-parametric Mann–Whitney U test was employed to determine whether differences existed only between adjacent age categories (U9 vs. U10, U10 vs. U11, U11 vs. U12, U12 vs. U13). To investigate differences within the same age category, the Kruskal–Wallis test for independent samples was used to assess differences among all subgroups. For parameters showing significant differences, post hoc comparisons between subgroups (Y vs. O) within each age category (e.g., U9Y vs. U9O, U10Y vs. U10O, etc.) were conducted using the Mann–Whitney U test. Statistical significance was set at $p \leq 0.05$. The same statistical procedure was then applied to detect significant differences between the subgroups classified according to birth quarter.

3. Results

3.1. Differences Between Age Groups

Kruskal–Wallis test showed significant differences among groups in all measured variables ($p < 0.01$); thus, the Mann–Whitney post hoc test between categories of adjacent ages was performed for each parameter. The p-values and their effect size [28] are reported for significant results. For CMJ, a significantly greater jump height in U12 was observed compared to U11, with a small-to-medium effect size ($p = 0.032$, $\eta^2 = 0.052$) (Figure 1a). In the CMJA, a significantly better performance of medium effect size was observed in U10 compared to U9 ($p = 0.045$, $\eta^2 = 0.074$), and in U12 compared to U11 ($p = 0.022$, $\eta^2 = 0.059$), suggesting that age accounts for a moderate proportion of the variability in CMJA for these groups (Figure 1b). In the 15m LS test, U10 showed significantly faster sprint times than U9 ($p = 0.01$, $\eta^2 = 0.124$) and U13 outperformed U12 ($p < 0.01$, $\eta^2 = 0.388$), indicating a medium-to-large effect size (Figure 1c). In the 15m LSB test, significant differences in medium-to-large effect size were observed in the oldest groups, with faster sprint times in U12 compared to U11 ($p < 0.01$, $\eta^2 = 0.199$) and in U13 compared to U12 ($p = 0.01$, $\eta^2 = 0.087$) (Figure 1d). In the AT, significantly better performance was observed in U10 compared to U9 ($p < 0.01$, $\eta^2 = 0.199$) and in U13 compared to U12 ($p < 0.01$, $\eta^2 = 0.284$); both effects were large, indicating that group differences were substantial (Figure 1e). In the ATB, a significantly faster time of medium-to-large effect size was found in U10 compared to U9 ($p = 0.01$, $\eta^2 = 0.12$), in U12 compared to U11 ($p < 0.01$, $\eta^2 = 0.133$) and in U13 compared to U12 ($p = 0.016$, $\eta^2 = 0.075$); indicating that the group differences were meaningful (Figure 1f). Finally, in the SeR test, a significantly greater flexibility was observed in U9 compared to U10 ($p < 0.01$, $\eta^2 = 0.126$), and in U11 compared to U12 ($p = 0.049$, $\eta^2 = 0.043$), indicating a medium effect for the first comparison and a small effect for the second one (Figure 1g). The median values and interquartile ranges of all groups are shown in Table 1.

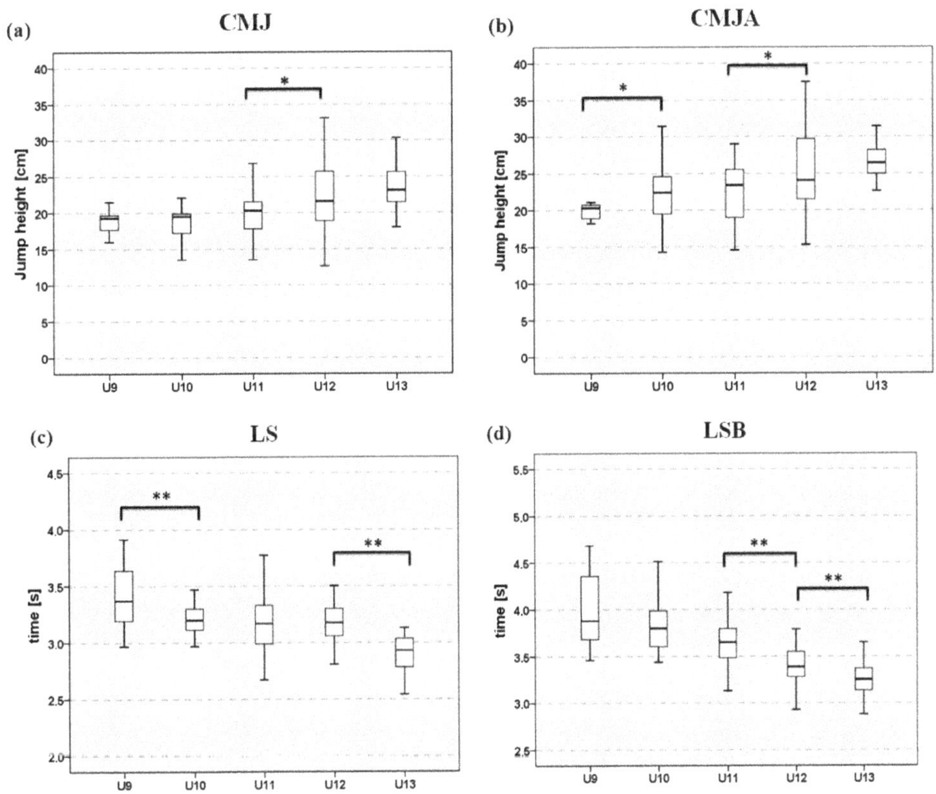

Figure 1. *Cont.*

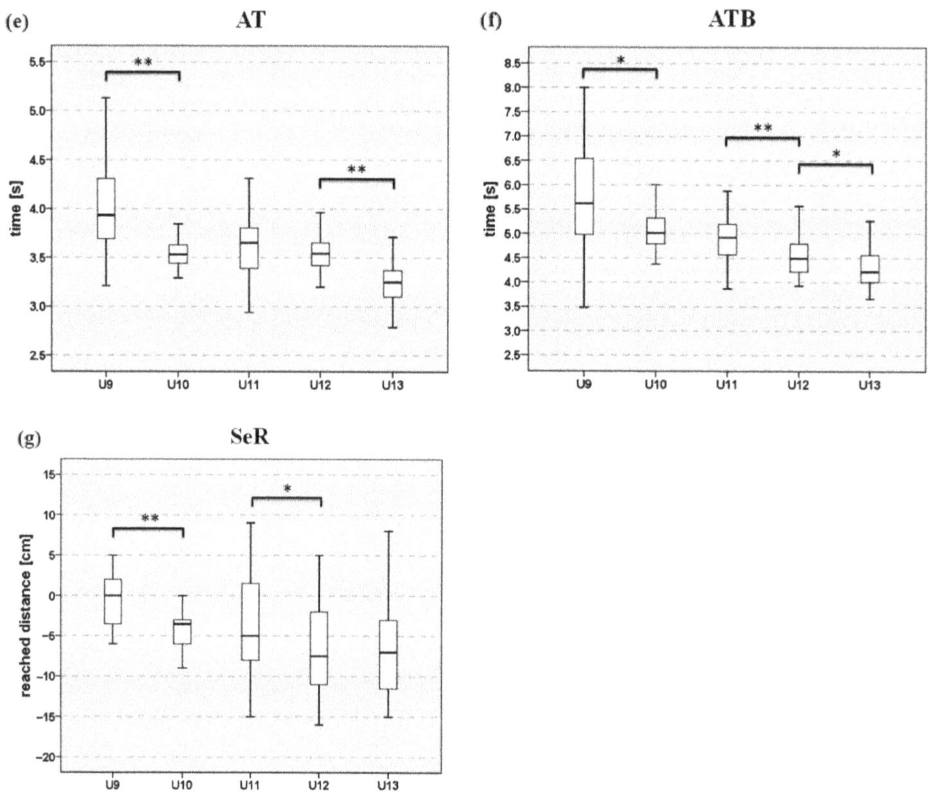

Figure 1. Median values and interquartile range of the five age groups. (**a**) CMJ with blocked arms. (**b**) CMJ with arm swing; (**c**) 15 m linear sprint without ball; (**d**) 15 m linear sprint with ball; (**e**) Agility test without ball; (**f**) Agility test with ball; (**g**) Sit and Reach test. Significant differences between adjacent age groups: * $p \leq 0.05$; ** $p \leq 0.01$.

Table 1. Median and interquartile range values of age groups.

Groups	CMJ [cm]	CMJA [cm]	LS [s]	LSB [s]	AT [s]	ATB [s]	SeR [cm]
U9	19.3 [17.5–19.7]	**20.3 [18.7–20.7]** *	**3.37 [3.16–3.64]** *	3.88 [3.66–4.4]	**3.93 [3.66–4.33]** *	**5.62 [4.82–6.85]** *	**0 [−4–+2]** *
U10	19.5 [17.1–19.9]	22.4 [19.5–24.6]	3.2 [3.11–3.31]	3.8 [3.59–3.99]	3.53 [3.44–3.64]	5.01 [4.75–5.38]	−3 [−6–−2]
U11	**20.3 [17.5–21.6]** *	**23.4 [18.7–25.6]** *	3.2 [3.0–3.3]	**3.65 [3.48–3.8]** *	3.65 [3.38–3.86]	**4.92 [4.52–5.25]** *	**−5 [−8–+2]** *
U12	21.6 [18.8–26.0]	24.1 [21.4–29.8]	**3.18 [3.06–3.3]** *	**3.39 [3.28–3.55]** *	**3.54 [3.4–3.65]** *	**4.49 [4.21–4.79]** *	−7.5 [−11.3–−2]
U13	23.1 [21.4–25.7]	26.4 [24.7–28.2]	2.93 [2.77–3.04]	3.25 [3.1–3.37]	3.25 [3.09–3.37]	4.22 [4.0–4.61]	−7 [−12–−3]

CMJ = Countermovement Jump; CMJA = Countermovement Jump with arm swing; LS = Linear Sprint; LSB = Linear Sprint with ball; AT = Agility test; ATB = Agility test with ball; SeR = Sit and Reach.
* $p \leq 0.05$ compared to the subsequent older age category.

3.2. Differences Within Age Subgroups

The Kruskal–Wallis test showed significant differences among subgroups in all measured variables ($p \leq 0.01$); thus, for each parameter, a Mann–Whitney post hoc test was performed between subgroups of the same age group.

In the youngest age group (U9), significant differences were observed in the CMJA test (Figure 2b), with subgroup U9O showing significantly higher scores compared to U9Y ($p = 0.040$, $\eta^2 = 0.18$), while no differences were found in the other tests. Among all age groups, U10 athletes showed the greatest number of differences between the two age subgroups. Specifically, subgroup U10O showed significantly better performance in both the CMJ (Figure 2a) ($p = 0.019$, $\eta^2 = 0.175$) and CMJA tests (Figure 2b) ($p = 0.033$, $\eta^2 = 0.144$) compared to U10Y. Moreover, U10O athletes also showed significantly better sprint times in the LSB (Figure 2d) test than those in U10Y ($p = 0.033$, $\eta^2 = 0.144$). In the U11 group, differences between subgroups were found only in the LS test (Figure 2c), with athletes in subgroup U11Y achieving better sprint times than those in subgroup U11O ($p = 0.016$, $\eta^2 = 0.147$). Overall, the effect sizes observed across these significant comparisons were consistently large, reflecting meaningful differences between subgroups. In the oldest age groups (U12 and U13), no significant differences were found between subgroups for any of the assessed parameters. In general, no significant differences between subgroups were detected in AT (Figure 2e), in ATB (Figure 2f), and in the SeR test (Figure 2g). The median values and interquartile ranges of all subgroups are shown in Table 2.

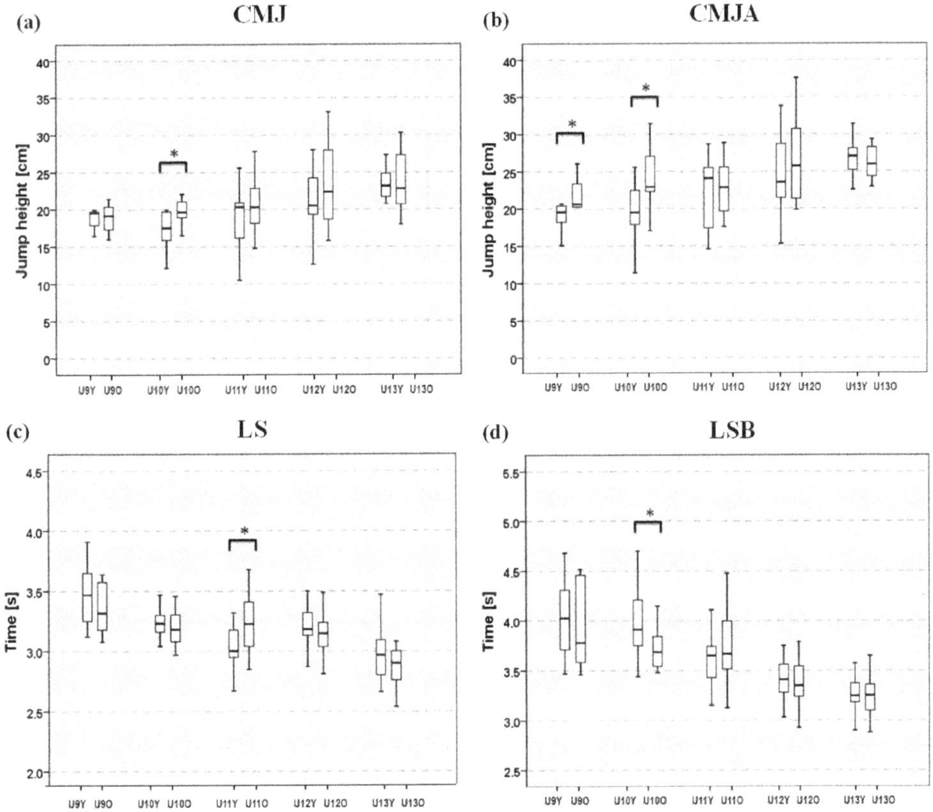

Figure 2. *Cont.*

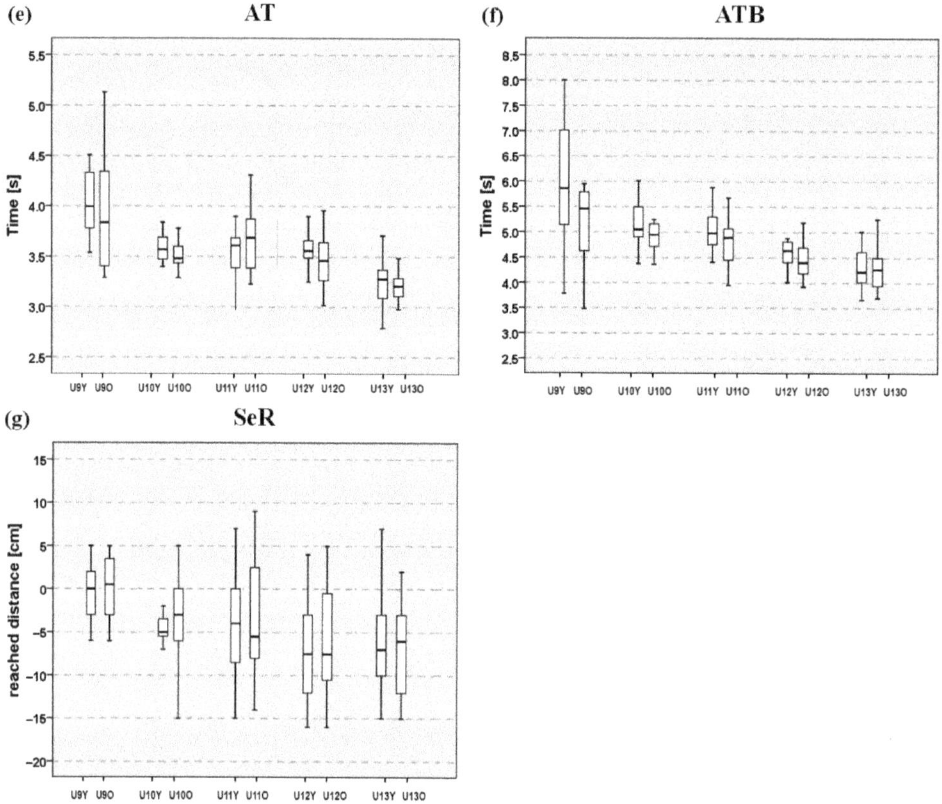

Figure 2. Median values and interquartile range of the ten age subgroups. (**a**) CMJ with blocked arms. (**b**) CMJ with arm swing; (**c**) 15 m linear sprint without ball; (**d**) 15 m linear sprint with ball; (**e**) Agility test without ball; (**f**) Agility test with ball; (**g**) Sit and Reach test. Significant differences between adjacent age groups: * $p \leq 0.05$.

Table 2. Median and interquartile range values of age subgroups.

Groups	Subgroups	CMJ [cm]	CMJA [cm]	LS [s]	LSB [s]	AT [s]	ATB [s]	SeR [cm]
U9	U9Y (n = 14)	19.6 [17.5–19.7]	19.9 [18.2–20.4]	3.39 [3.16–3.65]	4.02 [3.71–4.31]	3.93 [3.72–4.33]	5.86 [5.14–7.01]	0.0 [−4.0–+2.0]
	U9O (n = 9)	19.2 [17.2–21.0]	**20.75 [20.3–24.7]** *	3.32 [3.16–3.61]	3.78 [3.55–4.49]	3.84 [3.40–4.43]	5.46 [4.58–5.87]	0.5 [−3.5–+3.8]
U10	U10Y (n = 15)	17.5 [15.6–19.8]	19.5 [17.5–22.6]	3.23 [3.15–3.31]	3.91 [3.70–4.24]	3.57 [3.46–3.71]	5.05 [4.83–5.56]	−5 [−6.0–−3.0]
	U10O (n = 16)	**19.7 [18.8–21.1]** *	**22.9 [22.3–28.0]** *	3.18 [3.07–3.31]	**3.69 [3.54–3.86]** *	3.48 [3.43–3.60]	4.95 [4.72–5.18]	−3 [−7.5–0.0]
U11	U11Y (n = 15)	20.3 [16.1–21.0]	24.1 [17.3–25.6]	3.0 [2.92–3.18]	3.65 [3.38–3.74]	3.61 [3.28–3.70]	4.98 [4.72–5.31]	−4 [−9.0–0.0]
	U11O (n = 24)	20.3 [18.1–22.9]	23.0 [19.7–26.2]	**3.23 [3.04–3.42]** *	3.67 [3.51–4.01]	3.69 [3.39–3.88]	4.9 [4.46–5.10]	−5.5 [−8.0–+2.8]
U12	U12Y (n = 22)	20.5 [19.0–24.3]	23.6 [21.3–28.8]	3.18 [3.12–3.34]	3.41 [3.28–3.57]	3.56 [3.48–3.66]	4.64 [4.40–4.83]	−7.5 [−12.8–−2.8]
	U12O (n = 20)	22.4 [18.6–28.0]	25.7 [21.2–31.0]	3.15 [3.03–3.24]	3.35 [3.22–3.55]	3.465 [3.27–3.65]	4.405 [4.19–4.75]	−7.5 [−12.8–−0.3]
U13	U13Y (n = 22)	23.2 [21.7–25.0]	27.1 [25.1–28.2]	2.97 [2.79–3.09]	3.25 [3.16–3.39]	3.28 [3.08–3.37]	4.215 [4.02–4.62]	−7 [−10.3–−2.3]
	U13O (n = 13)	22.8 [20.5–22.8]	25.9 [24.2–28.8]	2.9 [2.74–3.0]	3.25 [3.08–3.39]	3.21 [3.06–3.36]	4.27 [3.95–4.72]	−6 [−13.0–−3.0]

CMJ = Countermovement Jump; CMJA = Countermovement Jump with arm swing; LS = Linear Sprint; LSB = Linear Sprint with ball; AT = Agility test; ATB = Agility test with ball; SeR = Sit and Reach. Subgroup Y is younger than subgroup O. * $p \leq 0.05$ compared to the corresponding subgroup of the same age category.

No significant differences were detected from the explorative analyses based on birth quarter, except for the LSB (U12-born Q4 (n = 12) vs. U11-born Q1 (n = 14): 3.41 ± 0.33 vs. 3.78 ± 0.38; p = 0.006, η^2 = 0.27), indicating a very large effect size. However, given the limited sample size, these results should be treated with caution.

4. Discussion

The findings of this research indicate age-related differences in motor tests with medium to large between-group effects for all adjacent ages for speed and agility, while improvements in ball-involving tasks appear only in later ages. These outcomes are consistent with other studies in the literature, demonstrating that some performance markers follow a relatively predictable pattern of improvement, yet are modulated by factors such as motor control, training adaptation, and biological maturation [3,6]. Indeed, for linear sprint and agility tests without the ball, adjacent age-group comparisons showed medium-to-large effects, whereas the ball-involving tasks version shifted these effects only toward older groups (U10–U11, U11–U12). On the other hand, jump performance generally improved with a smaller magnitude of effects. These, taken together, support the non-linear pattern in early adolescence consistent with other longitudinal studies accounting for accelerations and plateaus regarding pre-adolescence [3,6,29,30]. Semester subgrouping analyses revealed meaningful differences primarily in the younger categories (e.g., from 9 to 11 years old, differences in several tests have a large magnitude with η^2 comprised between 0.14 and 0.18), while no differences were observed in U12-U13. On the other hand, trimester analysis was explorative to verify the magnitude of changes. Indeed, the absence of consistency in the analysis suggest the non-linear trajectory changes that are more evident at the semester level. However, due to the sample size limitation and the contextual factors possible interference with the skill development path, trimester results should be interpreted cautiously [29].

In the considered sample, the within-age pattern is consistent with the over-representation of earlier-born athletes reported in youth soccer [20,21]. That is consistent with the literature, where a six-month age gap is associated with detectable differences only for non-complex explosive tasks among the youngest categories. However, due to subgroup sizes being modest and effects not being uniform, these differences should be interpreted cautiously. Moreover, the yearly semester division comparisons showed that the older categories outperformed the younger, in accordance with the Italian elite benchmarks [20]. Indeed, in Italy, RAEs are pronounced in top youth categories, tending to attenuate toward Serie A, which is consistent with our pattern [20,21]. This picture supports the interpretation that in younger groups, maturational advantages could induce early selection bias that then will cushion with age [21]. Despite that, differences were measure-specific and not consistent across all outcomes. Indeed, beyond maturational timing, semester-based differences might reflect selection and opportunity mechanisms that advantage relatively older players within the cut-off system. Accordingly, soccer evidence shows an over-representation of early born athletes, with magnitudes peaking during adolescence, being consistent with greater exposure, competitive minutes and perceived competence, reinforcing development over time [31,32]. On the other hand, within U11, the younger subgroup was faster in the linear sprint test than the older counterpart. This pattern could be interpreted in light of the non-linear variation typical of early adolescence that is characterized by spurts and plateau in terms of physical skills maturation, especially in easier tasks [6,29]. Accordingly, this difference might reflect the contextual influences that can modulate performance appearance and RAE prevalence [33].

To account for this mismatch between age groups, several authors propose other grouping strategies, challenging conventional cutoffs. For instance, Lovell [15] proposed using markers of physical maturity (height, weight, and body composition), while Perroni [34] and Malina [35] emphasize skeletal or pubertal assessments to refine groupings. Others, such as Malina [36], suggest classification based on skill level, and Sierra-Díaz with colleagues [32] propose introducing a quota system for later-born players to ensure equal opportunities. These approaches may help clubs promote talent discovery and tailor training to individual skills development. Nevertheless, power and speed development, including object control (e.g., dribbling), appear to benefit from significant differences between the ages of 10 and 12. These findings are consistent with models hypothesizing that strength and endurance often precede the emergence of fine coordination skills [29,30]. With adequate muscle capacity, players may be better equipped to adapt to drills demanding complex footwork, rapid decision-making, and sensorimotor integration [37].

Together, the results reported here should help to contextualize the group considered: large quarter/semester gaps in pre-adolescence are typical in competitive pathways but should be managed to avoid talent loss among relatively younger players. Potentially, in daily practical work, athletes' selection could be influenced more by multiple checkpoints and development trajectories rather than absolute values, given the athlete-specific skill improvements during adolescence [3,6]. Indeed, given that senior-level RAE focuses during career beginning, reducing early selection pressure in preadolescence may help contextualize evaluation in similar settings.

Limitations

Subgrouping strategy (i.e., half-year cohorts and birth quarters) reduced the size of each subgroup, which may have masked additional differences. Moreover, the cross-sectional design provides only a snapshot of each athlete's development, limiting the possibility to identify individualized trajectories over time. The lack of maturation markers (e.g., height, weight, skeletal age, etc.) has to be addressed as a barrier for generalizability. This study did not assess passing, shooting, or tactical decision-making, with ball-involving tests being considered as dribbling-related tests appropriate for 8 to 12-year-old groups. Finally, findings must be interpreted in light of the single-club male-only, cross-sectional design.

5. Conclusions

This study shows a progressive, though not strictly linear, path of motor development in youth soccer. Indeed, despite motor performance improving between each consecutive age group, the gain magnitude was not linear (e.g., ball-involving tasks tend to consolidate later) [3]. Semester grouping revealed meaningful differences in younger categories, while trimester contrasts were mainly trivial. When involving the ball, skills tend to consolidate later than easier speed and power. Therefore, potential practical implications should be modest and context-specific for clubs and academies.

Future Directions

To clearly map growth-related changes, a longitudinal design with larger samples should be adopted to track within-player paths and quantify how motor performance and the RAE evolve over time. It would also be valuable to account for the role of external factors such as training consistency, injury history, training disruptions when interpreting these outcomes [33]. Finally, future studies should include validated technical skills (e.g., passing, shooting) and game-based measures (e.g., decision-making tools) to delineate object involvement in these fields. With this strategy accounting for longer times and greater samples, a better understanding of motor-skill progression will be achieved.

Author Contributions: Conceptualization, L.M., F.P. and D.C.; methodology, L.M. and G.D.P.; software, F.S. and A.C.; validation, L.M., F.S. and G.D.P.; formal analysis, L.M. and F.M.; investigation, L.M. and F.S.; resources, L.M. and F.M.; data curation, F.S., A.C. and F.M.; writing—original draft preparation, F.S., G.D.P. and A.C.; writing—review and editing, M.C.G. and L.G.; visualization, M.C.G., L.G. and F.P.; supervision, F.P. and D.C.; project administration, F.P. and D.C.; funding acquisition, M.C.G. and L.G. All authors have read and agreed to the published version of the manuscript.

Funding: This research received no external funding.

Institutional Review Board Statement: The institutional ethics committee of Niccolò Cusano University (protocol number MO 8-22, approval date: 15 September 2022) granted ethical approval in accordance with the 1964 Helsinki Declaration and its subsequent amendments or comparable ethical standards.

Informed Consent Statement: Participants were informed of the study design and its requirements, as well as the possible benefits and risks, and gave their consent prior to the start of the study in accordance with the principles of the Declaration of Helsinki for the study of humans. Informed consent was obtained from all subjects and their guardians involved in the study.

Data Availability Statement: Data are available under request to the corresponding author. To preserve the integrity of the ongoing work, the dataset cannot be openly shared at this stage.

Conflicts of Interest: The authors declare no conflicts of interest.

References

1. Amatori, S.; Pintus, A.; Corsi, L.; Bensi, R.; Zanini, L.; Rocco, V.; Guidetti, L.; Baldari, C.; Rocchi, M.B.L.; Sisti, D.; et al. Chronological age, relative age, pubertal development, and their impact on countermovement jump performance in adolescent football players: An integrative analysis. *Heliyon* **2024**, *10*, e36879. [CrossRef]
2. Fernandez-Gonzalo, R.; De Souza-Teixeira, F.; Bresciani, G.; García-López, D.; Hernández-Murúa, J.A.; Jiménez-Jiménez, R.; De Paz, J.A. Comparison of Technical and Physiological Characteristics of Prepubescent Soccer Players of Different Ages. *J. Strength Cond. Res.* **2010**, *24*, 1790–1798. [CrossRef]
3. Saward, C.; Hulse, M.; Morris, J.G.; Goto, H.; Sunderland, C.; Nevill, M.E. Longitudinal Physical Development of Future Professional Male Soccer Players: Implications for Talent Identification and Development? *Front. Sports Act. Living* **2020**, *2*, 578203. [CrossRef] [PubMed] [PubMed Central]
4. Pienaar, A.E.; Gericke, C.; Plessis, W.D. Competency in Object Control Skills at an Early Age Benefit Future Movement Application: Longitudinal Data from the NW-CHILD Study. *Int. J. Environ. Res. Public Health* **2021**, *18*, 1648. [CrossRef]
5. Zhang, D.; Soh, K.G.; Chan, Y.M.; Zaremohzzabieh, Z. Effect of intervention programs to promote fundamental motor skills among typically developing children: A systematic review and meta-analysis. *Child. Youth Serv. Rev.* **2024**, *156*, 107320. [CrossRef]
6. Leyhr, D.; Kelava, A.; Raabe, J.; Höner, O. Longitudinal motor performance development in early adolescence and its relationship to adult success: An 8-year prospective study of highly talented soccer players. *PLoS ONE* **2018**, *13*, e0196324. [CrossRef] [PubMed] [PubMed Central]
7. Barnett, L.M.; Lai, S.K.; Veldman, S.L.C.; Hardy, L.L.; Cliff, D.P.; Morgan, P.J.; Zask, A.; Lubans, D.R.; Shultz, S.P.; Ridgers, N.D.; et al. Correlates of Gross Motor Competence in Children and Adolescents: A Systematic Review and Meta-Analysis. *Sports Med.* **2016**, *46*, 1663–1688. [CrossRef] [PubMed]
8. Duncan, M.J.; Eyre, E.L.J.; Noon, M.R.; Morris, R.; Thake, C.D.; Clarke, N.D.; Cunningham, A.J. Actual and perceived motor competence mediate the relationship between physical fitness and technical skill performance in young soccer players. *Eur. J. Sport Sci.* **2022**, *22*, 1196–1203. [CrossRef]
9. Hermassi, S.; Hayes, L.D.; Bartels, T.; Schwesig, R. Differences in body composition, static balance, field test performance, and academic achievement in 10–12-year-old soccer players. *Front. Physiol.* **2023**, *14*, 1150484. [CrossRef] [PubMed]
10. Selmi, M.A.; Sassi, R.H.; Yahmed, M.H.; Giannini, S.; Perroni, F.; Elloumi, M. Normative Data and Physical Determinants of Multiple Sprint Sets in Young Soccer Players Aged 11–18 Years: Effect of Maturity Status. *J. Strength Cond. Res.* **2020**, *34*, 506–515. [CrossRef]
11. Bolckmans, S.; Starkes, J.L.; Towlson, C.; Barnes, C.; Parkin, G.; Helsen, W.F. Leveling the Playing Field: A New Proposed Method to Address Relative Age- and Maturity-Related Bias in UK Male Academy Soccer Players. *Front. Sports Act. Living* **2022**, *4*, 847438. [CrossRef]

12. Gonçalves, C.E.B.; Rama, L.M.L.; Figueiredo, A.B. Talent Identification and Specialization in Sport: An Overview of Some Unanswered Questions. *Int. J. Sports Physiol. Perform.* **2012**, *7*, 390–393. [CrossRef]
13. Meylan, C.; Cronin, J.; Oliver, J.; Hughes, M. Talent identification in soccer: The role of maturity status on physical, physiological and technical characteristics. *Int. J. Sports Sci. Coach.* **2010**, *5*, 571–592. [CrossRef]
14. Roberts, S.J.; Boddy, L.M.; Fairclough, S.J.; Stratton, G. The Influence of Relative Age Effects on the Cardiorespiratory Fitness Levels of Children Age 9 to 10 and 11 to 12 Years of Age. *Pediatr. Exerc. Sci.* **2012**, *24*, 72–83. [CrossRef]
15. Lovell, R.; Towlson, C.; Parkin, G.; Portas, M.; Vaeyens, R.; Cobley, S. Soccer Player Characteristics in English Lower-League Development Programmes: The Relationships between Relative Age, Maturation, Anthropometry and Physical Fitness. *PLoS ONE* **2015**, *10*, e0137238. [CrossRef] [PubMed] [PubMed Central]
16. Cumming, S.P.; Lloyd, R.S.; Oliver, J.L.; Eisenmann, J.C.; Malina, R.M. Bio-banding in Sport: Applications to Competition, Talent Identification, and Strength and Conditioning of Youth Athletes. *Strength Cond. J.* **2017**, *39*, 34–47. [CrossRef]
17. Perroni, F.; Vetrano, M.; Rainoldi, A.; Guidetti, L.; Baldari, C. Relationship among explosive power, body fat, fat free mass and pubertal development in youth soccer players: A preliminary study. *Sport Sci. Health* **2014**, *10*, 67–73. [CrossRef]
18. Jakobsson, J.; Julin, A.L.; Persson, G.; Malm, C. Darwinian Selection Discriminates Young Athletes: The Relative Age Effect in Relation to Sporting Performance. *Sports Med. Open* **2021**, *7*, 16. [CrossRef] [PubMed]
19. Fortunato, Á.; Gonçalves, C.; Lopes, V.P. Relationship Between Motor Competence and Soccer-Specific Skills: A Longitudinal Study With Young Players. *J. Mot. Learn. Dev.* **2024**, *12*, 455–468. [CrossRef]
20. Brustio, P.R.; Lupo, C.; Ungureanu, A.N.; Frati, R.; Rainoldi, A.; Boccia, G. The relative age effect is larger in Italian soccer top-level youth categories and smaller in Serie A. *PLoS ONE* **2018**, *13*, e0196253. [CrossRef]
21. Lupo, C.; Boccia, G.; Ungureanu, A.N.; Frati, R.; Marocco, R.; Brustio, P.R. The Beginning of Senior Career in Team Sport Is Affected by Relative Age Effect. *Front. Psychol.* **2019**, *10*, 1465. [CrossRef]
22. Quagliarella, L.; Sasanelli, N.; Belgiovine, G.; Accettura, D.; Notarnicola, A.; Moretti, B. Evaluation of counter movement jump parameters in young male soccer players. *J. Appl. Biomater. Biomech.* **2011**, *9*, 40–46. [CrossRef]
23. Heishman, A.D.; Daub, B.D.; Miller, R.M.; Freitas, E.D.S.; Frantz, B.A.; Bemben, M.G. Countermovement Jump Reliability Performed With and Without an Arm Swing in NCAA Division 1 Intercollegiate Basketball Players. *J. Strength Cond. Res.* **2020**, *34*, 546–558. [CrossRef] [PubMed]
24. Slinde, F.; Suber, C.; Suber, L.; Edwen, C.E.; Svantesson, U. Test retest reliability of three countermovement jumping tests. *J. Strength Cond. Res.* **2008**, *22*, 640–644. [CrossRef]
25. Mujika, I.; Santisteban, J.; Impellizieri, F.M.; Castagna, C. Fitness determinants of success in men's and women's football. *J. Sport Sci.* **2009**, *27*, 107–114. [CrossRef] [PubMed]
26. Altmann, S.; Ringhof, S.; Neumann, R.; Woll, A.; Rumpf, M.C. Validity and reliability of speed tests used in soccer: A systematic review. *PLoS ONE* **2019**, *14*, e0220982. [CrossRef]
27. Nikolaidis, P.; Ziv, G.; Lidor, R.; Arnon, M. Inter-individual Variability in Soccer Players of Different Age Groups Playing Different Positions. *J. Hum. Kinet.* **2014**, *40*, 213–225. [CrossRef] [PubMed]
28. Cohen, J. *Statistical Power Analysis for the Behavioral Sciences (Rev. ed.)*; Lawrence Erlbaum Associates: Mahwah, NJ, USA, 1988. [CrossRef]
29. Abarghoueinejad, M.; Baxter-Jones, A.D.G.; Gomes, T.N.; Barreira, D.; Maia, J. Motor Performance in Male Youth Soccer Players: A Systematic Review of Longitudinal Studies. *Sports* **2021**, *9*, 53. [CrossRef] [PubMed] [PubMed Central]
30. Kokstejn, J.; Musalek, M.; Wolanski, P.; Murawska-Cialowicz, E.; Stastny, P. Fundamental Motor Skills Mediate the Relationship Between Physical Fitness and Soccer-Specific Motor Skills in Young Soccer Players. *Front. Physiol.* **2019**, *10*, 596. [CrossRef] [PubMed] [PubMed Central]
31. Bozděch, M.; Agricola, A.; Zháněl, J. The Relative Age Effect at Different Age Periods in Soccer: A Meta-Analysis. *Percept. Mot. Skills* **2023**, *130*, 2632–2662. [CrossRef] [PubMed]
32. Sierra-Díaz, M.J.; González-Víllora, S.; Pastor-Vicedo, J.C.; Serra-Olivares, J. Soccer and Relative Age Effect: A Walk among Elite Players and Young Players. *Sports* **2017**, *5*, 5. [CrossRef] [PubMed] [PubMed Central]
33. Keemss, J.; Sieland, J.; Pfab, F.; Banzer, W. Effects of COVID-19 Lockdown on Physical Performance, Sleep Quality, and Health-Related Quality of Life in Professional Youth Soccer Players. *Front. Sports Act. Living* **2022**, *4*, 875767. [CrossRef] [PubMed] [PubMed Central]
34. Perroni, F.; Amatori, S.; Corsi, L.; Bensi, R.; Guidetti, L.; Baldari, C.; Rocchi, M.B.L.; Castagna, C.; Gobbi, E.; Sisti, D.; et al. Assessment of Performance in Youth Soccer Players: Should We Consider the Maturation Status? *J. Hum. Kinet.* **2024**, *93*, 119–131. [CrossRef] [PubMed] [PubMed Central]
35. Malina, R.M.; Coelho-E-Silva, M.J.; Figueiredo, A.J.; Philippaerts, R.M.; Hirose, N.; Peña Reyes, M.E.; Gilli, G.; Benso, A.; Vaeyens, R.; Deprez, D.; et al. Tanner-Whitehouse Skeletal Ages in Male Youth Soccer Players: TW2 or TW3? *Sports Med.* **2018**, *48*, 991–1008. [CrossRef] [PubMed]

36. Malina, R.M.; Ribeiro, B.; Aroso, J.; Cumming, S.P. Characteristics of youth soccer players aged 13–15 years classified by skill level. *Br. J. Sports Med.* **2007**, *41*, 290–295; discussion 295. [CrossRef] [PubMed] [PubMed Central]
37. Koopmann, T.; Faber, I.; Baker, J.; Schorer, J. Assessing Technical Skills in Talented Youth Athletes: A Systematic Review. *Sports Med.* **2020**, *50*, 1593–1611. [CrossRef] [PubMed] [PubMed Central]

sports

MDPI

Article

Relationships Between Sport-Specific Anaerobic Tests, Interlimb Asymmetry, and Bilateral Deficit as Measured from Vertical Jump Performances in Highly Trained Taekwondo Athletes

Ibrahim Ouergui [1,2,*], Slaheddine Delleli [3,4], Gennaro Apollaro [5,6], Hamdi Messaoudi [3,4], Rafael Lima Kons [7], Craig Alan Bridge [8], Hamdi Chtourou [3,4], Emerson Franchini [9], Emanuela Faelli [6,10] and Luca Paolo Ardigò [11,*]

1. High Institute of Sport and Physical Education of Kef, University of Jendouba, El Kef 7100, Tunisia
2. Research Unit, Sports Science, Health and Movement, University of Jendouba, El Kef 7100, Tunisia
3. High Institute of Sport and Physical Education, University of Sfax, Sfax 3038, Tunisia; sdelleli2018@gmail.com (S.D.); hamdimessaoudihamdi@gmail.com (H.M.); hamdi.chtourou@isseps.usf.tn (H.C.)
4. Physical Activity, Sport, and Health, UR18JS01, National Observatory of Sport, Tunis 1003, Tunisia
5. Department of Neuroscience, Rehabilitation, Ophthalmology, Genetics and Maternal Child Health, University of Genoa, 16132 Genoa, Italy; gennaro.apollaro@edu.unige.it
6. Centro Polifunzionale di Scienze Motorie, University of Genoa, 16132 Genoa, Italy; emanuela.faelli@unige.it
7. Department of Physical Education, Faculty of Education, Federal University of Bahia, Salvador 40170-110, Brazil; rafakons0310@gmail.com
8. Sports Performance Research Group, Department of Sport & Physical Activity, Edge Hill University, Lancashire L39 4QP, UK; bridgec@edgehill.ac.uk
9. Martial Arts and Combat Sports Research Group, Sport Department, School of Physical Education and Sport, University of São Paulo, Sao Paulo 05508-060, Brazil; efranchini@usp.br
10. Department of Experimental Medicine, Section of Human Physiology, University of Genoa, 16132 Genoa, Italy
11. Department of Teacher Education, NLA University College, Linstows Gate 3, 0166 Oslo, Norway

* Correspondence: brahim.ouerghi@issepkef.u-jendouba.tn (I.O.); luca.ardigo@nla.no (L.P.A.)

Abstract: The present study investigated the effect of inter-limb asymmetry and bilateral indexes (BLIs) in power performance, assessed by squat jump (SJ) and countermovement jump (CMJ), on sport-specific anaerobic performance. Forty-eight taekwondo athletes (24 males and 24 females; mean ± SD, age: 19.8 ± 2.1 years) performed randomly, in separate sessions, SJ and CMJ tests using the right, left, and both legs to determine the asymmetry and BLI, the 10 s Frequency Speed of Kick Test ($FSKT_{10s}$), and its multiple version ($FSKT_{mult}$). $FSKT_{10s}$ was positively correlated with CMJ asymmetry ($\rho = 0.299$, $p = 0.039$, low) and SJ BLI ($r = 0.596$, $p < 0.001$, large), and negatively correlated with CMJ BLI ($r = -0.472$, $p = 0.001$, moderate). Similarly, $FSKT_{mult}$ was positively correlated with SJ BLI ($\rho = 0.632$, $p < 0.001$, large), and negatively correlated with CMJ BLI ($\rho = -0.532$, $p < 0.001$, large). CMJ and SJ BLI explained 45.9% of the variance of the $FSKT_{10s}$ performance, whilst they explained 55.7% of the variance of $FSKT_{mult}$ performance. These results highlight the importance of managing both interlimb asymmetry and bilateral deficit indexes to achieve better performance by improving the strength of the non-dominant leg and using exercises that are performed bilaterally despite unilateral movements being predominant in taekwondo, which can potentially enhance the effectiveness in sport-specific actions

Keywords: asymmetry; performance; strength; correlation; combat sports

1. Introduction

Sports performance generally includes unilateral or bilateral motor tasks that may result in differences between limbs in terms of force and power output [1]. Inter-limb asymmetry—defined as the imbalance in performance between limbs—is a common phenomenon, which particularly characterizes athletes practicing unilateral sports [2]. Several factors were found to explain this asymmetry such as training routines that emphasize unilateral movements, inducing strength imbalances, altered movement patterns, and motor learning adaptations that favor the dominant limb [3]. These adjustments can result in enhanced muscle strength, flexibility, and coordination on the dominant limb, although the non-dominant side may continue to be undeveloped [3]. From a neuromuscular point of view, lateral dominance is considered to represent the functional specialization of the brain's left or right hemispheres [4]. Moreover, in addition to training factors, lateral dominance is influenced by contextual factors, task complexity, gender, genetics, and training factors [3].

Although some level of asymmetry is acceptable in athletes, values greater than 15% between limbs can negatively impact performance and increase the risk of injury [2]. Bishop, et al. [5], systematically reviewing the literature related to inter-limb asymmetries and their effects on physical performance, found that asymmetries in strength appeared to negatively affect performance activities including change of direction (COD), jumping, and sport-specific skills such as kicking accuracy. Instead, for jumping-based asymmetries, they found varied associations between jumps (vertical and horizontal) and CODS performance [5]. In a recent systematic review with meta-analysis [6], inter-limb asymmetries, quantified through unilateral jumping performance, were found to negatively impact COD and sprinting, but not jumping performance, in cohorts of athletes, supporting the realization that asymmetry is task-dependent and the need for multiple assessments to provide a broad profile of the athlete's asymmetry. Additionally, Buoite et al. [1] found that muscle asymmetries in male soccer players were associated with performance metrics such as the countermovement jump (CMJ) and tensiomyography, which could influence athletic performance and injury prevention strategies.

As well, the concept of bilateral index (BLI)—which determines whether force generated bilaterally is less than or larger than the sum of unilateral forces— also varies in its effect depending on the type of sport. Specifically, Železnik, et al. [7] reported that bilateral deficit (BLD) can induce positive effect in tennis, basketball, and volleyball, while it is undesirable in other sports like judo.

The implications of asymmetry and bilateral indexes are less well understood in combat sports. While taekwondo research has shown a strong correlation between body composition asymmetries and performance in high-intensity kick tests [i.e., the frequency speed of kick test (FSKT)] [8], judo studies have found that bilateral asymmetry has a negative impact on performance in the Special Judo Fitness Test (SJFT) [9]. For BLI, studies investigating its relationship with performance in combat sports are limited to judo [10,11]. Negative correlations were observed between bilateral deficit (BLD) in CMJ performance metrics and SJFT performance [10]. Conversely, the BLI in the maximal handgrip strength test was not found to be related to SJFT performance in judo athletes [11].

Taekwondo is a full-contact open combat between two athletes that generates the intermittency of the activity in which high-intensity actions (kicks and punches), low-intensity actions (such as skipping), and pauses alternate [12,13]. A wide variety of unilateral technical actions can be observed in current taekwondo combat [14,15]. In addition, athletes must move faster during the combat to keep up with the average match pace imposed by the opponents [16,17], and agility is required to quickly execute technical-tactical movements in multidirectional planes [18]. Thus, the presence of inter-limb asymmetry in power performance and sport-specific anaerobic performance could potentially compromise the athlete's competition performance considering the relationship between the ability to repeat short high-intensity efforts and scoring actions. In addition, it could lead to an increased risk of injury as taekwondo training largely assumes repetition of typical unilateral and multidirectional technical-tactical actions. In taekwondo, both asymmetry and bilateral indexes have never been investigated although its relationship to performance in other sports contexts is well documented [9,19–21].

In this sense, the aim of this study was to investigate the influence of inter-limb asymmetry and bilateral strength deficit in power performance, assessed by squat jump (SJ) and countermovement jump (CMJ), on sport-specific anaerobic performance, by performing the FSKT, in high-level taekwondo athletes. We hypothesized that anaerobic test performance, as measured by both ten seconds frequency speed of kick test ($FSKT_{10s}$) and its multiple version ($FSKT_{mult}$), could be affected negatively by both asymmetry and bilateral indexes measured by jumping tests.

2. Materials and Methods

2.1. Study Design

This is a cross-sectional study design in which taekwondo athletes were assessed using jumping and technique-specific tests to assess the asymmetry and bilateral (BLI) indexes and their relationship with anaerobic-specific taekwondo performance as assessed using the frequency speed of kick test (FSKT).

2.2. Participants

An a priori power analysis (G*Power 3.1.9.7; Heinrich Heine University in Düsseldorf, Germany) indicated that a total sample of 29 subjects would be required with the following settings: bivariate normal model test, two-tailed, power of 0.80, α-value of 0.05, and a correlation of r = 0.50. Forty-eight taekwondo athletes (24 males and 24 females; mean ± SD, age: 19.8 ± 2.1 years, body mass: 62.2 ± 9.4 kg, height: 179.3 ± 9.5 cm, training experience: 8 ± 1 years) volunteered to participate in the present study. To be eligible, athletes should met the following inclusion criteria: (i) they were training four to five times per week, (ii) they were competing regularly during the last 2 years, (iii) athletes were asked to follow the same diet, avoid strenuous exercises, and refrain from caffeine consumption (in drinks and supplements) or any other ergogenic resources during the 48 h before each session, (iv) athletes were not under any weight-loss protocol during the period of experimentation, and (v) for female athletes, only those who were in their follicular phase of the menstrual cycle with a regular cycle duration, defined as a variation lower than 3 days in the range of their menstrual cycles' length [22] for the previous 2 months, were included. After a detailed explanation of the study's aims and risks, both parents and athletes provided written informed consent. The study was conducted in accordance with the latest Declaration of Helsinki [23] for human experimentation, followed the ethical standards outlined in the *Publication Manual of the American Psychological Association* [24] and was approved by the Local Research Ethics Committee [Comité de Protection des Personnes SUD (CPP SUD) N°. 0332/2021] before data collection.

2.3. Procedures

Athletes were well familiarized with the testing procedures (72 h before starting the experiment) and all assessments were conducted at the end of season, at the same time of day as the training sessions (18:00–20:00 h) to avoid any diurnal variation in the performance. Athletes performed randomly, in separate sessions, the squat jump (SJ), countermovement jump (CMJ) tests using the right, left, and both legs, the 10 s frequency of speed kick test ($FSKT_{10s}$), and its multiple version ($FSKT_{mult}$). Before each testing session, athletes performed 10 min of a standardized warm-up session consisting of light runs followed by dynamic stretching and submaximal jumps/technical executions for jumping/kicking testing sessions, respectively (Figure 1).

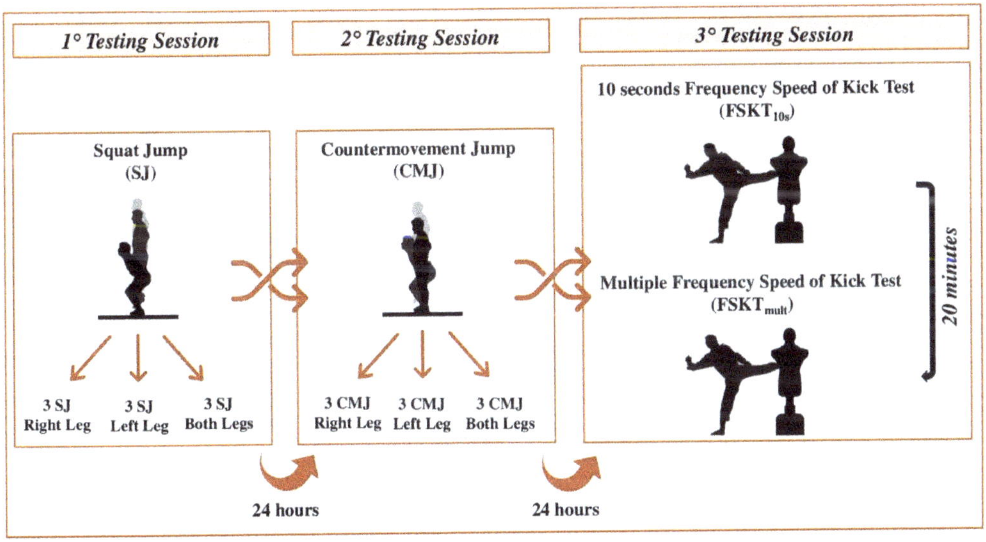

Figure 1. Schematic representation of the study design.

2.4. Measures

2.4.1. Squat Jump Test

From a stationary, semi-squatting position on the right (SJ^{R}), left (SJ^{L}), or both legs (SJ^{BL}), athletes jumped as maximum as possible without arm swing [25] using an infrared jump system (Optojump Next version 1.6.10, Microgate, Bolzano, Italy). Three tests were performed for each mode with 45 s as recovery interval between trials, and the best performance was retained for analysis. The intra-class correlation coefficient (ICC) for test–retest trial with the right, left, and both legs for the present study was 0.82, 0.84, and 0.93, respectively. The coefficient of variation (CV) was 7.42, 6.21, and 4.75%, respectively.

2.4.2. Countermovement Jump Test

From a standing position on the right (CMJ^{R}), left (CMJ^{L}), or both legs (CMJ^{BL}), athletes performed a quick downward movement by flexing the knees and hips immediately followed by a rapid extension of these joints while keeping their hands on their waists. No lower limb flexion or arm swing in the upward phase was allowed [25,26]. The CMJ test was performed using an infrared jump system (Optojump Next version 1.6.10, Microgate, Bolzano, Italy). Three tests were performed for each mode with 45 s as the recovery interval between trials, and the best performance was retained for analysis. The ICC for test–retest trial with the right, left, and both legs for the present study was 0.83, 0.79, and 0.91, respectively. Moreover, CV was 5.86, 5.27, and 7.33%, respectively.

2.4.3. Ten s Frequency Speed of Kick Test

The test consisted of performing the maximum number of bandal-chagi, executed against a bag at the trunk height by alternating legs for ten seconds [27,28]. The ICC and CV for test–retest trial for the present study were 0.90 and 7.81%, respectively.

2.4.4. Multiple Frequency Speed of Kick Test

Each athlete performed five sets of $FSKT_{10s}$ alternating both legs, with a ten-second rest interval between repetitions [27,28], and the total number of techniques was used for subsequent analysis. The ICC and CV for test–retest trial for the present study were 0.88 and 8.02%, respectively.

2.4.5. Interlimb Asymmetry and Bilateral Indexes from Jumping Tests

Interlimb asymmetry was quantified as the percentage of difference between the stronger and weaker limb using Equation (1) previously proposed [29]:

$$\text{Interlimb asymmetry (\%)} = (\text{Stronger limb} - \text{Weaker limb})/\text{Stronger limb} \times 100 \quad (1)$$

The bilateral index (BLI), expressed as a percentage, was calculated using Equation (2) as previously proposed [30]:

$$\text{BLI (\%)} = 1 - (\text{bilateral}/(\text{right} + \text{left})) \times 100 \quad (2)$$

A positive percentage score indicates the presence of a bilateral facilitation (BLF) where the bilateral performance is superior to the summed unilateral performances, whereas a negative percentage is indicative of a bilateral deficit (BLD) [31].

2.5. Statistical Analyses

Statistical analysis was performed using SPSS 20.0 statistical software (SPSS Inc., Chicago, IL, USA). The normality of datasets was checked and confirmed using the Shapiro–Wilk test. Spearman's correlation coefficient (ρ) was used between $FSKT_{10s}$ performance and the asymmetry indexes from CMJ and SJ, and between $FSKT_{mult}$ and the asymmetry and bilateral strength indexes from CMJ and SJ. Pearson's product-moment correlation coefficient (r) was used to examine relationships between $FSKT_{10s}$ performance and bilateral strength indexes from CMJ and SJ. Magnitude of correlation was determined as trivial when $r < 0.1$, low 0.1–0.3, moderate 0.3–0.5, large 0.5–0.7, very large 0.7–0.9, nearly perfect > 0.9, or perfect = 1 [32]. Multiple regression analyses were used to establish the relationship between the dependent variables ($FSKT_{10s}$ and $FSKT_{mult}$) and the independent variables (SJ and CMJ asymmetry indexes and SJ and CMJ bilateral strength indexes), based on collinearity principles [33]. The correlation coefficient value was determined and the coefficient of determination (R^2) was calculated to determine the proportion of the variability in the independent variables explained by the dependent variables. The standard error of estimate (SEE) of each equation is also presented. Statistical significance was set at $p < 0.05$.

3. Results

Figure 2 presents the correlations between technical performance, asymmetry, and bilateral indexes during jumping tests.

Regression analyses showed that ten seconds frequency speed of kick test ($FSKT_{10s}$) performance could be partially predicted from CMJ and SJ bilateral indexes using the following Equation (3):

$$FSKT_{10s}\ (n^{\circ}) = 19.16 - 0.109\ (\text{CMJ-BLI in cm}) + 0.081\ (\text{SJ-BLI in cm}),\ r = 0.677,\ R^2 = 0.459,\ \text{SEE} = 1.909,\ \text{and}\ p < 0.001 \quad (3)$$

Regression analyses showed that multiple sets of frequency speed of kick test ($FSKT_{mult}$) performance could be partially predicted from CMJ and SJ bilateral indexes using the following Equation (4):

$$FSKT_{mult}\ (n^{\circ}) = 93.008 - 0.587\ (\text{CMJ-BLI in cm}) + 0.428\ (\text{SJ-BLI in cm}),\ r = 0.747,\ R^2 = 0.557,\ \text{SEE} = 7.966,\ \text{and}\ p < 0.001 \quad (4)$$

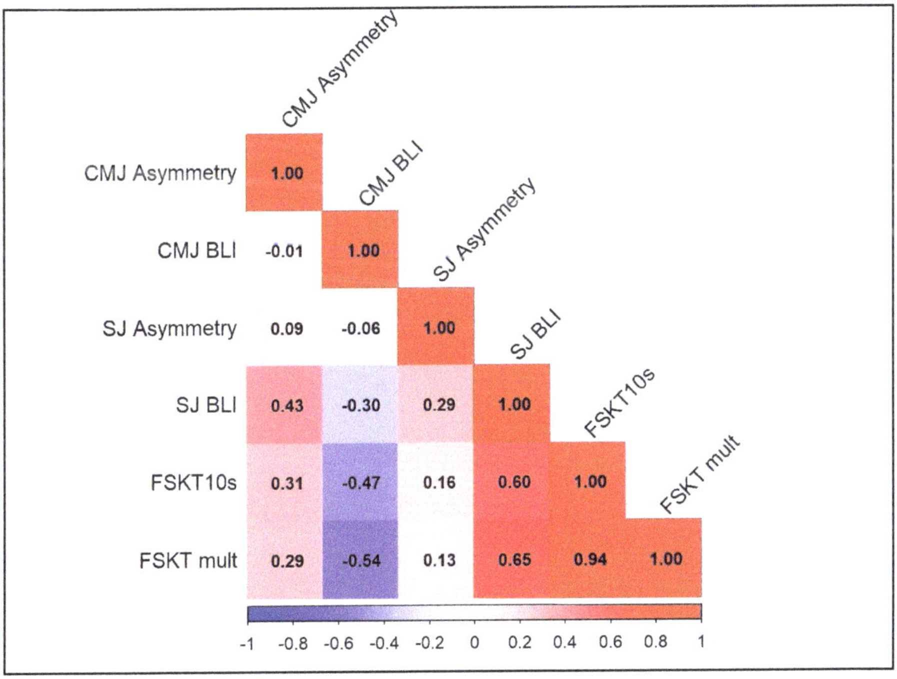

Figure 2. Correlations between technical performance, asymmetry, and bilateral indexes (BLIs) during squat jump (SJ) and countermovement jump (CMJ) tests. FSKT: frequency speed of kick test.

4. Discussion

This study explored the relationship between taekwondo-specific tests [ten seconds of frequency speed of kick test ($FSKT_{10s}$) and its multiple sets version ($FSKT_{mult}$)], interlimb asymmetry, and bilateral strength deficit (BLD) assessed by vertical jump tests (i.e., CMJ and SJ) in high-level taekwondo athletes. The main findings showed that CMJ and SJ BLI explained 45.9% of the variance of the $FSKT_{10s}$ performance, whilst they explained 55.7% of the variance of $FSKT_{mult}$ performance confirming the hypothesis of the present study.

The FSKT is an important test, which has been explored over the last few years, considering performance in taekwondo based on construct classificatory tables [34], reliability, sensitivity, and construct validity [27], group discrimination between competitive levels [35], post-activation potentiation conditioning [36,37], and correlated with performance in the CMJ [38]. Based on these aspects, the FSKT is an excellent alternative to assess the anaerobic fitness of taekwondo athletes in an intermittent and sport-specific mode. The FSKT (10 s and multiple) performance could be partially predicted from CMJ and SJ bilateral strength indexes. The neural responses, reflecting the imbalance between unilateral and bilateral performance, can be explained by the CMJ and SJ tests. This relationship is evident in the specific equations derived from the $FSKT_{mult}$ and $FSKT_{10s}$ performance.

The use of vertical jump tests as an indicator of interlimb asymmetry, based on the jump height metric [39], is a good alternative to assess the imbalance between limbs in high-level athletes [5,40], considering different sports modalities [5], and more recently, combat sports athletes [9,41]. The relationship between $FSKT_{10s}$ and $FSKT_{mult}$ and interlimb asymmetry demonstrated that the high number of kicks performed at high intensity is related to the high values of interlimb asymmetry assessed by the CMJ and SJ tests. This suggests that the repetitive nature of kicking with one leg can lead to greater strength and performance discrepancies between the dominant and non-dominant legs.

It is well known that due to the nature of the taekwondo modality, athletes are expected to present structural and functional asymmetries due to long-term specialized training since the kicks performed during specific tasks are performed unilaterally [40,42]. In this sense, the aspect of dominance significantly influences taekwondo performance giving that athletes normally have one side stronger than the other and consequently superior strength and power on the dominant kicking side.

From a psychopathological perspective, various factors can contribute to asymmetry and bilateral deficit in motor performance by disrupting the brain's ability to coordinate and control movement symmetrically [43]. Neurological conditions, such as those resulting from previous injuries, can impair the brain's control over one side of the body more than the other, leading to imbalances in tasks that require bilateral coordination [44]. This imbalance might manifest in taekwondo as uneven kicking power or poor balance when performing moves that rely on both sides. Additionally, psychological factors, including anxiety or stress, can also affect motor performance by increasing muscle tension or disrupting fluid movement [45], which may result in uneven performance between the left and right sides of the body. Furthermore, cognitive dysfunctions related to conditions like depression can impact executive functions such as focus, task-switching, and decision-making [46] which are crucial in high-intensity sports like taekwondo. Consequently, these psychopathological factors can provide valuable insight into the correlation between asymmetry and bilateral deficit in jumping performance and specific performance in taekwondo by influencing both the motor and cognitive systems essential for executing symmetric movements.

In specific performance, Liu et al. [42] reported that during a double roundhouse kick in sub-elite taekwondo athletes, there was a difference between dominant and non-dominant side in term of maximum knee flexion angle and the peak linear velocity of attack of the foot in the vertical hitting direction for the attacking leg and the peak hip extension moment for the supporting leg. Furthermore, in terms of strength, studies have shown significant differences between preferred and non-preferred legs in female taekwondo athletes [47] and in a mixed sample of athletes [48]. Similarly, Harbili et al. [49] reported that, in elite male and female taekwondo athletes, isometric hamstring strength was greater in the dominant leg by 15% for male athletes and 11% for female athletes aligning with the expected outcomes of unilateral training. However, the same study reported no significant differences in isokinetic and isometric knee strength between the dominant and non-dominant legs in male and female athletes reporting the absence of bilateral knee strength asymmetry.

Conversely, in terms of body composition, Ojeda-Aravena et al. [8] showed a negative relationship between body composition asymmetry and performance in FSKT; however, the values of body composition asymmetry were very low and did not reflect the asymmetry observed in unilateral physical tests in this study for example.

The bilateral index of strength measures force production in both unilateral and bilateral performance [7] across various tasks, such as isometric leg extension [50], vertical jump tests [10], and isometric handgrip strength tests [11]. Negative values in these tests indicate a bilateral deficit, whilst positive values suggest neuromuscular facilitation [7]. In this study, a negative relationship was found between the bilateral index and FSKT performance in both protocols. Specifically, a high negative bilateral index in CMJ negatively impacted FSKT performance. Practically, this suggests that taekwondo athletes need to be strong, stable, and powerful in both limbs to maximize their chances of successful defense and attacks during taekwondo-specific actions [42]. Therefore, it may be advantageous to reduce the bilateral deficit (i.e., improve bilateral jumping relative to unilateral jumping) to optimize taekwondo-specific performance, like the findings observed recently in judo [10].

Based on the results of the present study, coaches and strength and conditioning trainers should consider incorporating unilateral training exercises focusing not only to enhance the strength of the dominant leg but also to address the non-dominant leg to reduce interlimb asymmetry and thus maintain a balanced athletic profile and optimize overall specific performance. Additionally, conditioning training programs should be oriented to address the bilateral strength deficit by using exercises that are performed bilaterally (e.g., implementing bilateral strength exercises and ensuring that both legs are equally engaged and capable of generating force during training) irrespective of unilateral movements. This can improve the symmetry in terms of force production across both legs which may enhance performance in taekwondo-specific movements and may potentially enhance their kicking power and overall effectiveness.

Limitations and Future Perspectives

Although our study offers novel information, several limitations must be acknowledged. Firstly, during CMJ and SJ tests, only jump height was used to calculate asymmetry and bilateral indexes. In this sense, other metrics (e.g., power, velocity) might be measured to increase the amount of relevant information and insights that can be derived from the tests. Secondly, Fox et al. [6] indicated that asymmetry is task-dependent and there is a need for multiple assessments to provide a broad profile of the athlete's asymmetry. Therefore, it might be important to expand the present investigation by also using another taekwondo sport-specific test, such as the TSAT, as during combat, agility is required to quickly execute technical-tactical movements in multidirectional planes [18]. Finally, a limitation in studying asymmetry and bilateral deficit in this study is the lack of taking sex factor into consideration. Sex plays a crucial role in muscle properties, including differences in muscle mass, strength, and endurance between males and females. These variations may influence the degree of asymmetry and bilateral deficit observed in athletes. Future studies can be conducted using electromyography and tensiomyography to explore the neuromuscular mechanisms underlying the observed relationships between jump asymmetries/bilateral indexes and anaerobic kicking performance in taekwondo athletes. This may help to explore whether this difference between the dominant and non-dominant leg during jumping is due to neural mechanisms (e.g., muscle activation timing, recruitment patterns) or contractile muscles' characteristics (e.g., stiffness, contraction time, and relaxation time).

5. Conclusions

The present study showed that performance in $FSKT_{10s}$ was positively correlated with CMJ asymmetry and SJ BLI and negatively correlated with CMJ BLI, and that $FSKT_{mult}$ was positively correlated with SJ BLI, and negatively correlated with CMJ BLI. In addition, CMJ and SJ BLI explained 45.9% of the variance of the $FSKT_{10s}$ performance, whilst they explained 55.7% of the variance of $FSKT_{mult}$ performance. These results highlight the importance of managing both interlimb asymmetry and bilateral indexes to achieve better performance.

Author Contributions: Conceptualization, I.O. and L.P.A.; methodology, I.O., S.D. and L.P.A.; validation, I.O., S.D. and L.P.A.; formal analysis, I.O., S.D. and H.M.; investigation, I.O., S.D. and H.M.; resources, I.O., S.D. and H.M.; data curation, I.O., S.D. and H.M.; writing—original draft preparation, I.O., S.D., G.A. and R.L.K.; writing—review and editing, I.O., G.A., C.A.B., H.C., E.F. (Emerson Franchini), E.F. (Emanuela Faelli) and L.P.A.; visualization, I.O., S.D. and G.A.; supervision, I.O. and H.C.; project administration, I.O., H.C. and L.P.A. All authors have read and agreed to the published version of the manuscript.

Funding: This research received no external funding.

Institutional Review Board Statement: This study was conducted in accordance with the Declaration of Helsinki and approved by the Local Research Ethics Committee (Comité de Protection des Personnes SUD (CPP SUD N°. 0332/2021).

Informed Consent Statement: Informed consent was obtained from all subjects involved in the study.

Data Availability Statement: The datasets presented in this article are not readily available [the data are part of an ongoing study]. Requests to access the datasets should be directed to the corresponding author.

Acknowledgments: The authors thank the athletes who participated in this study.

Conflicts of Interest: The authors declare no conflicts of interest.

Abbreviations

BLI	Bilateral index
SJ	Squat jump
CMJ	Countermovement jump
FSKT10s	Ten s Frequency Speed of Kick Test
FSKTmult	Multiple Frequency Speed of Kick Test
FSKT	Frequency Speed of Kick Test
TSAT	Taekwondo-Specific Agility Test
COD	Change of direction
SJ^R	Squat jump with right leg
SJ^L	Squat jump with left leg
SJ^{BL}	Squat jump with both legs
CMJ^R	Countermovement jump with right leg
CMJ^L	Countermovement jump with left leg
CMJ^{BL}	Countermovement jump with both legs
ICC	Intra-class correlation coefficient
CV	Coefficient of variation
BLF	Bilateral facilitation
BLD	Bilateral deficit
ρ	Spearman's correlation coefficient
R^2	Coefficient of determination

References

1. Buoite Stella, A.; Galimi, A.; Martini, M.; Di Lenarda, L.; Murena, L.; Deodato, M. Muscle Asymmetries in the Lower Limbs of Male Soccer Players: Preliminary Findings on the Association between Countermovement Jump and Tensiomyography. *Sports* **2022**, *10*, 177. [CrossRef] [PubMed]
2. Maloney, S.J. The Relationship Between Asymmetry and Athletic Performance: A Critical Review. *J. Strength Cond. Res.* **2019**, *33*, 2579–2593. [CrossRef]
3. Carpes, F.P.; Mota, C.B.; Faria, I.E. On the bilateral asymmetry during running and cycling—A review considering leg preference. *Phys. Ther. Sport* **2010**, *11*, 136–142. [CrossRef] [PubMed]
4. Hebbal, G.V.; Mysorekar, V.R. Evaluation of Some Tasks Used for Specifying Handedness and Footedness. *Percept. Mot. Ski.* **2006**, *102*, 163–164. [CrossRef] [PubMed]
5. Bishop, C.; Turner, A.; Read, P. Effects of inter-limb asymmetries on physical and sports performance: A systematic review. *J. Sports Sci.* **2018**, *36*, 1135–1144. [CrossRef]
6. Fox, K.T.; Pearson, L.T.; Hicks, K.M. The effect of lower inter-limb asymmetries on athletic performance: A systematic review and meta-analysis. *PLoS ONE* **2023**, *18*, e0286942. [CrossRef]
7. Železnik, P.; Slak, V.; Kozinc, Ž.; Šarabon, N. The Association between Bilateral Deficit and Athletic Performance: A Brief Review. *Sports* **2022**, *10*, 112. [CrossRef]
8. Ojeda-Aravena, A.; Warnier-Medina, A.; Brand, C.; Morales-Zúñiga, J.; Orellana-Lepe, G.; Zapata-Bastias, J.; Tuesta, M. Relationship between Body Composition Asymmetry and Specific Performance in Taekwondo Athletes: A Cross-Sectional Study. *Symmetry* **2023**, *15*, 2087. [CrossRef]

9. Kons, R.L.; Diefenthaeler, F.; Orssatto, L.B.R.; Sakugawa, R.L.; da Silva Junior, J.N.; Detanico, D. Relationship between lower limb asymmetry and judo-specific test performance. *Sport Sci. Health* **2020**, *16*, 305–312. [CrossRef]
10. Kons, R.L.; Ache-Dias, J.; Gheller, R.G.; Bishop, C.; Detanico, D. Bilateral deficit in the countermovement jump and its associations with judo-specific performance. *Res. Sports Med.* **2023**, *31*, 638–649. [CrossRef]
11. Turnes, T.; Silva, B.A.; Kons, R.L.; Detanico, D. Is Bilateral Deficit in Handgrip Strength Associated With Performance in Specific Judo Tasks? *J. Strength Cond. Res.* **2022**, *36*, 455–460.
12. Barrientos, M.; Saavedra-García, M.A.; Arriaza-Loureda, R.; Menescardi, C.; Fernández-Romero, J.J. An Updated Technical–Tactical Categorisation in Taekwondo: From General Tactical Objectives to Combat Situations. *Sustainability* **2021**, *13*, 10493. [CrossRef]
13. Apollaro, G.; Sarmet Moreira, P.V.; Herrera-Valenzuela, T.; Franchini, E.; Falcó, C. Time-motion analysis of taekwondo matches in the Tokyo 2020 Olympic Games. *J. Sports Med. Phys. Fit.* **2023**, *63*, 964–973. [CrossRef]
14. Gamero-Castillero, J.A.; Quiñones-Rodríguez, Y.; Apollaro, G.; Hernández-Mendo, A.; Morales Sánchez, V.; Falcó, C. Application of the Polar Coordinate Technique in the Study of Technical-Tactical Scoring Actions in Taekwondo. *Front. Sports Act. Living* **2022**, *4*, 877502. [CrossRef]
15. Menescardi, C.; Falcó, C.; Hernández-Mendo, A.; Morales-Sánchez, V. Analysis of Different Key Behavioral Patterns to Score in Elite Taekwondoists According to the Weight Category and Gender. *Front. Psychol.* **2021**, *12*, 713869. [CrossRef]
16. Janowski, M.; Zieliński, J.; Ciekot-Sołtysiak, M.; Schneider, A.; Kusy, K. The Effect of Sports Rules Amendments on Exercise Intensity during Taekwondo-Specific Workouts. *Int. J. Environ. Res. Public Health* **2020**, *17*, 6779. [CrossRef]
17. Janowski, M.; Zieliński, J.; Kusy, K. Exercise Response to Real Combat in Elite Taekwondo Athletes Before and After Competition Rule Changes. *J. Strength Cond. Res.* **2021**, *35*, 2222–2229.
18. Chaabene, H.; Negra, Y.; Capranica, L.; Bouguezzi, R.; Hachana, Y.; Rouahi, M.A.; Mkaouer, B. Validity and Reliability of a New Test of Planned Agility in Elite Taekwondo Athletes. *J. Strength Cond. Res.* **2018**, *32*, 2542–2547.
19. Arboix-Alió, J.; Buscà, B.; Busquets, A.; Aguilera-Castells, J.; de Pablo, B.; Montalvo, A.M.; Fort-Vanmeerhaeghe, A. Relationship between Inter-Limb Asymmetries and Physical Performance in Rink Hockey Players. *Symmetry* **2020**, *12*, 2035. [CrossRef]
20. Bishop, C.; Brashill, C.; Abbott, W.; Read, P.; Lake, J.; Turner, A. Jumping Asymmetries Are Associated With Speed, Change of Direction Speed, and Jump Performance in Elite Academy Soccer Players. *J. Strength Cond. Res.* **2021**, *35*, 1841–1847.
21. Loturco, I.; Pereira, L.A.; Kobal, R.; Abad, C.C.; Rosseti, M.; Carpes, F.P.; Bishop, C. Do asymmetry scores influence speed and power performance in elite female soccer players? *Biol. Sport* **2019**, *36*, 209–216. [CrossRef]
22. Lara, B.; Gutiérrez-Hellín, J.; García-Bataller, A.; Rodríguez-Fernández, P.; Romero-Moraleda, B.; Del Coso, J. Ergogenic effects of caffeine on peak aerobic cycling power during the menstrual cycle. *Eur. J. Nutr.* **2020**, *59*, 2525–2534. [CrossRef] [PubMed]
23. World Medical, A. World Medical Association Declaration of Helsinki: Ethical Principles for Medical Research Involving Human Subjects. *JAMA* **2013**, *310*, 2191–2194. [CrossRef]
24. American Psychological Association. *Publication Manual of the American Psychological Association*, 7th ed.; American Psychological Association: Washington, DC, USA, 2020. [CrossRef]
25. Markovic, G.; Dizdar, D.; Jukic, I.; Cardinale, M. Reliability and Factorial Validity of Squat and Countermovement Jump Tests. *J. Strength Cond. Res.* **2004**, *18*, 551–555. [PubMed]
26. Bishop, C.; Read, P.; Lake, J.; Chavda, S.; Turner, A. Interlimb Asymmetries: Understanding How to Calculate Differences From Bilateral and Unilateral Tests. *Strength Cond. J.* **2018**, *40*, 1–6.
27. Ferreira da Silva Santos, J.; Lopes-Silva, J.P.; Loturco, I.; Franchini, E. Test-retest reliability, sensibility and construct validity of the frequency speed of kick test in male black-belt taekwondo athletes. *Ido Mov. Culture. J. Martial Arts Anthropol.* **2020**, *20*, 38–46.
28. Apollaro, G.; Ouergui, I.; Rodríguez, Y.Q.; Kons, R.L.; Detanico, D.; Franchini, E.; Ruggeri, P.; Falcó, C.; Faelli, E. Anaerobic Sport-Specific Tests for Taekwondo: A Narrative Review with Guidelines for the Assessment. *Sports* **2024**, *12*, 278. [CrossRef]
29. Impellizzeri, F.M.; Rampinini, E.; Maffiuletti, N.; Marcora, S.M. A vertical jump force test for assessing bilateral strength asymmetry in athletes. *Med. Sci. Sports Exerc.* **2007**, *39*, 2044. [CrossRef]
30. Rejc, E.; Lazzer, S.; Antonutto, G.; Isola, M.; di Prampero, P.E. Bilateral deficit and EMG activity during explosive lower limb contractions against different overloads. *Eur. J. Appl. Physiol.* **2010**, *108*, 157–165. [CrossRef]
31. Bishop, C.; McAuley, W.; Read, P.; Gonzalo-Skok, O.; Lake, J.; Turner, A. Acute Effect of Repeated Sprints on Interlimb Asymmetries During Unilateral Jumping. *J. Strength Cond. Res.* **2021**, *35*, 2127–2132. [CrossRef]
32. Hopkins, W.; Marshall, S.; Batterham, A.; Hanin, J. Progressive statistics for studies in sports medicine and exercise science. *Med. Sci. Sports Exerc.* **2009**, *41*, 3–13. [CrossRef] [PubMed]
33. Hair, J.; Black, W.; Babin, B.; Anderson, R.; Tatham, R. Multiple Regression Analysis. In *Multiple Regression Analysis*, 7th ed.; Pearson Prentice Hall: Upper Saddle River, NJ, USA, 2009; Volume 96, pp. 231–312.
34. Ferreira da Silva Santos, J.; Herrera-Valenzuela, T.; Franchini, E. Establishing frequency speed of kick test classificatory tables in male and female taekwondo athletes. *Kinesiology* **2019**, *51*, 213–218. [CrossRef]

35. Santos, J.F.d.S.; Franchini, E. Frequency Speed of Kick Test Performance Comparison Between Female Taekwondo Athletes of Different Competitive Levels. *J. Strength Cond. Res.* **2018**, *32*, 2934–2938. [CrossRef] [PubMed]
36. da Silva Santos, J.F.; Herrera-Valenzuela, T.; Ribeiro da Mota, G.; Franchini, E. Influence of half-squat intensity and volume on the subsequent countermovement jump and frequency speed of kick test performance in taekwondo athletes. *Kinesiology* **2016**, *48*, 95–102. [CrossRef]
37. da Silva Santos, J.F.; Valenzuela, T.H.; Franchini, E. Can Different Conditioning Activities and Rest Intervals Affect the Acute Performance of Taekwondo Turning Kick? *J. Strength Cond. Res.* **2015**, *29*, 1640–1647. [CrossRef]
38. Albuquerque, M.R.; Tavares, L.D.; Longo, A.R.; Caldeira Mesquita, P.H.; Franchini, E. Relationship between Indirect Measures of Aerobic and Muscle Power with Frequency Speed of Kick Test Multiple Performance in Taekwondo Athletes. *Int. J. Sports Med.* **2021**, *43*, 254–261. [CrossRef]
39. Bishop, C.; de Keijzer, K.L.; Turner, A.N.; Beato, M. Measuring Interlimb Asymmetry for Strength and Power: A Brief Review of Assessment Methods, Data Analysis, Current Evidence, and Practical Recommendations. *J. Strength Cond. Res.* **2023**, *37*, 745–750. [CrossRef]
40. Keogh, J.A.J.; Waddington, E.E.; Masood, Z.; Mahmood, S.; Palanisamy, A.C.; Ruder, M.C.; Karsan, S.; Bishop, C.; Jordan, M.J.; Heisz, J.J.; et al. Monitoring lower limb biomechanical asymmetry and psychological measures in athletic populations—A scoping review. *Scand. J. Med. Sci. Sports* **2023**, *33*, 2125–2148. [CrossRef]
41. Kons, R.L.; Pupo, J.D.; Gheller, R.G.; Costa, F.E.; Rodrigues, M.M.; Bishop, C.; Detanico, D. Effects of successive judo matches on interlimb asymmetry and bilateral deficit. *Phys. Ther. Sport* **2021**, *47*, 15–22. [CrossRef]
42. Liu, L.; Jia, M.; Ma, Y.; Lin, S.; Peng, Q.; Xiong, J.; Zheng, W. Biomechanics research on laterality effect between dominant and non-dominant during double roundhouse kick in the competitive taekwondo. *Heliyon* **2023**, *9*, e20843. [CrossRef]
43. Davidson, R.J. Asymmetric brain function, affective style, and psychopathology: The role of early experience and plasticity. *Dev. Psychopathol.* **1994**, *6*, 741–758. [CrossRef]
44. Zuleger, T.M.; Slutsky-Ganesh, A.B.; Anand, M.; Kim, H.; Warren, S.M.; Grooms, D.R.; Barber Foss, K.D.; Riley, M.A.; Yuan, W.; Gore, R.K.; et al. The effects of sports-related concussion history on female adolescent brain activity and connectivity for bilateral lower extremity knee motor control. *Psychophysiology* **2023**, *60*, e14314. [CrossRef]
45. Heller, W.; Etienne, M.A.; Miller, G.A. Patterns of perceptual asymmetry in depression and anxiety: Implications for neuropsychological models of emotion and psychopathology. *J. Abnorm. Psychol.* **1995**, *104*, 327–333. [CrossRef] [PubMed]
46. Pačesová, P. Cognitive and Executive Functions of Young Men regarding Sport Activity and Personality Traits. *Sustainability* **2021**, *13*, 11752. [CrossRef]
47. Yilmaz, A.K.; Yilmaz, C.; Karaduman, E.; Mayda, M.H.; Erail, S.; Bostanci, Ö.; Kabadayi, M. Correlation of bilateral and ipsilateral strength ratios with balance in female taekwondo athletes. *Rev. Artes Marciales Asiat.* **2021**, *16*, 67–79. [CrossRef]
48. Čular, D.; Miletić, Đ.; Miletić, A. Influence of dominant and non-dominant body side on specific performance in taekwondo. *Kinesiology* **2010**, *42*, 184–193.
49. Harbili, S.; Harbili, E.; Aslankeser, Z. Comparison of bilateral isokinetic and isometric strength differences in elite young male and female taekwondo athletes. *J. Exerc. Rehabil.* **2022**, *18*, 117–122. [CrossRef]
50. Nicholson, G.; Masini, D. Bilateral deficit: Relationships with training history and functional performance. *Kinesiology* **2021**, *53*, 86–94. [CrossRef]

MDPI AG
Grosspeteranlage 5
4052 Basel
Switzerland
Tel.: +41 61 683 77 34

Sports Editorial Office
E-mail: sports@mdpi.com
www.mdpi.com/journal/sports

www.ingramcontent.com/pod-product-compliance
Lightning Source LLC
Chambersburg PA
CBHW061458210926
51850CB00008B/1756
* 9 7 8 3 7 2 5 8 7 6 5 3 2 *